Cancer and Aging

Editors

Alvaro Macieira-Coelho, M.D., D.Sc.

INSERM
Paris, France

and

Bo Nordenskjöld, M.D., Ph.D.

Professor of Oncology
University of Linköping
Linköping, Sweden

CRC Press
Boca Raton   Ann Arbor   Boston

Library of Congress Cataloging-in-Publication Data

Cancer and aging / A. Macieira-Coelho and B. Nordenskjöld, editors.
    p.   cm.
    Includes bibliographies and index.
    ISBN 0-8493-6878-2
    1. Cancer--Age factors. I. Macieira-Coelho, Alvaro, 1932-
II. Nordenskjöld, B. (Bo)
    [DNLM: 1. Aging. 2. Neoplasms--in old age.   QZ 200 C21502]
RC262.C267 1990
616.99'4—dc20
DNLM/DLC
for Library of Congress   90-2158
                                  CIP

Direct all inquires to CRC Press, Inc., 2000 Corporate Blvd., N.W., Boca Raton, Florida, 33431.

© 1990 by CRC Press, Inc.

International Standard Book Number 0-8493-6878-2

Library of Congress Card Number 90-2158
Printed in the United States

THE EDITORS

Alvaro Macieira-Coelho, M.D., D.Sc., is Research Director at the French National Insitute of Health (INSERM) and Head of the Division for Cell Aging Rsearch at the Department of Cell Biology, University of Paris VII.

He obtained his M.D. degree in 1958 from the University of Lisbon, Portugal, and a D.Sc. degree from the University of Uppsala, Sweden, in 1967. From 1958 to 1961 he was an intern at the Lisbon University Hospital and a research associate at the Wistar Institute of the University of Pennsylvania (1961 to 1964) and in the Department of Pathology at the University of Uppsala (1964 to 1967). He was head of the Department of Cell Pathology at the Institute of Cell Pathology at the Insitute for Cancerlogy and Immunogenetics, Villejuif, France (1967 to 1986) and Visiting Professor at the Department of Cell Biology at the University of Linköping, Sweden (1987 to 1989).

Dr. Macieira-Coelho has taught at the Universities of Paris and Linköping, has given over 100 invited lectures at international meetings and guest lectures at various universities and institutes, has published more than 100 research papers, wrote one book, and is on the editorial board of four international gerontology journals.

Dr. Macieira-Coelho received the Johananoff International Visiting Professorship from the Mario Negri Institute (Milano) in 1982 and the Fritz-Verzàr Prize for Gerontology from the University of Vienna in 1988.

He is a member of the New York Academy of Sciences, American Society for Cell Biology, American Association for Cancer Research, American Tissue Culture Society, and the European Tissue Culture Society where he is an elected member of the Council.

His current research interests include the mechanisms of cellular aging and transformation.

Bo Nordenskjöld, M.D., Ph.D., is Professor of Oncology at the University of Linköping, Linköping, Sweden.

Professor Nordenskjöld obtained his M.D. and Ph.D. degrees in 1968 and 1971, respectively, from the Departments of Tumor Biology and Biochemistry at the Karolinska Institute in Stockholm. He was appointed Assistant Professor of Oncology at the Radiumhemmet in Stockholm in 1976 and became Professor of Oncology in Linköping in 1980.

He is a member of the Swedish Medical Society, the Swedish Cancer Society, the American Society of Clinical Oncology, the Scandinavian Breast Cancer Group, the Scandinavian Lymphoma Study Group, the EORTC Receptor Study Group, the Swedish Society of Therapeutical Radiology, the and European Society for Therapeutical Radiology.

Professor Nordenskjöld has been the recipient of research grants from the Swedish Cancer Society for studies of tumor virology, mechanisms of steroid hormone action, and the biology and therapy of breast cancer.

This volume was prepared during the time of my (AMC) visiting professorship at the University of Linköping. The assistance of the staff of the Cell Biology Department and of the librarians of that university is gratefully acknowledged.

CONTRIBUTORS

Bengt Björkstén, M.D., Ph.D.
Department of Pediatrics
University Hospital
Linkoping, Sweden

John A. Carmichael, M.D.C.M.
Professor
Department of Obstetrics and Gynecology
Queen's University
Kingston, ON, Canada

William Ershler, M.D.
Associate Professor
Department of Medicine
University of Wisconsin Medical Center
Madison, Wisconsin

Bengt Glimelius, M.D., Ph.D.
Department of Oncology
University Hospital
Akademiska Sjukhuset
Uppsala, Sweden

Makoto Goto, M.D.
Division of Rheumatic Diseases
Tokyo Metropolitan Otsuka Hospital
Tokyo, Japan

Tomas M. Heimann, M.D.
Department of Surgery
Mount Sinai School of Medicine
New York, New York

Kouki Inai, M.D., Ph.D.
Professor
Department of Pathology
Hiroshima University School of Medicine
Hiroshima, Japan

Paul R. Kaesberg, M.D.
Department of Medicine
University of Wisconsin
Madison, Wisconsin

Jacqueline Labat-Robert, Ph.D.
Faculte de Médecine
Laboratoire de Biochimie du Tissu
 Conjonctif
Université de Paris XII
Creteil, France

Marvin L. Lewbart, M.D., Ph.D.
Director, Steroid Laboratory
Crozer-Chester Medical Center
Chester, Pennsylvania

Alexei J. Likhachev, M.D.
Laboratory of Biophysics
N. N. Petrov Research Institute
 of Oncology
Leningrad, U.S.S.R.

Janet C. Mohle-Boetani, M.D.
Department of Internal Medicine
Stanford University Hospital
Stanford, California

C. M. Muir, M.B., Ph.D.
Deputy Director
International Agency for Research on
 Cancer
Lyon, France

Hiroshi Nagasawa, Ph.D.
Experimental Animal Research Laboratory
Meiji University
Kawasaki, Japan

Hakan Olsson, M.D., Ph.D.
Associate Professor
Department of Oncology
University Hospital
Lund, Sweden

Laura Pashko, Ph.D.
Laboratory Manager
Fels Research Institute
Temple University School of Medicine
Philadelphia, Pennsylvania

Stanislav Pejchl, M.D., Ph.D.
Assistant Professor
Department of Internal Medicine
Charles University
Prague, Czechoslovakia

Ladislas Robert
Faculte de Médecine
Laboratoire de Biochimie de Tissu
 Conjonctif
Université de Paris XII
Creteil, France

Arthur G. Schwartz, Ph.D.
Professor
Department of Microbiology
Fels Research Institute
Temple University School of Medicine
Philadelphia, Pennsylvania

Catarina Svanborg Eden, M.D., Ph.D.
Department of Clinical Immunology
University of Gothenburg
Gothenburg, Sweden

Lyly Teppo, M.D.
Director
Finnish Cancer Registry
Helsinki, Finland

Shoji Tokuoka, M.D., Ph.D. (retired)
Professor
Department of Pathology
Hiroshima University School of Medicine
Hiroshima, Japan

TABLE OF CONTENTS

IC: TIME AFTER EXPOSURE TO THE CARCINOGEN

PART II: CANCER INCIDENCE AND PROGRESSION

INTRODUCTION

A. Macieira-Coelho

There is a general belief that aging favors the development of cancer. With rare exceptions, this belief is expressed repeatedly in the scientific literature and at meetings and symposia.

Although cancer may become clinically apparent, in most cases, only in the later part of the life span, the events favoring its development are present all along the life of the organism from the embryonic stage on. The relationship between cancer and age can only be understood through a global comprehensive analysis of the natural history of the disease, so it should not be a surprise that a book on cancer and aging does not deal only with tumors of the late part of the animal life span.

The idea that aging is a potentiating factor for cancer comes in part from the ways of collecting data. One of them is the plotting of incidence curves for all human cancers combined. The curves combine pathological entities that are not comparable since they initiate and progress through different mechanisms, raise different host responses, have silent phases of different duration, and have different incidences. Even in cases where the pathologist may not be able to make distinctions, there can be tumors which from the clinical point of view are in fact different pathological entities. Such is the case for instance for breast cancers where those occurring in premenopausal and postmenopausal women have a different physiopathology.[1]

Many incidence curves are based on mortality from neoplasia, raising additional heterogeneity. The time between the initiation of neoplastic growth and the time when it kills the host is extremely variable. Survival depends upon factors such as time of diagnosis, type of treatment, host response, associated diseases, age at incidence, tendency of the tumor to spread, and also on the influence it has on the organism at large through the secretion of humoral factors causing paraneoplastic syndromes[2] which can debilitate the host. These aspects of the disease can be extremely variable.

Some tumors do not alter survival. Reviews by Cairns[3] on epidemiological studies performed in Norway showed that for women with colon cancer the survival of 30% of the patients was not affected by the disease. Actually about one third of all Norwegian cancer patients in that survey had no loss of life span. This emphasizes the errors that can be introduced by combining what are thought to be identical tumors and one aspect of the limitations of mortality curves. Hence mortality curves are irrelevant for the problem of the age-incidence of cancer.

The complexity of the relationship between cancer and age becomes apparent when the data is analyzed critically. In many respects, data are not even available to answer the questions that can be raised. This is the case, for instance, concerning the influence of the incidence of cancer on the life span of a species. Since neoplasia can curtail the life span, do species with a shorter life span have a higher incidence of cancer? This does not seem to be the case for the Wistar SPF Tox rat where the high tumor incidence seems to be due to their long life expectancy.[4] Hence it is possible that in some cases the factor time allows for more of the conditions leading to cancer to be met.

An interesting aspect of the relationship between cancer prevalence and species life span is discussed in the chapter on cancer and aging at the cellular level; it relates to the easier induction of cancers in some shorter lived animals and the higher susceptibility of their cells to transformation *in vitro*. Another interesting aspect is the inverse relationship between the capacity of cells to activate chemical carcinogens and the life span of the respective species.[5]

On the other hand, one should consider the possible effects of cancer on aging. Can cancer in itself accelerate the aging process? Predictions from epidemiological studies made by the U.S. Bureau of Statistics[6] point out that if cancer could be eliminated at birth or at age 65, life span would only increase by 2.3 and 1.2 years, respectively. This in itself suggests that cancer is not a main event in the aging syndrome since the increase would be less if the disease were eliminated later in life. It also suggests that the role of cancer on the human life span carries little weight.

A critical analysis of the information available on cancer incidence emphasizes the multifactorial determinants and favors an age relationship rather than the view that cancer is part of the aging syndrome. This is so not only for childhood cancers but also for tumors of adulthood such as testicular cancer which is reviewed in this volume. Chondrosarcomas are another type of tumor where the mean age-incidence is found to be 37 years of age.[7]

In other adulthood cancers, the incidence can increase during the second half of the human life span, but interesting enough, it may decline or level off late in life. This occurs for incidence curves for all cancers combined[8] and for cigarette smokers and nonsmokers in regard to the incidence of cancers related to smoking.[9] Is this a cohort effect, the individuals with a longer life span being more resistant to cancer? Could it be that aging itself opposes the development of some cancers? If aging favors the development of cancer, the incidence should increase continuously to the end of the life span.

It is interesting to compare the age-specific incidence for cancer of the colon and rectum in white Americans.[10] For the former there is a decline in incidence late in life, while for the latter the incidence increases progressively. Some events may occur later during the life span, interfering with the development of colonic cancer that do not interfere with rectal cancer. This again illustrates the fallacy of plotting incidence curves for all cancers combined.

Other puzzling data concern the incidence of lung cancer caused by nickel. Epidemiological studies showed that there is no regular change in susceptibility with age at first exposure and that the risk decreased significantly with the passage of time after the carcinogen was removed from the environment.[11] These results differed from those obtained for nasal sinus cancer which could reflect a difference in the way the two diseases are produced.[11] The relative risk of pulmonary cancer in retired smelter workers was also found to decrease with increasing age or time since retirement.[12]

Premature aging syndromes are often given as an example favoring a relationship of causality between cancer and aging. In this case, a close analysis raises more questions than answers. In Werner's Syndrome for instance, there is an unusual number of mesenchymal tumors which, in the general population, tend to appear earlier.[13] Furthermore, prostatic and pancreatic cancers which are more common in the later part of the human life span, are absent in Werner's Syndrome.[13] Could it be that mechanisms developing during aging, which determine the decline in the morbidity from some cancers late during the life span, are more prevalent in Werner's Syndrome patients and cause the absence of those tumors that are typical of the later period but eventually decline or level off in the general population?

There are other difficulties in interpreting the data:

1. The definition of incidence itself is fallacious
2. The determination of the real incidence is quite difficult to establish in humans.

It can be close to reality in the case of skin or cervical cancers, where the beginning of the neoplastic process can be determined with a good approximation, in the former by direct examination, and in the latter through the Papanicolau test. In many cancers, however, the time between the first clinical manifestations and the beginning of the neoplastic growth is anybody's guess.

Some events show how systematic screening can detect earlier the presence of a tumor. This is exemplified with the 1974 peak incidence of breast cancer in the U.S., which corresponded to the increased screening following the disclosures that the wives of President Ford and Vice President Rockefeller had breast cancer.[14]

Another parameter that can interfere with the exact determination of the age incidence is regression. It can occur rather frequently in pregnant women with carcinoma *in situ*.[15] How often cancer regresses is impossible to guess but "at least in the skin and breast, there are several paths to a fully developed carcinoma and on each of them there are repeated choices between regression, persistence and progression".[15]

Cancer progression is frequently slow and it can take several years for the tumor to become clinically apparent. Hence in many instances, the data collected from the onset of the first symptom reveal a process that may have started many years before. For instance, the initiation of mammary neoplasia in women can precede clinical detection by 20 to 30 years,[15] the early stages starting probably at puberty and during adolescence.[16]

Breast cancer is an example often given to demonstrate an association with aging. However, other factors besides the long occult phase and the two peaks incidence question the possible influence of aging on its development. The distribution of the age incidence of postmenopausal breast cancer correlates with the presence of obesity, hypertension, and/or glucose tolerance.[1] It seems there are other conditions besides age which influence the incidence, such as diseases that are characteristic of the later part of the human life span. These conditions may constitute the risk factors and not aging per se.

The two peaks incidence during the human life span is well known for other cancers. Hodgkin's lymphoma, for instance, can have two distinct age peaks, at 18 and 48 years of age.[17] On epidemiological grounds there appear to be three different types of Hodgkin's lymphoma: childhood (0 to 14 years), young adult (15 to 34 years), and older adult (55+ years).[18] There are also geographic variations in incidence but they are different for the three age groups.[18]

Cancers can also remain silent so that the host dies with, but not from the cancer.[19] In 1300 autopsies on patients over 70 years old, McKeown[20] found 20% with malignant disease of which 20% were unsuspected during life and not responsible for death.

A remarkable cancer morbidity study has been performed in Sweden at the Malmö General Hospital.[19] Data have been obtained by the systematic examination of all organs during autopsies from all causes of death and included even those tumors that remained silent. The data also included patients which had been cured of their disease. These studies showed that the prevalence of tumors was never above 43% in a human population and that only prostate cancer increased progressively with age and did not level off. The prevalence of all other type of tumors is summarized in Figure 1. The prevalence of most types of tumors peaked sometime during the human life span but then declined. The prevalence of cancer of the colon, for instance, peaked in men between ages 30 to 34 and at 75; in women it was steady at all ages from the thirties on.

Epidemiological studies can give quite different results depending on whether they have been collected postmortem or *intra vitam*. A surprising result was obtained from the cancer incidence in England and Wales taken from the number of cancer registries for both sexes.[21] The percentage increase in cancer incidence showed a peak between 25 and 30 years of age for women and between 50 and 55 for men (Figure 2). Among other things, these data show how different the situation can be in each sex. The early age period was excluded in these studies since it would distort the picture because of the peak incidence found during childhood.

A parameter that can influence the age incidence is the genetic background. It was found that for almost any type of human cancer, there is a heritable and a nonheritable form, the former having an earlier onset;[22] the difference in onset can be of 2 to 3 decades.

Another aspect of the genetic influence is that reported for bladder cancer in workers exposed to carcinogenic amines (which started earlier in blacks).[23] Other factors besides the genetic background, such as different lifestyles, could also be implicated in this earlier onset. This may be one of the reasons why incidence can vary according to regional areas; intraoral carcinoma, for instance, occurs earlier in Nigeria than in Europe or North America.[24] Regardless of the possible interpretations, these examples suggest that the age factor may carry less weight than other determinants.

Different onsets, depending on the geographical distribution, are found with many types of

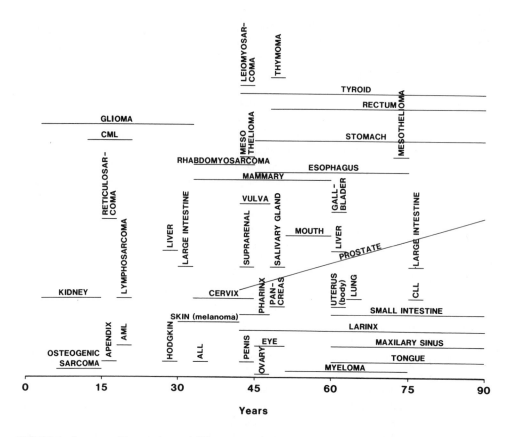

FIGURE 1.   Summary of the prevalence of different tumors in the autopsy studies from the Malmö General Hospital.[19] The length of the lines indicates the age span (bottom line) when the prevalence was maximal. Horizontal lines mean that the prevalence did not increase, the ascending line means an increase in the prevalence.

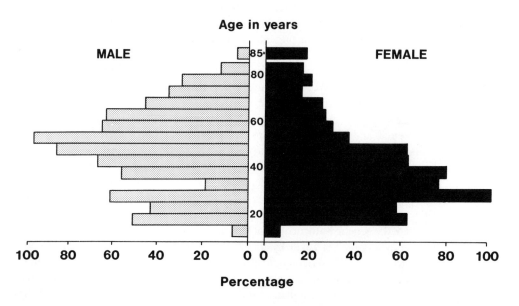

FIGURE 2.   Cancer incidence in England and Wales taken from the number of cancer registries for both sexes (cancer statistics: registrations, Her Majesty's Stationery Office, London). The histograms show the percentage of increase in incidence of cancer of each 5-year group over the previous one excluding the age groups 0 to 10. (From *Nature*, 261, 586, © 1976. With permission of Macmillam Magazines Ltd.)

cancer, including some that have been supposed to be associated with aging, such as breast cancer. Epidemiological studies have shown that the age profile for breast cancer is shifted toward younger ages in Cuba as compared to Sweden.[25]

The increased incidence of tumors in younger age groups observed recently speaks against the influence of aging on the development of some tumors. This has occurred *inter alia* for cervical cancer in different regions,[26-29] for Hodgkin's lymphoma,[30] and for breast cancer.[31]

Animal studies do not point to a simple straightforward relationship between cancer and aging; they show that as in humans, age incidence varies and depends upon many parameters.

Several types of tumors are characteristic of young rather than old animals,[32] in particular those caused by viruses such as leukemias in cat.[33] It shows that the variations in incidence can be related *inter alia,* with the different mechanisms that cause cancer and with the respective response of the host. Young animals seem indeed to be more susceptible to different oncogenic viruses.[34]

An interesting result with viral-induced tumors in animals was obtained by Copeland and Bigner.[35] Rats were injected at different ages with avian sarcoma virus; the incidence of animals developing tumors was 100% in all groups, but the incidence of multiple tumors declined with increasing age at inoculation. Neoplasias arising in older mice treated with urethane[36] were larger and more invasive. Also, mice with tumors induced by diethylnitrosamine died earlier with increasing age at the time of induction.[37]

With regard to spontaneous tumors in animals, the results do not favor a simple overall potentiating effect of aging on the incidence of cancer. In mice, the age incidence varies with the type of tumor and the animal strain.[38] In rats, although the incidence of most tumors increases as the population ages, "some tumors peak at a relatively young age so that older rats are at a much lower risk than their younger cohorts. Some rats die without tumors even in the oldest age groups; this is especially true for the BN/Bi rats."[39] The results led to the conclusion that the risk of developing an increased number of tumors with age is strain and sex dependent.[39] In the Wistar SPF Tox rat where the incidence is high, some tumor types occur early in life and others appear later.[4]

In some cases though, aging may be a potentiating factor; the incidence of chromatoblastoma in the goldfish was proportional to the third power of age.[40]

Another aspect of the relationship between cancer and age is the problem of the spreading of tumors in the organism. In many instances, spreading is slower in older hosts, described elsewhere in this volume. In the experiments cited,[35] with rats injected with avian sarcoma virus, survival was increased in old rats.

Progression of spontaneous tumors in rats varies strikingly with the strain. One strain (BL/BL females) had metastatic tumors in 16% of the animals because of the higher frequency of metastatic adrenal cortical carcinomas.[39] There was a positive correlation between age and metastatic cancer. In other strains, this evaluation was more difficult to make because of the low incidence of metastatic cancer (3 to 9% of the animals). Burek[39] concluded that if any trend was seen, it suggested a lack of any increased risk for the oldest rats to develop tumor metastases.

So the relationship between cancer and age depends upon multiple factors such as genetic determinants, time of exposure to carcinogens, the number of carcinogens, sex, lifestyles (e.g., diet), associated diseases, and developmental changes started during embryonic life and progressing through the animal life span. From fertilization of the egg up to old age, the organism is continuously remodeled at the molecular, cellular, tissue, organ, and organismal levels. These continuous modifications can be favorable at certain times for the initiation of some types of cancer, but can create adverse conditions for other types.

These are some of the questions raised when reviewing the cancer-age relationship. We can only wonder how the idea of the general potentiating effect of aging on cancer development became widely accepted and gave rise to global theories involving both phenomena. Cancer development during the animal life span is a dynamic process where new variables are continuously created. The linear eschatological view of the process is not supported by the appraisal of all the aspects involved.

The volume is organized so that the reader can become aware of the multiple phenomena that intervene in the cancer-age relationship, not to find answers to such a complex problem, but rather to raise questions.

To understand neoplastic disease, we must be aware of the molecular, cellular, tissue, physiopathological, epidemiological, and clinical aspects of the disease. For the sake of space, we have limited the choice of subjects, but enough are covered to make the reader realize that there is no place for simple-minded interpretations.

REFERENCES

1. **de Waard, F., Baanders-van Halewijn, E. A., and Huizinga, J.,** The bimodal age distribution of patients with mammary carcinoma, *Cancer,* 17, 141, 1964.
2. **Abeloff, M. D.,** Paraneoplastic syndromes. A window on the biology of cancer, *Lancet,* 2, 1598, 1987.
3. **Cairns, J.,** The treatment of diseases and the war against cancer, *Sci. Am.,* 253, 31, 1985.
4. **Kroes, R., Garbis-Berkvens, J. M., de Vries, T., and van Nesseboog, J. H. J.,** Histopathological profile of a Wistar rat stock including a survey of the literature, *J. Gerontol.,* 36, 259, 1981.
5. **Schwartz, A. G.,** Correlation between species life span and capacity to activate 7,12-dimethylbenzantracene to a form mutagenic to mammalian cells, *Exp. Cell Res.,* 94, 445, 1975.
6. National Center of Health Statistics, *Some Demographic Aspects of Aging in the United States,* U.S. Public Health Service and U.S. Bureau of the Census, Washington, D.C., 1973.
7. **Azzarelli, A., Gennari, L., Guagliuolo, V., Bonfanti, G., Cerasoli, S., and Bufalino, R.,** Chondrosarcoma-55 unreported cases: epidemiology, surgical treatment and prognostic factors, *Eur. J. Surg. Oncol.,* 12, 165, 1986.
8. **Cutler, S. J.,** Third National Cancer Survey-An overview of available information, *J. Natl. Cancer Inst.,* 53, 1565, 1974.
9. **Doll, R.,** An epidemiological perspective of the biology of cancer, *Cancer Res.,* 38, 3573, 1978.
10. **Wynder, E. L.,** The epidemiology of large bowel cancer, *Cancer Res.,* 35, 3388, 1975.
11. **Doll, R., Morgan, L., and Speitzer, F. E.,** Cancers of the lung and nasal sinuses in nickel workers, *Br. J. Cancer,* 24, 623, 1984.
12. **Pinto, S. S., Henderson, W., and Enterline, P. E.,** Mortality experience of arsenic-exposed workers, *Arch. Environ. Health,* 33, 325, 1978.
13. **Salk, D.,** Werner Syndrome: a review of recent research with an analysis of connective tissue metabolism, growth control of cultured cells and chromosomal aberrations, *Hum. Genet.,* 62, 1, 1982.
14. **Bailar J. C., III and Smith, E. M.,** Progress against cancer? *N. Engl. J. Med.,* 314, 1226, 1986.
15. **Foulds, L.,** The natural history of cancer, *J. Chronic Dis.,* 8, 2, 1958.
16. **de Waard, F. and Trichopoulos, D.,** A unifying concept of the aetiology of breast cancer, *Int. J. Cancer,* 41, 666, 1988.
17. **Mughal, T. I., Robinson, W. A., and Padmos, M. A.,** Adult Hodgkin's disease in Saudi Arabia, *Eur. J. Surg. Oncol.,* 11, 41, 1985.
18. **Grufferman, S. and Delzell, E.,** Epidemiology of Hodgkin's disease, *Epidemiol. Rev.,* 6, 76, 1984.
19. **Berge, T. and Lundberg, S.,** Cancer in Malmö 1958-1969. An autopsy study, *Acta Pathol. Microbiol. Scand.,* suppl. no. 260, 1977.
20. **Mc Keown, F.,** Malignant disease in old age, *Br. J. Cancer,* 10, 251, 1956.
21. **Kee, M.,** Cancer incidence in England and Wales, *Nature,* 302, 199, 1983.
22. **Anderson, D. E.,** Familial susceptibility, in *Persons at High Risk of Cancer, An Approach to Cancer Etiology and Control,* Fraumeni, J.F., Jr., Ed., Academic Press, New York, 1975, 43.
23. **Schulte, P. A., Ringen, K., Hemstreet, G .P., Altekruse, E. B., Gullen, W. H., Patton, M. G., Allsbrook, W. C., Crosby, J. H., West, S. S., Witherington, R., Koss, L., Bales, C. E., Tillet, S., Rooks, S., Stern, F., Stringer, W., Schmidt, V. A., and Brubaker, M. M.,** Risk assessment of a cohort exposed to aromatic amines, *J. Occup. Med.,* 27, 115, 1985.
24. **Adekeye, E. O., Asamoa, E., and Cohen, B.,** Intraoral carcinoma in Nigeria: a review of 137 cases, *Ann. R. Coll. Surg. Engl.,* 67, 180, 1985.

25. **Skoog, L., Wallgren, A., Pascula, M. R., Macías, A., Pérez, R., and Lage, A.,** Factors associated with prognosis in human breast cancer. VII. A comparison between a Cuban and a Swedish study, *Neoplasma,* 34, 587, 1987.
26. **Green, G. H.,** Cervical cancer and cytology screening in New Zealand, *Br. J. Obstet. Gynecol.,* 85, 881, 1978.
27. **Carmichael, J. A., Clarke, D. H., Moher, D., Ohlke, I. D., and Karchmar, E. J.,** Cervical carcinoma in women aged 34 and younger, *Am. J. Obstet. Gynecol.,* 154, 264, 1986.
28. **Bourne, R. G. and Grove, W. D.,** Invasive carcinoma of the cervix in Queensland. Change in incidence and mortality, *Med. J. Aust.,* 1, 156, 1983.
29. **Armstrong, B. and Holman, D'A.,** Increasing mortality from cancer of the cervix in young Australian women, *Med. J. Aust.,* 1, 460, 1981.
30. **Aozasa, K., Ueda, T., Tamai, M., and Tsujimura, T.,** Hodgkin's disease in Osaka, *Eur. J. Cancer Clin. Oncol.,* 22, 1117, 1986.
31. **White, E., Daling, J. R., Norsted, T. L. and Chu, J.,** Rising incidence of breast cancer among young women in Washington State, *J. Natl. Cancer Inst.,* 79, 239, 1987.
32. **Cotchin, E.,** Spontaneous tumors in young animals, *Proc. R. Soc. Med.,* 68, 653, 1975.
33. **Hardy, W. D., Old, L. J., Hess, P. W., Essex, M., and Cotter, S.,** Horizontal transmission of feline leukemia virus, *Nature,* 244, 266, 1973.
34. **Gross, L.,** Spontaneous leukemia developing in C3H mice following inoculation in infancy with AK-leukemic extracts or AK-embryos, *Proc. Soc. Exp. Biol. Med.,* 76, 27, 1951.
35. **Copeland, D. D. and Bigner, D. D.,** Influence of age at inoculation on avian oncornavirus-induced brain tumor incidence, tumor morphology and postinoculation survival in F344 rats, *Cancer Res.,* 37, 1657, 1977.
36. **Anderson, V. N. and Budinger, J. M.,** Qualitative histological differences between transplacentally-induced lung tumors in young and aging mice, *Cancer Lett.,* 11, 285, 1981.
37. **Clapp, N. K., Perkins, E. H., Klima, W. C., and Cacheiro, L. H.,** Temporal advancement of diethylnitrosamine carcinogenesis in aging mice, *J. Gerontol.,* 36, 158, 1981.
38. The Staff of the Jackson Laboratory, *Biology of the Laboratory Mouse,* Green, E.L., Ed., Dover Publications, New York, 1975, 523.
39. **Burek, J. D.,** *Pathology of Aging Rats,* CRC Press, Boca Raton, Florida, 1978, 170.
40. **Etoh, H., Hyodo-taguchi, Y., Aoki, K., Murata, M., and Matsudaira, H.,** Incidence of chromatoblastomas in aging goldfish (*Carassius auratus*), *J. Natl. Cancer Inst.,* 70, 523, 1983.

Part I:
Factors Affecting the
Age Incidence of Cancer

IA: Developmental Cell and Tissue Determinants

Chapter 1

CANCER AND AGING AT THE CELLULAR LEVEL

A. Macieira-Coelho

TABLE OF CONTENTS

The unknown in the occult phase of neoplastic disease is one of the reasons for difficulty in ascertaining the relationship between cancer and age. In order to grasp the variables involved in the occult phase, it is necessary to understand how neoplasia progresses at the cellular level.

I. NEOPLASTIC DEVELOPMENT AT THE CELLULAR LEVEL

A. *IN VIVO* STUDIES

The complexity of the events at the cellular level leading to a clinically detectable tumor have become apparent from the comparative study of the natural history of cancer.[1]

As described by Foulds,[1] the development of neoplasia in an organ is not necessarily followed by a relentless invasion of the tissue and later metastases, killing of the host. Foulds reviewed, in a convincing way, the evidence that neoplasia is discontinuous in space and time. The discontinuity is unpredictable for any type of tumor and also within the same type of tumors. Tumor progression can stop for a variable period of time or may even be completely arrested until the animal dies of old age without any obvious relationship of causality between the tumor and death. Progression can also proceed by intermittent steps with variable times spent at each stop. According to Foulds,[1] "Neoplasia needs studying from beginning to end as a dynamic process advancing along many different pathways and through qualitatively different stages at which there is a choice between regression, persistence without qualitative change, and progression by irreversible qualitative change, involving the manifestation of properties not formerly present." Hence, one can find several types of situations during cancer initiation and progression. This is so because of the various number of new properties a cell population has to acquire to spread in the organism and also because the latter has to change to facilitate the spreading; these processes can take several years.

Neoplasia is the result of multiple changes occurring in a cell through the action of a variety of agents. The escape from homeostasis implies changes in the cells directly implicated in neoplastic growth, changes in the microenvironment, and changes in the organism as a whole. "In many forms of neoplasia there is evidence of a wide field of prepared tissue within which neoplasia develops focally."[1]

Locally it can mean *inter alia* the capacity to accumulate through division, to invade neighboring cell systems, to overcome basal membranes that limit cellular territories, to create its own blood supply, and to overcome immune surveillance. To achieve this, the cells that start to deviate from normalcy must secrete new enzymes capable of digesting membranes that constitute barriers for cell migration. The cell membranes must be modified so that they can get loose from their normal anchorage. Sometimes the cells create a cocoon of fibrin protecting them from the response of the organism.[2] In other tumors, on the contrary, the cells develop fibrinolytic activity. They may secrete factors stimulating their migration or growth; substances capable of neovascularization, and immune suppressors facilitating their migration and survival in lymphatic vessels. They also must go through modifications allowing them to survive in the vascular system in a state of anchorage independence, etc.

The neoplastic cells must also be modified in their response to external signals (humoral and cellular) that normally restrain cell systems to their physiological role. Many of these signals are just beginning to be understood, but it is well known that interactions between different cell systems are crucial for tissue homeostasis. The development of a cancer cell population depends not only upon changes in the cells directly implicated, but also on deviations of the internal milieu caused by modifications of other cells. Indeed, there is experimental evidence now favoring Foulds'[1] view, that, at least in some cases, neoplasia from the beginning is a generalized disease where somatic cells create a field effect that favors its development.[3,4] The stromal cells of the neoplastic tissue for instance, are particularly important for the survival of the cancer cells. Within the stroma there are also modifications in macromolecules like proteoglycans, structural glycoproteins, collagen, and elastic fibers, in other words the extracellular matrix, that plays a role as a supporting structure.

According to Foulds, "tumors in general are not composed of random conglomeration of cells, but of organized tissues with characteristic histologic patterns".[5] The idea of The Cancer Cell, which originated from experimental anaplastic tumors that have been carried in laboratories through serial transplantations, is incompatible with the observations made on spontaneous tumors.[5]

Later the modified cells may acquire the capacity to anchor in a distant organ and grow in the new environment. Another important aspect of the neoplastic disease is that related to modifications induced in the whole organism.[6] The cells can start secreting substances that cause repercussions in distant organs. Examples of this are the bone resorption accompanied by hypercalcemia,[7] the Cushing Syndrome present in some cancer patients,[8] and the tumor producing cachexia.[9] These features give a perception of the multiple changes that have to occur in the genome, from the beginning of the neoplastic process to the time it kills the host.

It should be emphasized that the cellular, tissue, and organismal changes leading to neoplastic disease can be absent or present in different combinations in an unpredictable pattern. Those who are aware of what neoplastic disease is can only wonder how such simple-minded ideas as cancer caused by one gene or initiated by two events could "have had the day". The same is true of the concept that the incidence of cancer increases with senescence. The relationship between cancer and age is as complex as neoplastic disease itself and it cannot be appraised without keeping in mind the complexity of the evolution of the latter.

B. *IN VITRO* STUDIES

The cultivation of cells *in vitro* has been a valuable tool to study the cellular changes leading to cancer. In particular, the experiments analyzing the relationship between cancer and aging at the cellular level contributed strongly to a better understanding of the pathogenesis and physiopathology of neoplastic disease and to the experimental demonstration of the discontinuity of tumor progression.

Our understanding has been possible through the observation of how normal cells behave *in vitro*, which has then allowed the understanding of deviations from normalcy, e.g., transformation. It has been a laborious task which has been met with misunderstanding. Indeed, many investigators did not realize the limits of normal cell behavior which led in many cases to the use of cell systems thought to be normal, but which in fact presented deviations from normal growth control. It is for this reason that the word "transformation" has been so misinterpreted and misused in cell biology. The study of transformation *in vitro* has helped us understand the biology of the cancer cell, rendering apparent the multiple steps a cell population has to go through until a clinically detectable tumor develops.

Transformation is supposed to encompass the spontaneous or induced changes occurring in a cell population *in vitro*, having analogies with what occurs *in vivo* during the development of a neoplastic growth. Those changes should follow a pattern analogous to the ones leading to cancer and express at least some of the steps allowing a cell population *in vivo* to escape homeostasis. These steps are extremely complex and *in vitro*, we can probably analyze just a fraction.

Transformation is the progressive acquisition of growth autonomy, such that a cell population becomes less dependent upon the different mechanisms which restrain the growth of normal cells. Duing transformation, a cell population goes through a series of steps whose succession is unpredictable and which can stop anywhere along the path to full autonomy. Transformation represents the opposite of what occurs during *in vitro* senescence where cells on the contrary become more sensitive to the various mechanisms that limit growth and eventually stop proliferating.[10]

A cell population cultivated *in vitro* has characteristics that can be measured to evaluate deviations from normalcy. It should be stressed, however, that like any phenomenon in biology, the limits are often subtle and assume a gradient-like pattern without a clear borderline. The final evaluation must be the result of a multiparameter analysis. What follows is an enumeration of the different steps of transformation that can be measured in cultivated cells.

A monolayer of confluent normal cells in resting phase usually assumes a pattern characteristic for a given cell system and results from the "social" organization of the cell population. It is caused by the restraint of cell-cell overlapping and proliferation during cell crowding and leads to resting phase at a given cell density. The arrest of cell division may not be absolute but is more pronounced when compared with transformed cell populations.[11]

The growth requirements of transformed cells can change in the sense that they become less dependent upon the serum supplement of the medium to reach high densities.[12] This seems to be due to the secretion of autocrine growth factors which can partially replace the growth-promoting activity of serum.[13,14]

The restraint from cell overlapping, i.e., from mutual invasion due to contact inhibition of movement, can be measured.[15] It is more or less pronounced depending on the cell type; in some, like endothelial or brain derived cells, overlapping is almost nonexistent, in others, such as fibroblasts, it can take place in normal cell populations but the social order is respected. In other words, it occurs in a regular pattern without anarchy. In fibroblast populations, overlapping decreases during senescence.

In some cases transformation can be accompanied by a reduction of cell overlapping[12] due to other events that become predominant. In other cases, cell overlapping can be so extensive that cells tend to pile up and form foci which can be counted and this way express transformation quantitatively.[16]

It is due to these variable changes in the loss of contact inhibition of movement and of growth that transformation at this stage can be expressed in different ways depending on the cell type and upon the carcinogen:[11,12] sometimes the cells are only able to grow to higher densities but eventually division stops; other times division does not stop, either because the cells are capable to grow on top of each other or because cells detach, leaving space for other cells to grow. The latter is analogous to what happens with some tumors *in vivo* where cell loss can be very significant and is certainly an event that retards the killing of the host but can also create the conditions for metastasis. When cell loss is important during transformation *in vitro,* maximal cell densities are low. These different expressions of transformation at this stage have a common denominator, i.e., the fraction of dividing cells at the density where the controls reach resting phase, is higher in the transformed cells. This gave rise to a quantitative test of this transformation step.[11] These different behaviors of transformed cells are representative of the paths a cell population can follow during the escape from growth control and is analogous to the pleiotropism of tumor progression *in vivo.*

The potential of cells to grow on top of each other depends on how far the cells have gone along the path of transformation and upon the extracellular matrix.[17] At certain stages of transformation, some cells will pile up and survive without proliferation; at more advanced stages of transformation the cells will also multiply.[17]

Another characteristic of normal cells (with the exception of those of the hematoopoetic system) is the need for survival and division of a substratum to which to attach, i.e., they are anchorage dependent.[18] This gave rise to a useful test where cells are suspended in an agarose semisolid medium and checked for the growth of colonies.[19] Again, it should be remembered that this criterion is not absolute and that in a normal cell population one can find cells that are able to form colonies under those conditions, but that the fraction of colony forming cells and the size of the colonies they originate are smaller than in the case of transformed cells.

The capacity to grow in a semisolid medium can also present a progressive pattern in the sense that some cells will grow in suspension only if supplied with a particular nutritional environment and others will do it without any special nutrient requirements.[20] Growth in a semisolid medium does not depend only upon external factors; it is also correlated to such different events as the secretion of a cell surface proteoglycan[21] or the utilization of purines via the salvage pathway.[22] This gives an idea of the multiple events involved in this transformation step.

Some cells which have progressed further along the path of transformation can grow in suspension in a liquid medium, i.e., they become completely anchorage independent. This is analogous to what happens *in vivo* when tumor cells get loose from the tissue where they originated and acquire the capacity to survive when transported in the peripheral blood.

Another feature revealing modifications of the cell membrane and which can be quantitated is the tendency of some transformed cell populations to form aggregates.[23] This is also analogous to the biology of some tumors which have been reported to form large aggregates in an agitation system.[24] It may represent a step where tumor cells acquire a selective advantage through cooperation.

Normal cells are endowed with a limited division potential and the acquisition of unlimited growth is another stop in the progression toward autonomy,[25] but there are intermediate steps where the cells acquire an increased growth potential, albeit finite.[26] The time of occurrence of the immortalization step was studied during the progression of breast cancer;[27] it was found to take place at a late stage.

Another feature that can also occur along the path of transformation is the loss of the capacity to attach and retract a plasma clot. This has been developed into a quantitative method and has a bearing with the disturbed cell-fibrin interactions occurring during neoplastic development *in vivo*.[28]

The plasma clot retraction depends upon the attachment of the cells to fibrin and the pulling of the clot. The loss of the capacity to retract is related *inter alia* with the altered distribution of actin-containing cables that can be observed during transfomation.[29] A reorganization of actin is also a feature of mesenchymal cells from some patients at high risk of cancer[30] and seems to be due to a reduced half-life of actin[31] and to modifications in the synthesis of actin binding molecules such as tropomyosin.[32] Germane to this modification during transformation is the finding that a human oncogene contains sequences coding for tropomyosin.[33]

Changes in the organization of actin filaments and of other elements of the cytoskeleton also occur during cell senescence;[34] they are different, however, from those that occur during transformation. Their functional implications are also different in these two situations, since in the latter it is associated with an increased motility, as opposed to senescence where the cell loses its conformational flexibility.

This feature has implications for, on one hand, the decreased capacity to divide during senescence, and on the other, the loss of growth control during transformation. Indeed, several experiments support the view that membrane movements are propagated through the cytoskeleton to the nuclear matrix where they help to create the chromatin conformation favorable for gene expression and to initiating sites the right steric configuration for DNA synthesis.[34] The pleiotropic changes occurring in the membrane and in the cellular scaffold during transformation favor an unregulated flow of this information from the cell periphery to the nucleus, which increases the probability of engaging into the division cycle. On the contrary, during senescence, the flow of information is hindered,[34] thus decreasing the probability of initiating DNA synthesis.

Another characteristic of normal cells is to avoid the invasion of normal tissues. A test has been developed where the cells attach to an organ explant left in nutrient medium during a few days, which is then fixed for histological examination to check for invasion of the tissue.[35] Growth in chicken embryonic skin is also a good assay of this transformation step.[36] It has the same significance as the invasion of the organ explant.

Several attempts were made to find a correlation between each of these different steps and tumorigenicity. This was obviously a hopeless task since the latter is the sum of these different events and many more such as the response of the host, that progressively liberate the cells from the control of growth in the organism. Hence, when a correlation was found, it was just fortuitous.

The invasion of tissues *in vivo* and the killing of the host after injecting the cells into laboratory animals is an advanced stage of transformation. Here, one can use the term "malignant transformation" since malignancy has only meaning *in vivo*.

The capacity to invade a host can also be acquired to different degrees. Mice are the animals used in most cases; some cell populations can form only local tumor masses that eventually stop growing. Other cells can kill only immune depressed hosts or animals where the thymus does not develop. There are transformed cells that can form progressive tumors in nontreated animals if the latter are of the same strain from which the transformed cells were derived. Finally, some cell populations have evolved *in vitro* to such an extent that they can form tumors and kill any strain of mice, i.e., they have become isogenic.

In every one of these tests a progressive accumulation of subtle differences identical to the evolution has become obvious from the study of the natural history of cancer. The differences illustrate the multiple events that must occur at the molecular and cellular levels during cancer progression.

Like spontaneous cancers, the appearance of these deviations from the norm, their association, and mutual relationship are random and unpredictable. This means that tumor cell populations are heterogeneous not only between tumors but also within the tumor where there is a complete heterogeneity with respect to the different biological properties described above. The heterogeneity is manifest in regard to many traits such as drug resistance,[37] antigen expression,[38] metastatic potential,[39] karyotype,[40] and oncogene expression.[41] This explains why the search for universal biochemical markers of transformation has been elusive as has been the search for similar markers for cancer.

Some molecular events occur more frequently than others. This is the case for the lack of fixation of fibronectin at the cell surface.[42] A disturbance in fibronectin-membrane interactions also occurs in tumors *in vivo*. It also takes place during cell senescence[43] and it would be interesting to know if it has any implications for the increased susceptibility of aged human fibroblasts to virus transformation.[44] This is discussed below in more detail.

An increased fibrinolytic activity due to the increased synthesis of plasminogen activator occurs rather frequently during transformation by different agents.[45] Normal human embryonic fibroblasts, however, also produce plasminogen activator in large amounts and one might wonder if in the transformed cells, it corresponds to a regression to the embryonic phenotype.

Another interesting marker is the acquisition of resistance to xanthines. It has been reported during transformation of human embryonic liver cells by carcinogens that became resistant to theophylline[46] (for the real origin of these cells, see Reference 47) and during spontaneous immortalization of mouse fibroblasts which became resistant to caffeine.[48] Its implications are for the moment obscure; the elucidation of the underlying mechanisms, though, could be useful in the identification of some metabolic changes implicated in cell transformation.

Newly secreted phosphoproteins have been reported to be modified during transformation;[49] this is the reflection of a general change of phosphorylation during transformation.

The full understanding of the role of phosphorylation and dephosphorylation in cell metabolism has not been reached. It is known, however, that it is one of the tools developed by nature to switch a molecule between configurations that respond differently to substrates and regulator molecules.[50] This must certainly be finely tuned for homeostasis to prevail. It is no wonder, then, that phosphorylation is modified both during transformation and senescence. The deregulation of phosphorylation is probably one of the events responsible for the increased conformational flexibility of the transformed cell mentioned above.

The problem of oncogenes is related to that of protein phosphorylation. Indeed, oncogene products are direct or indirect effectors of different corners of the web where energy mobilization and transduction takes place. Their products can intervene in the phosphorylation of various proteins and thus, it should be expected that they play a role in such fundamental processes as development, growth, and differentiation.

On the other hand, alterations in the expression of oncogenes must inevitably lead to deviations of those processes since their products act at the most fundamental level of the life of a cell and are able to activate many different metabolic pathways. It should not be surprising to find them implicated in different pathological processes besides cancer.

This also explains that, contrary to what still shows up in much of the scientific literature, oncogenes cannot by themselves transform cells *in vitro* or trigger cancer, but just contribute to the deregulation of different matabolic pathways that create the conditions for the progressive escape from homeostasis. As discussed below, the effect of oncogenes seems to depend upon the susceptibility of the target cells to progress along the path of transformation.

The study of cell aging *in vitro*, reviewed in the following section, is seminal for understanding this fundamental aspect of the effect of oncogenes in transformation. Their exact role will only be known when the regulation of the pathways of energy mobilization and transduction are elucidated.

II. AGING AND TRANSFORMATION AT THE CELLULAR LEVEL

A. SUSCEPTIBILITY OF CELLS FROM DIFFERENT SPECIES TO ESCAPE SENESCENCE AND TO TRANSFORM

The possibility of studying aging at the cellular level was extended considerably by the use of tissue culture techniques. The aspect of cell senescence that is more relevant to the subject dealt with herein, concerns the division potential of cells.

Early in the 1960s, it was shown that during development and aging, mesenchymal cells lose their division potential, a phenomenon which can be detected by serially subcultivating the cells *in vitro*.[51,52]

Additional evidence that serial divisions of cells *in vitro* cause changes identical to those taking place during development, came from the finding that the kinetics of proliferation occurring in embryonic cells at the end of their proliferative potential are identical to those found in postnatal cells, early during their *in vitro* life span.[53]

Other authors have also found a correlation between the long-term doubling potential of human cells *in vitro* and donor's age. This was so not only for mesenchymal cells of different tissues,[54-60] but also for lens,[61] arterial smooth muscle,[62,63] keratinocytes,[64] chondrocytes,[65] and a population of T lymphocytes.[66]

An interesting test of the hypothesis that this is an aging phenomenon[51] was made by Ryan et al.[67] who cultivated skin fibroblasts from pairs of monozygotic twins. The results showed a similar poliferation and replicative life span within each twin pair. Among the twin pairs with different ages, however, the cells differed in these respects.

A decline in the cell growth potential with age was also found for fibroblasts from tortoise[68] and hamster,[69] for smooth muscle cells from two murine species,[70] and for chondrocytes from dog and rabbit.[71,72]

Parameters other than the long-term division potential have also been tested. Thus, human epidermal keratinocytes from newborn donors proliferate more rapidly and attain a higher concentration at confluence than those from aged donors.[73] Also during development and aging, there is an increase in the concentration of PDGF required for optimal growth *in vitro*.[74-77]

Further support for the relationship between aging and division potential came from studies with cells originated from patients with Werner's syndrome of premature aging. These cells have a decreased doubling potential when compared with those of age-matched normal donors.[78] Another disease with features of premature aging where fibroblasts were found to senesce earlier *in vitro* than age-matched controls is cystic fibrosis.[79]

Obviously it would be naïve to think that in old age our somatic cells have lost their capacity to divide. This has been a misinterpretation due in part to the approach of some investigators who have considered senescent cells only as those in the terminal stage of their life span. One of the contributions of the cell culture model is that it has shown that although some terminal cells are produced from the mass population at each doubling, long before the cell population reaches the terminal stage, subtle changes can be detected in the initiation of the division cycle and in the transit through the cycle.[80,81] It is this progressive evolution that can explain events such as delayed wound healing[82] and the disturbed proliferation in the salivary gland[83] observed during aging *in vivo*. They are certainly the expression of the modifications created in the cell through division, apparent long before a cell reaches the terminal postmitotic state. In other words, events taking place during the division cycle, which modify the cells, create a permanent drift that leads to heterogeneity and to changes in the response of the cells to growth stimuli long before a cell population reaches the terminal nondividing stage.

There is an important implication for the pathogeny of cancer resulting from the disturbance in the regulation of growth taking place with time in some dividing cell compartments. Homeostasis at the tissue level depends upon an equilibrium between different cell systems resulting from cell-cell interactions. In particular, mesenchymal cells play an important role in creating a microenvironment through the secretion of large tissue-supporting macromolecules such as structural glycoproteins, elastine, and collagen,[84] or through the synthesis of small soluble diffusable molecules such as growth factors[85,86] and prostaglandins[87] that are important for the regulation of the homeostasis of the tissue. The deregulation of the response to division is accompanied by changes of the cell metabolism causing a disruption of the equilibrium with other cell systems. This must be responsible in part to hyperplastic proliferations taking place with time in the organism, which could be a favorable ground for neoplastic development.

This concept of cellular aging is important in other regards for the relationship we are reviewing herein; it has to be understood within a historical perspective. The paradigm accepted by the scientific community at the time the hypothesis was postulated[88] was that under adequate culture conditions it should be possible to propagate *in vitro* an immortal cell population maintaining all characteristics of normalcy. Two investigators,[89] however, had obtained data suggesting that some cells may be endowed with a limited number of doublings, while others are able to divide indefinitely.

What finally became clear, though not for all, is that cells differ in their ability to acquire an unlimited growth potential,[90] but that in any case the acquisition of the latter is an abnormal characteristic. Furthermore, it became apparent that the probability of escaping senescence has a bearing on the susceptibility to be transformed by all types of carcinogens and oncogenes.[91]

The failure to grasp this important conclusion led to the indiscriminate use of cells for the study of the effect of carcinogens and wrong interpretations of their mechanism of action due to the misunderstanding of the biology of the target cell.

Indeed, much of the work on transformation *in vitro* led to the study of the action of carcinogens on cells that had already gone through some steps of the transformation process. It contributed to the terrible confusion surrounding the word "transformation", to simple-minded concepts such as that cancer is a two-step event, or that one gene can induce malignancy.

One of the interesting windfalls of the concept of aging *in vitro* and of its opposite, cell immortalization, was to have shown evolutionary differences between species that also have a bearing on cancer and aging *in vivo*.

When comparing fibroblasts from different species according to the probability of yielding spontaneously a population with unlimited growth potential, a scale is found going from a very low to a 100% probability (Figure 1). The latter is found with mouse fibroblasts regardless of the animal strain.[92,93] In general, murine fibroblasts tend to have a higher probability of yielding permanent cell lines than, for instance, human and bovine. This has led to the claim that one [94] or two genes[95] are necessary for the transformation of murine cells. In fact, these cells evolve spontaneously through the different transformation steps[96,97] and the introduction of those genes just accelerates a latent potential.

Several results described below support the view that this phenomenon is not an artifact of *in vitro* subcultivation. One aspect relevant to the cancer-aging relationship is the fact that it is

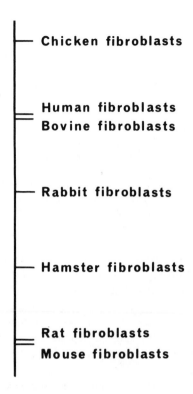

FIGURE 1. Scale representing from the top to the bottom, the increasing probability of obtaining spontaneous immortalization from fibroblast-like cells of different species. (Reprinted by permission from *Gerontology,* 26, 276, 1980, S. Karger AG, Basel.)

easier to induce cancers in those species (e.g., murine) whose fibroblasts have a higher probability of escaping *in vitro* senescence.[98] Indeed, anything can induce tumors in mice, even the implantation of pieces of plastic. This is not so in humans where there are no reports concerning tumor development at sites of implantation of prostheses used in surgery.

The species whose fibroblasts immortalize easily seem also to be more short lived. Is there any relationship of cause and effect between cell instability and short life span? The question remains open but the relationship seems reasonable, even more when it is realized that the cellular instability seems to be related to some particularities of the genome that are described below.

The other results showing that the probability of *in vitro* immortalization is not an artifact, concern the response to carcinogens. Transformation of chicken fibroblasts, which are at one end of the scale, by Rous sarcoma virus (RSV), for instance, yields cells which go through some transformation steps e.g., piling up and loss of contact inhibition of growth, but which in general do not immortalize and indeed have a shorter life span than the noninfected cells.[98] Tumors developed in chickens after RSV infection also do not have a clonal type of growth;[98] the spread of these tumors is due to increased cell proliferation after viral infection. The infected cells die after a few divisions and the virus is propagated to new cells which then become recruited into the proliferative compartment, probably due to the release of autocrine growth factors.[13,14]

Mouse cells, on the contrary, are easily transformed by viruses. The cell population rapidly goes through many of the steps of transformation.

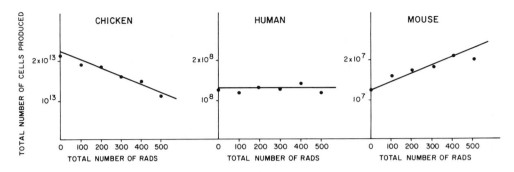

FIGURE 2.   Plot of the total number of cells produced *in vitro* by control cultures and cultures that received the indicated number of rads. In mouse cultures, the total number of cells produced was calculated up to the 20th passage, that is, at the time the cultures were immortalized. (Reprinted by permission from *Nature,* 261, 586, ©1976, Macmillan Magazines, Ltd.)

Human and bovine fibroblasts, which have an intermediate position on the scale, when infected for instance with SV40 virus, go through some steps of transformation such as morphological changes, loss of contact inhibition of growth,[11] and prolonged life span,[99] but stop short of full transformation since they generally phase out.[100] More recently, however, it has been claimed that a small-plaque SV40 variant can immortalize human fibroblasts with a 100% efficiency.[101] The latter work does not change the feature of the particular resistance of human fibroblasts to progress along the path of transformation, since it is manifested in response to all oncogenic viruses tested so far.

Identical responses can be obtained with chemical carcinogens. They easily make mouse cells progress along different transformation steps,[102] but in general only partially transform human fibroblasts.[47,103]

The response to low dose rate ionizing radiation also fits the relative probability of the fibroblasts from the species shown on the scale of Figure 1 to spontaneously escape senescence. Thus, this type of radiation shortens the life span of chicken embryo fibroblasts,[104,105] it has no effect or can prolong the division potential of human embryonic fibroblasts,[106,107] and it accelerates the immortalization of mouse fibroblasts[105,108] (Figure 2).

These data suggest that all carcinogens, regardless of their nature (viral, chemical, or physical) act on the fibroblasts of these different species, as activators of a latent potential. Again, the effect of oncogenes is related to the relative position of these cells on the scale of Figure 1. They transform without the immortalization of chicken cells,[109] can induce in human fibroblasts some transformation steps such as focus formation and anchorage independence[110] but rarely immortalize them,[111,112] and easily immortalize murine fibroblasts,[94,95] a phenomenon which occurs spontaneously with these cells.[96,97] The problems concerning the human species are discussed in more detail below.

The susceptibility to transformation is not only influenced by the origin of the fibroblasts, but also by their age in terms of the residual proliferative potential. This is so for different types of carcinogens but the time when the cell susceptibility is more pronounced is not the same for all carcinogens.

In regard to SV40 transformation, three different groups have reported that human fibroblasts are more susceptible after having exhausted most of their division potential.[44,113,114] Transformation occurred either in the immortalization step or only in the formation of foci against a monolayer background. Matsumura et al.,[115] however, reported that infection with SV40 virus induces DNA synthesis in terminal postmitotic cells but does not induce proliferation. The different results could be due to the use of either preterminal cells with a small residual proliferation potential or terminal postmitotic cells.

Young, low population doubling level human fibroblasts are susceptible to chemical carcinogens; old higher doubling level cells are refractory to the insult.[103] The requirement for DNA synthesis during treatment is a necessary condition for transformation; this could be the reason why old cells, where it is more difficult to induce DNA synthesis, are refractory. The young, carcinogen treated cells have a prolonged life span and a higher rate of colony formation in agar, are invasive on embryonic chicken skin, and have a cell surface antigen also found on human sarcoma cells, but are not immortalized.[103]

A different response of young and old cells to a tumor promoter has also been reported. Early passage cells are susceptible to the inhibition of queuine uptake by a tumor promoter.[116] Queuine is a nucleoside found in the first position of the anticodon for some tRNAs. Late passage cells, however, become refractile to this induced inhibition of the nucleoside uptake. This property of early passage cells seems to be due to a factor secreted by young fibroblasts. Furthermore, the growth factor stimulation of queuine uptake is also inhibited by the tumor promoter in young cells and is enhanced in the old cells. The kinase activities of growth factor receptors and of phorbol ester-stimulated protein kinase C suggest that phosphorylation is a crucial control event in the uptake of queuine.[116]

The susceptibility to the transforming action of low dose rate ionizing radiation also varies with cell age. It is greater in young cells. Radiation can prolong the life span, induce foci, and increase the proliferative activity of human fibroblasts when applied on young cells;[26,106,107,117] on older cells, it shortens their life span.[106] On the contrary, the susceptibility to ultraviolet (UV) radiation seems to be identical throughout the life span of a human fibroblastic cell population.[47]

B. SUSCEPTIBILITY OF CELLS FROM DIFFERENT HUMAN DONORS TO ESCAPE SENESCENCE AND TO TRANSFORM

The interspecies diversity in the probability of escaping senescence and transforming is analogous to that found in the response to carcinogens of cells from different human donors.

This problem was raised for the first time in a report that fibroblasts obtained from two patients with Fanconi's anemia (FA), infected with SV40 virus, gave rise to ten times more colonies of piling up cells than the fibroblasts from normal donors.[118] The number of colonies in cells from heterozygous cultures was intermediate to those of the control cultures and of the homozygous. The way, however, the viral DNA is presented to the cells seems to influence the outcome.[119]

Further evidence suggesting an instability of fibroblasts from FA patients was obtained with another carcinogen. When the cells were treated with low dose rate ionizing radiation, their division potential increased by 58%.[26] A significant increase in the number of doublings was also obtained by keeping the cultures 25 d in resting phase and resuming growth after this period.[120] It is interesting that an increased radioresistance was also found for other genetically linked cancer prone diseases.[117,121-125]

An increased susceptibility to UV light and chemical and viral transformation was reported for cells from several genetically determined cancer prone diseases. These included Down Syndrome,[126] xeroderma pigmentosum,[127-130] Bloom's Syndrome, ataxia-telangiectasia,[131-133] and hereditary adenomatosis of the colon and rectum.[134-136] A prolongation of the human fibroblast growth potential by an oncogene has also been obtained with cells from cancer prone patients.[137]

It became apparent that fibroblasts from cancer patients without any known genetically determined predisposition to the disease could present spontaneous deviations from normal senescence.[3] As expected, an inverse correlation was found between the doubling potential of fibroblasts in vitro and the donor's age for the controls (patients with benign lesions or having undergone plastic surgery). No correlation was found, though, with the cultures obtained from the cancer patients (Figure 3).

The cells from donors with breast cancer also responded abnormally to other biological parameters: they displayed increased anchorage independence, formed colonies on monolayers of normal epithelial cells, and when subcultivated at high inocula, could reach higher densities.

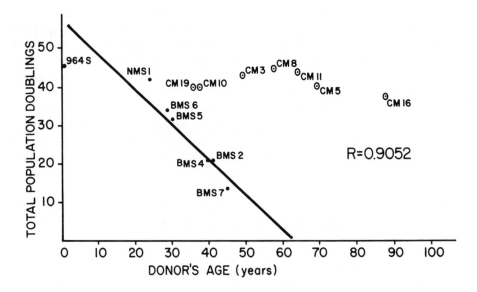

FIGURE 3. Correlation between the age of the donors and the doubling potential of the respective fibroblast-like cells obtained from control donors (◐) and from patients with breast cancer (●). (Reprinted by permission from *Int. J. Cancer,* 33, 759, 1988, Alan R. Liss, New York.)

Multiple subcultivations in overcrowded conditions allowed the selection of a fibroblastic cell subset with greater growth potential which could invade foreign tissues *in vitro*. This selected cell population also had a reduced capacity to retract a plasma clot and to anchor on fibrin, had an increased sensitivity to gelsolin (an actin-binding protein which blocks the fast-growing end of actin), a modified pattern of fibronectin secretion during spreading, and displayed a higher cloning efficiency.[28]

In one 30-year-old patient with a benign mammary tumor, the detection of deviations from normalcy in her skin fibroblasts cultivated *in vitro* anticipated by 3 years the appearance of a clinically detectable cancer in the same breast.[3] Thus, it seems that the deviations from the normal pattern of aging of the somatic cells may precede the development of the neoplasia by a long period.

Since at least some types of breast cancers seem genetically linked, patients with other tumors were also screened in regard to the behavior of their fibroblasts cultivated *in vitro*.[138] Deviations from normalcy could thus be detected in skin fibroblasts from patients with melanoma, hepatoma, and osteosarcoma. Hence, the higher susceptibility to progress along a few of the transformation steps observed in the somatic cells of some cancer patients may not be limited to genetically linked cancers.

Various investigators also ascertained other type of deviations from normalcy in fibroblasts from the normal skin of breast cancer patients. Shor et al.[139] identified a defect in the migratory behavior of the cells on a collagen gel: the fibroblasts from the cancer patients displayed a fetal-like behavior. The authors suggested that this is due to a leftover embryonic phenotype in the mesenchymal cells of the cancer patients which would create a field effect that facilitates the transformation of epithelial cells. The same group could identify the secretion of a migratory factor by embryonic fibroblasts and by those of cancer patients, but not by the cells from normal adults.[140]

The possibility of reversion of mesenchymal cells to an embryonic phenotype was tested by checking the expression of two antigens (4F2 and IL2) which can be detected in human embryonic fibroblasts and in sarcoma cells, but not in normal adult fibroblasts.[28] The cells from breast cancer patients, however, did not express the antigen. It is interesting, however, that the skin fibroblasts from patients with adenomatosis of the colon and rectum were 4F2 positive. Hence, the extent of reversion may vary and may be expressed only in relation to some markers.

Other investigators have also observed spontaneous transformation of fibroblasts obtained from the normal skin of a patient with primary malignant melanoma.[141] In this case, the cells went through the immortalization step, constituting the only example of spontaneous immortalization of human fibroblasts where the origin of the transformed cells was ascertained.[47]

Regardless of the problem of the mechanisms involved, one may wonder why mesenchymal cells express *in vitro* these properties having a bearing with the cancer-aging relationship, not only in regard to interspecies differences, but also within the human species. This is understandable in the face of the present-day knowledge concerning the role of mesenchymal-epithelial cell interactions in development and in homeostasis.

It should be remembered that mesenchymal cells are ubiquitous in the organism and have the task of creating a microenvironment through the secretion of soluble substances and large insoluble molecules of the interstitial tissue. This property gives them a fundamental role during development through inductive interactions with other cell systems. Indeed, development of the thymus, for instance, depends on an interaction between mesenchyme and epithelium[142] and mouse embryo mammary rubiments fail to develop in the absence of mesenchyme.[143] These are just two examples of the functions of mesenchymal cells during development, for which there is an almost endless list of experimental evidence available. The influence of mesenchymal cells on other cell compartments proceeds in the mature organism and its disturbance can lead to disease.[144]

The expression of those different behaviors of fibroblast cell populations *in vitro*, mentioned above, must be the expression of their regulatory task in the homeostasis of the organism and thus reveals some fundamental properties of that milieu where they originate. In regard to neoplasia, as was already mentioned, there is clinical evidence in many cases of a field effect favorable for the development of tumor growth. There is also good evidence showing that fibroblasts from the stroma of tumors have developed new properties relevant for interactions with the neoplastic cells; the mesenchyme is not only important for the initiation of neoplasia, but also for its maintenance and propagation.[145,146]

III. MECHANISMS IMPLICATED IN THE DIFFERENT PROBABILITIES OF ESCAPING CELL SENESCENCE AND TO TRANSFORM

One of the steps of transformation is the acquisition of the capacity to replicate indefinitely. The data suggest that the probability of cell immortalization is related to physiopathologic characteristics of the species or of the donors within the human species from which the mesenchymal cells originate.

The belief, however, that normal cells can divide forever is by no means dead and the conflict between "nature" and "nurture" goes on in the scientific community. Some investigators still argue that cell populations that senesce *in vitro*, i.e., that exhaust their division potential, do so because of deficiencies in the nutrient medium. On the contrary, the tissue culture media available would be adequate for those cell populations that can divide indefinitely. In addition to the evidence described above, against those that are prone to support the effect of the *in vitro* environment, other data buttress the presence of intrinsic cell properties as a determinant of the susceptibility to escape senescence and to transform. We would like to stress that these phenomena have been particularly well studied in mammalian and avian species; we do not know yet if the same rules apply for lower species.

An experiment performed by Dell'Orco et al.[147] strongly suggests that the available nutrient media are adequate for the maintenance of human fibroblasts. These investigators kept human fibroblast populations in medium supplemented with 0.5% fetal calf serum, which maintained them in a near-resting stage. The cells can be kept under these conditions for several months and when resubcultivated and serially replicated in medium with 10% serum, they will go through the same number of doublings as identical cultures that had been maintained constantly in a replicating state. This would not happen if the nutrient medium would have been deficient.

However, adherents to the role of nurture have hypothesized[148] that senescence of dividing cell compartments is an artifact of *in vitro* maintenance; the immortal cells would be present in the primary culture, but due to cultivation methods, would not grow out. Cells committed to senescence would segregate at the division of the immortal ones, but serial subcultivations would dilute out the immortal cells so that after serial passages, the population would consist only of cells committed to senescence.

The hypothesis was claimed to be supported by a so-called "bottleneck experiment" where cells were plated at very low inocula at different population doubling levels (PDL). The procedure reduced the total number of doublings only when performed at early PDL and not at late stages of the cells life span.[148]

Other investigators, however, did not obtain the same results. Maintaining the cells by serially plating them at low inocula yielded the same number of doublings as identical cultures plated at higher inocula.[51,149]

The present author, on the other hand, obtained a higher number of doublings with the same type of experiments. Cells maintained at a 1:16 split ratio (each new bottle inoculated with $^1/_{16}$ of the previous maximal density) yielded more doublings than when maintained at a 1:2 split ratio (unpublished).

Other data support the idea that the immortal cells develop through new properties acquired *in vitro*. Indeed, the extrapolation of cumulative growth curves of mouse fibroblastic cultures suggested that the immortal cells are not present in the primary culture.[92] The same conclusion was reached from direct observation with time lapse cinematography of the geneologies of clones of rat fibroblastic cells.[150]

The kinetics of cell proliferation analyzed with bromodeoxyuridine (BrdU) labeling also suggested that the immortalized cells develop *in vitro*.[93] The experiments showed that in the primary culture, the dividing population is essentially constituted of cells which perform three divisions during 48 h without any cells making only one division. The pool of rapidly dividing cells decreased when approaching the growth crisis, while at the same time a sharp increase in the fraction of slowly dividing cells was observed. When growth resumed, the slowly dividing cells (one division within a 48-h period) disappeared and the fraction of dividing cells was constituted by an identical percentage of cells which had performed two and three divisions within 48 h. When the fibroblasts immortalized, all mitoses corresponded to cells that had performed three divisions within 48 h. If the immortal cells were already present in the primary culture, one would expect that rapidly dividing cells increase progressively from the start.

It was found that during immortalization of mouse fibroblastic cultures, the cells become progressively resistant to caffeine without the need for the cultures to be previously exposed to the drug.[48] Before immortalization the cell population dies in the presence of caffeine; resistant cells appear only after the recovery from the growth crisis. If resistant cells were present from the beginning, in the presence of the drug, they would outgrow the sensitive cells. These experiments show that caffeine resistance is not a selection phenomenon but is rather a new, spontaneously acquired property occurring in parallel with immortalization.

Several experiments suggest possible explanations for the different susceptibility of cells *in vitro* to escape from senescence and to immortalize; they concern observations at the cytogenetic level during serial divisions of these cell populations. These data suggest that the long-term doubling potential of cells is directly related to the potential for continuous rearrangements — in other words, with the plasticity of the genome.

Human embryonic fibroblasts, when cultivated *in vitro*, go through continuous chromosomal rearrangement without any definite pattern becoming predominant.[151,152] The data suggest that

TABLE 1

Number of Sister Chromatid Exchanges/Cell[a] in Human and Mouse Fibroblasts at Different Population Doubling Levels (PDL) after Two Division Cycles in the Presence of Bromodeoxyuridine

Human		Mouse	
PDL	SCE	PDL	SCE
33	7	1	11
37	5	3	11
41	8	4	17
46	6	12	12

[a] Mean of 100 cells.

multiple clones arise continuously and compete between each other without any one overgrowing the others. These cells have a longer division potential than postnatal fibroblasts which go through more stable clonal-type chromosomal rearrangements during serial divisions *in vitro*.[152] Moreover, fibroblasts from Werner's Syndrome patients, which have a reduced doubling potential when compared with cells from age-matched normal donors, present chromosomal rearrangements (variegated translocation mosaicism) which become fixed and remain predominant during the cell population *in vitro* life span.[153] These findings suggest that a "rigidity" of the genome is associated with a shorter doubling potential as opposed to a higher "plasticity" which would favor a longer doubling potential.

Another feature that points in the same direction is the finding that in human fibroblasts that have exhausted most of their doubling potential, it becomes more difficult to induce sister chromatid exchanges.[154] These results suggest that the loss of the division potential is associated with a loss of the potential for recombination of the genome.

On the other hand, the mouse genome seems to be endowed with the capacity to survive pronounced chromosome recombinations and reorganizations. The chromosomes of mouse fiboblasts cultivated *in vitro* show a very unusual capacity for recombination which is expressed by the presence of crossing overs and bridges between chromosomes.[93] Another difference between the mouse and the human genome is the higher rate of sister chromatid exchanges in the former (Table 1) and the rapidity with which mouse cells can switch from the diploid to the tetraploid state.[93] Furthermore, the chromatin lability which accumulates during cellular aging disappears in mouse cells during the chromosomal rearrangements which occur in the transition from senescence to immortalization.[155]

DNA elimination in mouse fibroblasts during the period preceding immortalization could be germane to the disappearance of the fragile chromatin sites. DNA measurements on cells in interphase after ethidium bromide staining showed that occasionally at early PDL, the DNA content of G2 cells is less than that expected from the G1 content.[93] This suggests that a process of DNA elimination goes on in these cells, as has been reported for other organisms.[156] Although DNA elimination also takes place during the division cycle of human cells, it is not of the same magnitude as in mouse cells.[157]

The potential for chromosomal recombinational events expressed by mouse fibroblasts *in vitro* also has a counterpart *in vivo*. Although 40 acrocentric chromosomes is the usual diploid number of the mouse species, localized races with 38 to 22 chromosomes resulting from robertsonian fusions have been found in the wild.[158] This property of the mouse genome could be responsible for

1. The high probability of escaping senescence and immortalizing[92]
2. The high frequency of spontaneous malignant transformation[159]

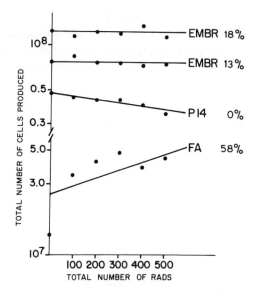

FIGURE 4.   Effect of low dose rate ionizing radiation
on the long-term division potential of embryonic lung
(embr) and postnatal skin human fibroblasts from a control donor (P14) and from a patient with Fanconi's anemia
(FA). The total number of cells produced *in vitro* by
control cultures and by cultures that received different
number of rad, was plotted. For details of the irradiation
procedure, see reference in Figure 2. The frequency (%) of
chromosome rearrangements through the life span of the
respective nonirradiated cell populations is indicated.

3.   The high susceptibility to viral, chemical, and physical carcinogens[98,102,105,108] and oncogenes[160]
4.   The facility with which one can induce tumors in mice[98]

The response of cells to low dose rate ionizing radiation also suggests a relationship of
causality between the capacity of the genome to recombine and the probability to excape
senescence. Human embryonic fibtoblasts, when treated with low dose rate radiation at low
PDL, can have their life span prolonged,[106] but if irradiated late during their life span, when the
potential number of chromosome rearrangements is reduced,[154] their doubling potential is
shortened.[106] The same type of radiation shortens the division potential of early passage
postnatal fibroblasts whose genome has a lower potential for chromosomal recombinations than
that of embryonic cells.[161] On the other hand, the same treatment can significantly prolong the
life span of human postnatal fibroblasts from donors with genetic diseases with a high rate of
chromosome recombinations which are at high risk of cancer.[26,117]

Some of these findings are illustrated in Figure 4 which shows the effect of different doses
of ionizing radiation on the doubling potential of human fibroblast populations and the
frequency (%) of chromosome rearrangements observed in the respective nonirradiated cells
through their *in vitro* life span. No chromosome rearrangements were observed in cells whose
life span was shortened by radiation. By contrast, a high level of rearrangements was observed
in the cell population whose doubling potential was increased by radiation (skin fibroblasts from
a Fanconi's anemia patient). Finally, the cells whose life span was not affected by radiation
(human embryonic lung fibroblasts) had an intermediate number of chromosome rearrangements.

TABLE 2
Percent Changes in Cell Population Doublings (CPD) in Skin Fibroblast Cultures from Retinoblastoma Patients that Received 2×100 rad and Frequency of Sister Chromatid Exchanges in the Respective Nonirradiated Cell Populations

Donor	%Change in CPD	Mean SCE/cell[a]
1	+89	19.6 (11—30)
2	+47	11.0 (4—20)
3	−36	9.4 (1—16)

[a] Mean of 20 cells; values within parentheses indicate the maximal and minimal number of SCE found in a cell.

These results suggest that the effect of radiation depends upon the potential of the cell populations for chromosome rearrangements and that ionizing radiation under the experimentl conditions used (low dose rate) accentuates the intrinsic growth potential of fibroblasts, perhaps by accelerating changes in the genome which normally take place during cell replication.

Another pertinent observation was the finding[161] that in the irradiated cells, most of the breaks involved in exchanges (53 out of 62) concerned the centromeric and telomeric regions. Thus, the intrachromosomal break distribution where exchanges took place was preferentially located at regions rich in repetitive DNA, which has been implicated in recombinational events.[162]

The present author also found that the prolongation of the doubling potential of skin fibroblasts from retinoblastoma patients by low dose rate ionizing radiation, showed a correlation with the potential for sister chromatid exchanges of the cells of the respective patients (Table 2).

In the face of these results it was proposed[90,163] that aging or transformation of dividing cell compartments depends on random reorganization of the cell genome and is determined by chance, intrinsic properties of the cell genome, and external factors. The capacity to overcome this reorganization differs between cell populations; the probability of creating a new genetic progressively autonomous program is higher for some cells than for others and is increased by external events that introduce de novo information.

Other interspecies differences are known that could be implicated in the response to carcinogens (described above). The capacity to activate a carcinogen into a mutagenic form and to metabolize the carcinogen into a water-soluble form differs in cells from species with different life spans and could be implicated in the susceptibility to transformation.[164] Another important difference concerns DNA repair. Both the initial rate and the maximum incorporation of ^{3}H-thymidine after UV irradiation were found to be higher in human and bovine than in hamster, rat, and mouse cells.[165]

Another type of repair where interspecies differences have been described is the removal of *Micrococcus luteus* UV-endonuclease susceptible sites. Human fibrtoblasts maintain this type of repair in contrast to rat cells which lose it during serial proliferation.[166] Mullaart et al. suggested that this characteristic may render the rat cells more dependent on postreplication repair systems which are error prone. It may lead to an increased frequency of genetic changes in rat cells, which could have a bearing on their susceptibility to transformation described above. On the other hand, mouse cells have a reduced capacity for excision repair as revealed by the low host-cell reactivation of UV-irradiated herpes simplex virus.[167,168]

Single strand break repair also differs; the relative increased efficiency of this type of repair is mouse<chicken<human fibroblasts.[169] The repair of potential lethal damage is also more efficient in human and chicken than in murine cells.[169]

Repair evaluated as a function of the colony forming ability was higher for chicken than for mouse cells and higher for mouse than for human cells.[169] However, so many functions are implicated in this type of assay that it is difficult to draw any conclusions.

DNA repair mechanisms have been studied in almost all human genetically determined diseases prone to cancer after the discovery of the defective repair in xeroderma pigmentosum cells,[170] and different types of repair defects have been described. DNA repair, however, although unquestionably important for the transformation process, must be only part of the picture.

Few other approaches have been used to identify differences at the molecular level between normal human fibroblasts and the same type of cells from cancer patients or from donors at high risk of cancer. An interesting finding concerned the presence of a higher level of DNA transcripts from a subgenomic fraction obtained from Fanconi's anemia and retinoblastoma skin fibroblasts, which is also preferentially expressed in all human tumor cells tested so far.[171] These results fit other findings, suggesting that fibroblasts from patients with some genetic diseases prone to cancer, are preneoplastic.[172]

A nutritional difference has also been reported between normal postnatal fibroblasts and identical cells from patients with Gardner's syndrome and familial colon cancer; the growth of the latter cells was more sensitive to methionine deprivation.[173]

Infection with SV40 virus has been extensively used to study the mechanisms involved in the escape from senescence. As mentioned above, in most cases, infection of human fibroblasts with SV40 causes changes in morphology and the loss of contact inhibition of growth,[11] but eventually the cells stop dividing and die.[100] Immortalized cells can be obtained but at a low frequency.[99] The SV40 antigen plays a role in the expression of some transformation steps such as morphological changes, focus-forming ability, loss of contact inhibition of growth, and anchorage independence, but it is not enough for cell immortalization.[99]

An efficient immortalization can be achieved if the cells are transfected with the SV40 early region encoding the T antigen and with the hypoxanthine-guanine phosphoribosyl transferase gene.[174] It is interesting that to achieve immortalization, the transformed cells have to go through the terminal senescent phase (phase IV) where division is arrested. This suggests that some fundamental change occurring in the terminal cell is needed for immortalization, which complements the changes induced by the virus and helps to modify the genetic information leading to unlimited divisions. It has been claimed, however, that human fibroblasts infected with a small-plaque variant of SV40, in many instances, do not go through a growth crisis.[101]

For the moment it is impossible to guess which are the changes occurring during phase IV that are important for immortalization. Aging of proliferative compartments is accompanied by a continuous reorganization of the genome;[157,175-180] this reorganization leads to profound changes which can be detected at different levels of DNA structure in the terminal stage. These modifications are so profound that one can only wonder which could be more impotant than the other.

Experiments with transformation of human fibroblasts by SV40 virus led to the suggestion that phase IV transformed, but not immortalized fibroblasts, contrary to normal cells, lose the ability to enter a G1 arrested state.[181] Both normal and transformed cells, however, lose the ability to respond to mitogens during senescence. Concomitantly, the rate of cell death increased steadily. It was hypothesized that the transformed cells undergo the same aging process as the normal fibroblasts, but they enter their life span in crisis because they continue their cycle traverse coupled with cell death.[181]

Experiments by Ide et al.[182] led to the conclusion that aging progresses in transformed cells as in normal ones. These investigators used a temperature-sensitive mutant virus to infect the cells. When cultured at 34°C, the life span of the cells was prolonged. When the transformed cells whose life span had been prolonged were shifted to 39.5°C, they immediately reached the end of their proliferative potential. A similar event occurs when the life span of human embryonic fibroblasts is prolonged by hydrocortisone.[183] When the hormone is removed from the medium of cultures that have grown beyond the limit observed in the controls, the cells soon stop dividing.

A factor implicated in the postmitotic terminal state of senescent fibroblasts that is reversed after SV40 immortalization, is the increase in the 5′-nucleotidase.[184,185] This enzyme hydrolyzes nucleotides and thus its increase hinders DNA synthesis. The enzyme levels go down after immortalization.[184]

Fusions between normal and immortalized cells were used to study the genetics of the escape from senescence and acquisition of an infinite growth potential. Muggleton-Harris and DeSimone[186] studied the replicative potentials of fusion products between normal WI-38 cells and identical cultures transformed by SV40. The replicative potential of the hybrids was similar to the control WI-38 cells in the majority of cases. Only less than 2% of the hybrids had a prolonged life span and possibly immortalized. Fusions between normal WI-38 cytoplasts and transformed karyoplasts did not show sustained replication. Mass culture hybridizations between Lesh Nyhan cells with finite life span (deficient in hypoxanthine-phosphoribosyl transferase) and HeLa cells showed that most hybrids had a limited life span slightly longer than Lesh Nyhan fibroblasts; only 1 in 10^5 cells were capable of indefinite replication.[187] Fusions of Lesh Nyhan cells with HeLa cytoplasts did not show transformation. Pereira-Smith and Smith[99] found that the majority of hybrids (70%) obtained between normal and SV40-transformed human fibroblasts did not make more than seven population doublings; the others had a more extensive proliferation but a finite life span. Thus, in these hybrids, senescence could only be partially reversed. Only 1 or 2 foci per 10^5 cells had indefinite growth. All hybrid clones, including those that exhibited a finite life span, expressed the viral T antigen. In the hybrids, the SV40 genome was integrated in the same region as in the parental SV40-transformed cells.[99]

Pereira-Smith and Smith[188] obtained hybrids between normal human fibroblasts and immortalized cell lines that either can induce DNA synthesis in heterokaryons with old nuclei or whose nuclei are inhibited by the nucleus of the postmitotic cell. A higher percentage of the hybrids with the former cell lines was capable of dividing more than eight times. Fusion with the other cells, those that are inhibited by the old nucleus, resulted in fewer than 10% of the hybrids capable of more than eight doublings. Surprisingly, in a number of fusions between immortal cell lines, the hybrids had a finite proliferative potential.[188] It was concluded that cellular immortality has a recessive nature.

These results have to be interpreted with the thought in mind that the data obtained by Martinez et al.[189] showed that clones from the HeLa tumor derived cell line display a nonproliferative and a proliferative pool. The fastest growing clones and subclones segregate daughter cells with different growth potentials, showing a shift in the distributions toward lower growth rates and an increase in the proportion of cells belonging to the nonproliferative pool. This phenomenon was called clonal attenuation. The same phenomenon exists in normal human fibroblast populations, but whereas the proliferating fraction disappears progressively in these cultures, in HeLa cells the two distinct pools are continuously produced.

In the fusions (described above) between immortalized and normal cells, some of the hybrids may have been obtained from cells committed to clonal attenuation. Furthermore, if HeLa cells display clonal attenuation, all other immortalized cell populations must have it to different degrees. It is possible that the different life spans obtained with the hybrids, depending on the type of immortalized parental cell line, depend on the degree of clonal attenuation displayed by the latter. On the other hand, the methods used for fusion may cause genetic changes which accentuate the phenomenon of clonal attenuation.

It should also be kept in mind that the product of fusion between two nuclei is unpredictable and that during serial divisions the remodeling in these genomes is probably random. Furthermore, immortalization is a complex genetic phenomenon which cannot be due to single genes and cannot be interpreted in terms of Mendelian genetics.

There are additional factors in such experiments which should be taken into account. Le

Borgne et al.[190] obtained results which are representative of the complexity of the genetic effects triggered by hybridizations between eukaryotic cells. Clones were obtained between normal fibroblasts and immortal cell populations and between immortal cell populations, both from human and mouse origin. Contact inhibition of growth was measured in the parental lines and in the hybrids. Hybrids between normal and transformed human cells, and between normal and transformed mouse cells were not contact inhibited. Fusion products between normal human and transformed mouse cells, and between transformed human and mouse cells were contact inhibited. Hence, the results suggested that the inhibition of division due to cell crowding in the hybrids was more dependent upon the species of the parental cell lines rather than on their normal or transformed character. In other words, growth inhibition seemed to be triggered by interspecies differences between the parental genomes. These experiments raise the problem of the role of species-related genetic determinants which may interfere with the expression of certain phenotypes. Similar events may take place in intraspecies hybridization. It is an interesting aspect that was for the first time reported in this work, and has been overlooked in the interpretation of other experiments along these lines.

In regard to future directions there are two important conclusions that can be drawn from the studies reviewed herein. One is that it seems crucial for the understanding of the mechanisms leading to neoplastic development to identify at the molecular level the differences in the genomes of cells with variable potentials for chromosomal recombinational events, associated with an increased susceptibility to transformation. It is no easy task, but it seems crucial in order to get to the core of the problem.

The second conclusion concerns the relevance of studying the mechanisms involved in the deviations from normalcy of mesenchymal cells distant from the organ where the tumor developed. They can probably shed more light on the process leading to neoplasia than the tumor cells themselves which have already gone through several steps of the evolution toward malignancy.

REFERENCES

1. **Foulds, L.,** The natural history of cancer, *J. Chron. Dis.,* 8, 2, 1958.
2. **Dvorak, H. F., Dickersin, G. R., Dvorak, A. M., Mansean, E. J., and Pyne, K.,** Human breast carcinoma: fibrin deposits and desmoplasia. Inflammatory cell type and distribution. Microvasculature and infarction, *J. Natl. Cancer Inst.,* 67, 335, 1981.
3. **Azzarone, B., Mareel, M., Billard, C., Scemama, P., Chaponnier, C., and Macieira-Coelho, A.,** Abnormal properties of skin fibroblasts from patients with breast cancer, *Int. J. Cancer,* 33, 759, 1984.
4. **Schor, S. L., Schor, A. M., Durning, P., and Rushton, G.,** Skin fibroblasts obtained from cancer patients display foetal-like migratory behaviour on collagen gels, *J. Cell Sci.,* 73, 235, 1985.
5. **Foulds, L.,** *Neoplastic Dev.,* Vol. 1, Academic Press, London, 1969, 160.
6. **Abeloff, M. D.,** Paraneoplastic syndromes. A window on the biology of cancer, *N. Engl. J. Med.,* 317, 1598, 1987.
7. **Ralston, S. H.,** The pathogenesis of humoral hypercalcaemia, *Lancet,* 2, 1443, 1987.
8. **Maton, P. N., Gardner, J. D., and Jensen, R. T.,** Cushing's syndrome in patients with the Zollinger-Ellison syndrome, *N. Engl. J. Med.,* 315, 1, 1986.
9. **Beck, S. A. and Tisdale, M. J.,** Production of lipolytic and proteolytic factors by a murine tumor-producing cachexia in the host, *Cancer Res.,* 47, 5919, 1987.
10. **Macieira-Coelho, A., Pontén, J., and Philipson, L.,** The division cycle and RNA synthesis in diploid human cells at different passage levels *in vitro, Exp. Cell Res.,* 42, 673, 1966.
11. **Macieira-Coelho, A.,** Relationship between DNA synthesis and cell density in normal and virus-transformed cells, *Int. J. Cancer,* 2, 297, 1967.
12. **Macieira-Coelho, A.,** Dissociation between inhibition of movement and inhibition of division in RSV transformed human fibroblasts, *Exp. Cell Res.,* 47, 193, 1967.

13. **Macieira-Coelho, A. and Pontén, J.,** Induction of the division cycle in resting stage human fibroblasts after RSV infection, *Biochem. Biophys. Res. Commun.,* 29, 316, 1967.

14. **Macieira-Coelho, A., Hiu, I. J., and Garcia-Giralt, E.,** Stimulation of DNA synthesis in resting stage human fibroblasts after infection with Rous sarcoma virus, *Nature,* 222, 1172, 1969.

15. **Abercrombie, M. and Heaysman, J.,** Observations on the social behaviour of cells in tissue culture. II. Monolayering of fibroblasts, *Exp. Cell Res.,* 6, 293, 1954.

16. **Manaker, R. A. and Groupé, V.,** Discrete foci of altered chicken embryo cells associated with Rous sarcoma virus in tissue culture, *Virology,* 2, 838, 1956.

17. **Macieira-Coelho, A., Berumen, L., and Avrameas, S.,** Properties of protein polymers as substratum for cell growth *in vitro, J. Cell. Phys.,* 83, 379. 1974.

18. **Stoker, M. G. P., O'Neil, C., Berryman, S., and Waxman, V.,** Anchorage and growth regulation in normal and virus-transformed cells, *Int. J. Cancer,* 3, 683, 1968.

19. **MacPherson, I. and Montagnier, L.,** Agar suspension culture for the selective assay of cells transformed by polyoma virus, *Virology,* 23, 291, 1964.

20. **Otsuka, H. and Moskowitz, M.,** Difference in transport of leucine in attached and suspended 3T3 cells, *J. Cell. Phys.,* 85, 665, 1975.

21. **Harper, J. R. and Reisfeld, R. A.,** Inhibition of anchorage-independent growth of human melanoma cells by a monoclonal antibody to a chondroitin sulfate proteoglycan, *J. Natl. Cancer Inst.,* 71, 259, 1983.

22. **Leavitt, J. C., Crawford, B. D., Barrett, J. C., and Ts'O, P. O. P.,** Regulation of requirements for anchorage-independent growth of Syrian hamster fibroblasts by somatic mutation, *Nature,* 269, 63, 1977.

23. **Steuer, A. F. and Ting, R. C.,** Formation of larger cell aggregates by transformed cells: an *in vitro* index of cell transformation, *J. Natl. Cancer Inst.,* 56, 1279, 1976.

24. **Moskowitz, M.,** Growth, differentiation and reproduction of aggregates of cultured mammalian cells, *Nature,* 203, 1233, 1964.

25. **Hayflick, L.,** Oncogenesis *in vitro, J. Natl. Cancer Inst. Monogr.,* 26, 355, 1967.

26. **Diatloff, C. and Macieira-Coelho, A.,** Effect of low-dose-rate irradiation on the division potential of cells *in vitro.* V. Human skin fibroblasts from donors with a high risk of cancer, *J. Natl. Cancer Inst.,* 63, 55, 1979.

27. **Smith, H. S., Wolman, S. R., Dairkee, S. H., Hancock, M. C., Lipman, M., Leff, A., and Hackett, A. J.,** Immortalization in culture: occurrence at a late stage in the progression of breast cancer, *J. Natl. Cancer Inst.,* 78, 611, 1987.

28. **Azzarone, B., Chaponnier, C., Krief, P., Mareel, M., Suarez, H., and Macieira-Coelho, A.,** Human fibroblasts from cancer patients: lifespan and transformed phenotype *in vitro* and role of mesenchyme *in vivo, Mutat. Res.,* 199, 313, 1988.

29. **Marshall, C. J., Humphreys, K. C., and Pollack, R. E.,** Microfilament bundles, LETS protein, and growth control in somatic cell hybrids, *J. Cell Sci.,* 33, 191, 1978.

30. **Kopelovich, L., Lipkin, M., Blattner, W. A., Fraumeni, J. F., Lynch, H. T., and Pollack, R. E.,** Organization of actin-containing cables in cultured skin fibroblasts from individuals at high risk of colon cancer, *Int. J. Cancer,* 26, 301, 1980.

31. **Antecol, M. H., Darveau, A., Sonenberg, N., and Mukherjee, B.,** Altered biochemical properties of actin in normal skin fibroblasts from individuals predisposed to dominantly inherited cancers, *Cancer Res.,* 46, 1867, 1986.

32. **Leavitt, J., Latter, G., Lutomski, L., Goldstein, D., and Burbeck, S.,** Tropomyosin isoform switching in tumorigenic human fibroblasts, *Mol. Cell. Biol.,* 6, 2721, 1986.

33. **Martin-Zanca, D., Hughes, S. H., and Barbacid, M.,** A human oncogene found by the fusion of truncated tropomyosin and protein tyrosine kinase sequences, *Nature,* 319, 743, 1986.

34. **Macieira-Coelho, A.,** Changes in membrane properties associated with cellular aging, *Intern. Rev. Cytol.,* 83, 183, 1983.

35. **Mareel, M., Kint, T., and Meyvish, C.,** Methods of study of the invasion of malignant C3H mouse fibroblasts into embryonic chick heart *in vitro, Virchow's Arch.,* B30, 95, 1979.

36. **Noguchi, P. D., Johnson, J. B., O'Donnell, R., and Petricciani, J. C.,** Chick embryonic skin as a rapid organ culture assay for cellular neoplasia, *Science,* 199, 980, 1978.

37. **Nowell, P. C.,** The clonal evolution of tumor cell populations, *Science,* 194, 23, 1976.

38. **Albino, A. P., Lloyd, K. C., Houghton, A. N., Oettgen, H. F., and Old, L. J.,** Heterogeneity in surface antigen and glycoprotein expression of cell lines derived from different melanoma metastases of the same patient, *J. Exp. Med.,* 154, 1764, 1981.

39. **Fidler, I. J. and Hart, I. R.,** Biological diversity in metastatic neoplasms: origins and implications, *Science,* 217, 998, 1982.

40. **Shapiro, J. R., Yung, W.-K. A., and Shapiro, W. R.,** Isolation, karyotype and clonal growth of heterogeneous subpopulations of human malignant gliomas, *Cancer Res.,* 41, 2349, 1981.

41. **Albino, A. P., Le Strange, R., Oliff, A. I., Furth, M. E., and Old, L. J.,** Transforming *ras* genes from human melanoma: a manifestation of tumour heterogeneity?, *Nature,* 308, 69, 1984.

42. **Hynes, R. O.,** Cell surface proteins and malignant transformation, *Biochim. Biophys. Acta,* 458, 73, 1976.
43. **Vogel, K. G., Kelley, R. O., and Steward, C.,** Loss of organized fibronectin matrix from the surface of aging diploid fibroblasts, *Mech. Ageing Dev.,* 16, 295, 1981.
44. **Jensen, F., Koprowski, H., and Pontén, J.,** Rapid transformation of human fibroblast cultures by simian virus 40, *Proc. Natl. Acad. Sci. U.S.A.,* 50, 343, 1963.
45. **Ossowski, L., Unkeless, J. C., Tobia, A., Quigley, J. P., Rifkin, D. B., and Reich, E.,** An enzymatic function associated with transformation of fibroblasts by oncogenic viruses, *J. Exp. Med.,* 137, 112, 1973.
46. **Namba, M., Nishitani, K., and Kimoto, T.,** Characteristics of WI-38 cells (WI-38 CT-1) transformed by treatment with Co-60 gamma rays, *Gann,* 71, 300, 1980.
47. **McCormick, J. J. and Maher, V. M.,** Towards an understanding of the malignant transformation of diploid human fibroblasts, *Mutat. Res.,* 199, 273, 1988.
48. **Icard, C. and Macieira-Coelho, A.,** Resistance to caffeine of mouse fibroblasts after acquisition of an infinite division potential, *Cell Biol. Int. Rep.,* 5, 9, 1983.
49. **Senger, D. R., Hasch, B. B., Smith, B. D., Perruzzi, C. A., and Dvorak, H. F.,** A secreted phosphoprotein marker for neoplastic transformation of both epithelial and fibroblastic cells, *Nature,* 302, 714, 1983.
50. **Cohen, P.,** The role of protein phosphorylation in neural and hormonal control of cellular activity, *Nature,* 296, 613, 1982.
51. **Hayflick, L.,** The limited *in vitro* lifetime of human diploid cell strains, *Exp. Cell Res.,* 37, 614, 1965.
52. **Martin, G. M., Sprague, C. A., and Epstein, C. J.,** Replicative life span of cultivated human cells. Effects of donor's age, tissue and genotype, *Lab. Invest.,* 23, 86, 1970.
53. **Macieira-Coelho, A. and Pontén, J.,** Analogy in growth between late passage human embryonic and early passage human adult fibroblasts, *J. Cell Biol.,* 43, 374, 1969.
54. **Le Guilly, Y., Simon, M., Lenoir, P., and Bourel, M.,** Long-term culture of human adult liver cells: morphologic changes related to *in vitro* senescence and effect of donor's age on growth potential, *Gerontologia,* 19, 303, 1973.
55. **Schneider, E. L. and Mitsui, Y.,** The relationship between *in vitro* cellular aging and *in vivo* human age, *Proc. Natl. Acad. Sci. U.S.A.,* 73, 3584, 1976.
56. **Vracko, R., McFarland, B. H., and Pecoraro, R. E.,** Seeding efficiency, plating efficiency and population doublings of human skin fibroblast-like cells: results of replicate testing, *In Vitro,* 19, 504, 1983.
57. **Mets, T., Bekaert, E., and Verdonk, G.,** Similarity between in vitro and in vivo cellular aging, *Mech. Ageing Dev.,* 22, 71, 1983.
58. **Azzarone, B. and Macieira-Coelho, A.,** Role of cytoskeletal elements in the retractile activity of human skin fibroblasts, *Exp. Cell Res.,* 155, 299, 1984.
59. **Lipschitz, D. A. and Udupa, K. B.,** Effect of donor age on long-term culture of bone marrow *in vitro, Mech. Ageing Dev.,* 24, 119, 1984.
60. **Bartold, P. M., Boyd, R. R., and Page, R. C.,** Proteoglycans synthesized by gingival fibroblasts derived from human donors of different ages, *J. Cell. Phys.,* 126, 37, 1986.
61. **Tassin, J., Malaise, E., and Courtois, Y.,** Human lens cells have an *in vitro* proliferative capacity inversely proportional to the donor age, *Exp. Cell Res.,* 123, 388, 1979.
62. **Bierman, E. L.,** The effect of donor age on the *in vitro* life span of cultured human arterial smooth-muscle cells, *In Vitro,* 14, 951, 1978.
63. **Volicer, L., West, C. D., Chase, A. R., and Greene, L.,** Beta-adrenergic receptor sensitivity in cultured vascular smooth muscle cells: effect of age and of dietary restriction, *Mech. Ageing Dev.,* 21, 283, 1983.
64. **Rheinwald, J. G.,** The role of terminal differentiation in the finite culture lifetime of the human epidermal keratinocyte, *Int. Rev. Cytol.,* Suppl. 10, 25, 1979.
65. **Evans, C. H. and Georgescu, H. J.,** Observations on the senescence of cells derived from articular cartilage, *Mech. Ageing Dev.,* 22, 179, 1983.
66. **Walford, R. L., Janvaid, S. Q., and Naeim, F.,** Evidence for *in vitro* senescence of T-lymphocytes cultured from normal human peripheral blood, *Age,* 4, 67, 1981.
67. **Ryan, J. M., Ostrow, D. G., Breaiceheld, X. O., Gershon, E. S., and Upchurch, L.,** *In Vitro,* 17, 20, 1981.
68. **Goldstein, S.,** Aging *in vitro:* growth of cultured cells from the Galapagos tortoise, *Exp. Cell Res.,* 83, 297, 1974.
69. **Bruce, S. A., Deamond, S. F., and Ts'O, P. O. P.,** *In vitro* senescence of Syrian hamster mesenchymal cells of foetal to aged adult origin. Inverse relationship between *in vivo* donor age and *in vitro* proliferative capacity, *Mech. Ageing Dev.,* 34, 151, 1986.
70. **Martin, G. M., Ogburn, G. E., and Wight, T. N.,** Comparative rates of decline in the primary cloning efficiencies of smooth muscle cells from the aging thoracic aorta of two murine species of contrasting maximum life span potentials, *Am. J. Pathol.,* 110, 236, 1983.
71. **Adolphe, M., Ronot, X., Jaffray, P., Hecquet, C., Fontagne, J., and Lechat, P.,** Effects of donor's age on growth kinetics of rabbit articular chondrocytes in culture, *Mech. Ageing Dev.,* 23, 191, 1983.
72. **Evans, C. H. and Georgescu, H. J.,** Observations on the senescence of cells derived from articular cartilage, *Mech. Ageing Dev.,* 22, 179, 1983.

73. **Liu, S. C. C., Parsons, C. S., and Hanawalt, P.,** DNA repair response in human epidermal keratinocytes from donors of different age, *J. Invest. Dermatol.,* 79, 330, 1982.

74. **Slayback, J. R. B., Cheung, L. W. G., and Geger, R. P.,** Comparative effects of human platelet growth factor on the growth and morphology of human fetal and adult diploid fibroblasts, *Exp. Cell Res.,* 110, 462, 1977.

75. **Plisko, A. and Gilchrest, B. A.,** Growth factor responsiveness of cultured human fibroblasts declines with age, *J. Gerontol.,* 38, 513, 1983.

76. **Nilsson, J., Ksiasek, T., Heldin, C. H., and Thyberg, J.,** Demonstration of stimulatory effects of platelet-derived growth factor on cultivated rat arterial smooth muscle cells, *Exp. Cell Res.,* 145, 231, 1983.

77. **Phillips, P. D., Kaji, K., and Cristofalo, V. J.,** Progressive loss of the proliferative response of senescing WI-38 cells to platelet derived growth factor, epidermal growth factor, insulin, transferrin and dexamethasone, *J. Gerontol.,* 39, 11, 1984.

78. **Salk, D., Au, K., Hoehn, H., and Martin, G. M.,** Cytogenetics of Werner's syndrome cultured skin: variegated translocation mosaicism, *Cytogen. Cell Genet.,* 30, 92, 1981.

79. **Shapiro, B., Lam, L. F., and Fast, L.,** Premature senescence in cultured skin fibroblasts from subjects with cystic fibrosis, *Science,* 203, 1251, 1979.

80. **Macieira-Coelho, A. and Taboury, F.,** A re-evaluation of the changes in proliferation in human fibroblasts during ageing *in vitro, Cell Tissue Kinet.,* 15, 213, 1982.

81. **Macieira-Coelho, A. and Azzarone, B.,** Aging of human fibroblasts is a succession of subtle changes in the cell cycle and has a final short stage with abrupt events, *Exp. Cell Res.,* 141, 325, 1982.

82. **Holm-Pedersen, P., Fenstad, A. M., and Folke, L. E. A.,** DNA, RNA and protein synthesis in healing wounds in young and old mice, *Mech. Ageing Dev.,* 3, 173, 1974.

83. **Roth, G. S., Karoly, K., Britton, V. J., and Adelman, R. C.,** Age-dependent regulation of isoproterenol-stimulated DNA synthesis in rat salivary gland *in vivo, Exp. Gerontol.,* 9, 1, 1974.

84. **Robert, B. and Robert, L.,** *Frontiers in Matrix Biology,* S. Karger, Basel, 1973, 1.

85. **Clemmons, D. R. and Shaw, D. S.,** Variables controlling somatomedin production by cultured human fibroblasts, *J. Cell. Phys.,* 142, 115, 1983.

86. **Kurobe, M., Furukawa, S., and Hayashi, K.,** Synthesis and secretion of an epidermical growth factor by human fibroblast cells in culture, *Biochem. Biophys. Res. Commun.,* 131, 1080, 1985.

87. **Hunter, S. A., Burstein, S., and Cedor, C.,** Stimulation of prostaglandin synthesis in WI-38 human lung fibroblasts following inhibition of phospholipid acylation by p-hydroxy-mercuribenzoate, *Biochim. Biophys. Acta,* 793, 202, 1984.

88. **Hayflick, L. and Moorhead, P. S.,** The serial cultivation of human diploid cell strains, *Exp. Cell Res.,* 25, 585, 1961.

89. **Swim, H. E. and Parker, R. F.,** Culture characteristics of human fibroblasts propagated serially, *Am. J. Hyg.,* 66, 235, 1957.

90. **Macieira-Coelho, A.,** Implications of the reorganization of the cell genome for aging or immortalization of dividing cells *in vitro, Gerontology,* 26, 276, 1980.

91. **Macieira-Coelho, A.,** Cancer and aging, *Exp. Gerontol.,* 21, 483, 1986.

92. **Todaro, G. and Green, H.,** Quantitative studies of the growth of mouse embryo cells in culture and their development into established lines, *J. Cell Biol.,* 17, 299, 1963.

93. **Macieira-Coelho, A. and Azzarone, B.,** The transition from primary culture to spontaneous immortalization in mouse fibroblast populations, *Anticancer Res.,* 8, 669, 1988.

94. **Spandidos, D. A. and Wilkie, N. M.,** Malignant transformation of early passage rodent cells by a single mutated human oncogene, *Nature,* 310, 469, 1984.

95. **Land, H., Parada, L. F., and Weinberg, R. A.,** Tumorigenic conversion of primary embryo fibroblasts requires at least two cooperating oncogenes, *Nature,* 304, 596, 1983.

96. **Freeman, A. E., Igel, H. J., and Price, P. J.,** Carcinogenesis *in vitro, In Vitro,* 2, 107, 1975.

97. **Kraemer, P. M., Travis, G. L., Ray, F. A., and Cram, L. S.,** Spontaneous neoplastic evolution of chinese hamster cells in culture: multistep progression of phenotype, *Cancer Res.,* 43, 4822, 1983.

98. **Pontén, J.,** *Spontaneous and Virus Induced Transformation In Cell Culture,* Springer-Verlag, New York, 1971, 25.

99. **Pereira-Smith, O. M. and Smith, J. R.,** Expression of SV40 T antigen in finite life-span hybrids of normal and SV40-transformed fibroblasts, *Som. Cell Genet.,* 7, 411, 1981.

100. **Gotoh, S., Gelb, L., and Schlessinger, D.,** SV40-transformed human diploid cells that remain transformed throughout their limited lifespan, *J. Gen. Virol.,* 42, 409, 1979.

101. **Miranda, A. F., Duigon, G. J., Hernandez, E., and Fisher, P. B.,** Characterization of mutant human fibroblast cultures transformed with simian virus 40, *J. Cell Sci.,* 89, 481, 1988.

102. **Mondal, S. and Heidelberger, C.,** Transformation of C3H/10T1/2 C18 mouse embryo fibroblasts by ultraviolet radiation and phorbol ester, *Nature,* 260, 710, 1977.

103. **Milo, G. E. and Casto, B. C.,** Conditions for transformation of human fibroblast cells: an overview, *Cancer Lett.,* 31, 1, 1986.

104. **Lima, L., Malaise, E., and Macieira-Coelho, A.,** Aging *in vitro.* Effect of low dose rate irradiation on the division potential of chicken embryonic fibroblasts, *Exp. Cell Res.,* 73, 345, 1972.

105. **Macieira-Coelho, A., Diatloff, C., and Malaise, E.,** Doubling potential of fibroblasts from different species after ionizing radiation, *Nature,* 261, 586, 1976.

106. **Macieira-Coelho, A., Diatloff, C., Billardon, C., Bourgeois, C. A., and Malaise, E.,** Effect of low dose rate ionizing radiation on the division potential of cells *in vitro.* III. Human lung fibroblasts, *Exp. Cell Res.,* 104, 215, 1977.

107. **Croute, F., Vidal, S., Soleihavoup, J. P., Vincent, C., Serre, G., and Planel, H.,** Effects of a very low dose rate of chronic ionizing radiation on the division potential of human embryonic lung fibroblasts *in vitro, Exp. Gerontol.,* 21, 1, 1986.

108. **Macieira-Coelho, A., Diatloff, C., and Malaise, E.,** Effect of low dose rate irradiation on the division potential of cells *in vitro.* II. Mouse lung fibroblasts, *Exp. Cell Res.,* 100, 228, 1976.

109. **Stehelin, D., Guntaka, R. V., Varmus, H. E., and Bishop, J. M.,** Purification of DNA complementary to nucleotide sequences required for neoplastic transformation of fibroblasts by avian sarcoma viruses, *J. Mol. Biol.,* 101, 349, 1976.

110. **Hurlin, P. J., Fry, D. G., Maher, V. M., and McCormick, J. J.,** Morphological transformation, focus formation, and anchorage independence induced in diploid human fibroblasts by expression of a transfected H-ras oncogene, *Cancer Res.,* 47, 5752, 1987.

111. **Hurlin, P. J., Maher, V. M., and McCormick, J. J.,** Malignant transformation of human fibroblasts caused by expression of a transfected T24HRas oncogene, *Proc. Natl. Acad. Sci. U.S.A.,* 86, 187, 1989.

112. **Sager, R., Tanaka, K., Lan, C. C., Ebina, Y., and Anisowicz, A.,** Resistance of human cells to tumorigenesis induced by cloned transforming genes, *Proc. Natl. Acad. Sci. U.S.A.,* 80, 7601, 1983.

113. **Todaro, G., Wolman, S. R., and Green, H.,** Rapid transformation of human fibroblasts with low growth potential into established cell lines by SV40, *J. Cell. Comp. Phys.,* 62, 257, 1963.

114. **Webb, T., Harnden, D. G., and Harding, M.,** The chromosome analysis and susceptibility to transformation by Simian Virus 40 of fibroblasts from Ataxia-Telangiectasia, *Cancer Res.,* 37, 997, 1977.

115. **Matsumura, T., Pfendt, E. A., Zerrudo, Z., and Hayflick, L.,** Senescent human diploid cells (WI-38). Attempted induction of proliferation by infection with SV40 and by fusion with irradiated continuous cell-lines, *Exp. Cell Res.,* 125, 453, 1980.

116. **Elliot, M. S., and Katze, J. R.,** Inhibition of queuine uptake in diploid human fibroblasts by phorbol-12,13-didecanoate, *J. Biol. Chem.,* 261, 13019, 1986.

117. **Diatloff-Zito, C., Turleau, C., Cabanis, M. O., Macieira-Coelho, A., and de Grouchy, J.,** Induction of growth stimulation in skin fibroblasts from retinoblastoma donors after ionizing radiation, *C. R. Acad. Sci.,* 297, 431, 1983.

118. **Todaro, G. J., Green, H., and Swift, M. R.,** Susceptibility of human diploid fibroblast strains to transformation, *Science,* 153, 1252, 1966.

119. **Zimmerman, R. J. and Cerutti, P. A.,** A comparison of markers of human fibroblast transformation induced by chemical carcinogen treatment or by transfection of an origin-defective SV40-containing plasmid, *Mutat. Res.,* 199, 449, 1988.

120. **Diatloff-Zito, C. and Macieira-Coelho, A.,** Effect of growth arrest on the doubling potential of human fibroblasts *in vitro:* a possible influence of the donor, *In Vitro,* 18, 606, 1982.

121. **Bech-Hansen, N. T., Sell, B. M., Lampkin, B. C., Blattner, W. H., McKeen, E. A., Fraumeni, J. F., Jr., and Paterson, M. C.,** Transmission of *in vitro* radioresistance in a cancer-prone family, *Lancet,* 2, 1335, 1981.

122. **Wang, Y., Kateley-Kohler, S., Maher, V. M., and McCormick, J. J.,** ^{60}Co radiation-induced transformation to anchorage independence of fibroblasts from normal persons and patients with inherited predisposition to retinoblastoma, *Carcinogenesis,* 7, 1927, 1986.

123. **Kopelovich, L. and Chapman, T.,** An imbalance in sex chromosomes alters cell survival of human skin fibroblasts exposed to ionizing radiation *in vitro, Cancer Genet. Cytogenet.,* 20, 115, 1986.

124. **Kopelovich, L. and Rich, R. F.,** Enhanced radiotolerance to ionizing radiation is correlated with increased cancer proneness of cultured fibroblasts from precursor states in neurofibromatosis patients, *Cancer Genet. Cytogenet.,* 22, 203, 1986.

125. **Chang, E. H., Pirollo, K. F., Zou, Z. Q., Cheung, H.-Y., Lawler, E. L., Garner, R., White, E., Bernstein, W. B., Fraumeni, J. W., Jr., and Blattner, W. A.,** Oncogenes in radio-resistant, noncancerous skin fibroblasts from a cancer-prone family, *Science,* 237, 1036, 1987.

126. **Todaro, G. J. and Martin, G. M.,** Increased susceptibility of Down's Syndrome fibroblasts to transformation by SV40, *Proc. Soc. Exp. Biol. Med.,* 124, 1232, 1967.

127. **Chang, K. S.,** Susceptibility of Xeroderma Pigmentosum cells to transformation by murine and feline sarcoma viruses, *Cancer Res.,* 36, 3294, 1976.

128. **Shimada, H., Shibuta, H., and Yoshikawa, M.,** Transformation of tissue-cultured Xeroderma Pigmentosum fibroblasts by treatment with N-methyl-N-nitro-N-nitrosoguanidine, *Nature,* 264, 547, 1976.

129. **McCormick, J. J., Kateley-Kohler, S., Watanabe, M., and Maher, V. M.,** Abnormal sensitivity of human fibroblasts from Xeroderma Pigmentosum variants to transformation to anchorage independence by ultraviolet radiation, *Cancer Res.,* 46, 489, 1986.

130. **Canaani, D., Naiman, T., Teitz, T., and Berg, P.,** Immortalization of Xeroderma Pigmentosum cells by SV40 DNA having a defective origin of DNA replication, *Som. Cell. Mol. Genet.,* 12, 13, 1986.

131. **Webb, T. and Harding, M.,** Chromosome complement and SV40 transformation of cells from patients susceptible to malignant disease, *Br. J. Cancer,* 36, 583, 1977.

132. **Doniger, J., Dipaolo, J. A., and Popescu, N. C.,** Transformation of Bloom's syndrome fibroblasts by DNA transfection, *Science,* 222, 1144, 1983.

133. **Shaham, M., Adler, B., and Chaganti, R. S. K.,** Transformation of chromosome breakage syndrome fibroblasts by SV40 DNA transfection, *Cancer Genet. Cytogenet.,* 20, 137, 1986.

134. **Pfeffer, L. M. and Kopelovich, L.,** Differential genetic susceptibility of cultured human skin fibroblasts to transformation by Kirsten murine sarcoma virus, *Cell,* 10, 313, 1977.

135. **Rasheed, S. and Gardner, M. B.,** Growth properties and susceptibility to viral transformation of skin fibroblasts from individuals at high genetic risk for colorectal cancer, *J. Natl. Cancer Inst.,* 60, 43, 1981.

136. **Friedman, E., Carnright, K., and Lipkin, M.,** Differential response of familial fibroblasts to two bifunctional alkylating agents, *Carcinogenesis,* 3, 1481, 1982.

137. **Shimada, T., Dowjat, W. K., Gindhart, T. D., Lerwan, M. J., and Colburn, N. H.,** Lifespan extension of basal cell nevus syndrome fibroblasts by transfection with mouse pro OR v-myc-genes, *Int. J. Cancer,* 39, 649, 1987.

138. **Azzarone, B. and Macieira-Coelho, A.,** Further characterization of the defects of skin fibroblasts from cancer patients, *J. Cell Sci.,* 87, 155, 1987.

139. **Schor, S. L., Schor, A. M., and Rushton, G.,** Foetal and cancer patient fibroblasts produce an autocrine migration-stimulating factor not made by normal adult cells, *J. Cell Sci.,* 90, 391, 1988.

140. **Shor, S. L., Shor, A. M., and Rushton, G.,** Fibroblasts from cancer patients display a mixture of both foetal and adult-like phenotype characteristics, *J. Cell Sci.,* 90, 401, 1988.

141. **Mukherji, B., MacAlister, T. J., Guha, A., Gillies, C. G., Jeffers, D. C., and Loeum, S. K.,** Spontaneous *in vitro* transformation of human fibroblasts, *J. Natl. Cancer Inst.,* 73, 583, 1981.

142. **Auerbach, R.,** Morphogenetic interactions in the development of the mouse thymus gland, *Dev. Biol.,* 2, 271, 1960.

143. **Kratochwill, K.,** Organ specificity in mesenchymal induction demonstrated in the embryonic development of the mammary gland of the mouse, *Dev. Biol.,* 20, 46, 1969.

144. **Elias, J. A., Zurier, R. B., Schreiber, A. D., Leff, J. A., and Danièle, R. P.,** Monocyte inhibition of lung fibroblast growth: relationship to fibroblast prostaglandin production and density defined monocyte subpopulations, *J. Leukocyte Biol.,* 37, 15, 1985.

145. **Hamada, J.-I., Takeichi, N., and Kobayashi, H.,** Inverse correlation between the metastatic capacity of cell clones derived from a rat mammary carcinoma and their intercellular communication with normal fibroblasts, *Jpn. J. Cancer Res. (Gann),* 78, 1175, 1987.

146. **Dabbous, M. Kh., Haney, L., Carter, L. M., Paul, A. K., and Reger, J.,** Heterogeneity of fibroblast response in host-tumor cell-cell interactions in metastatic tumors, *J. Cell. Biochem.,* 35, 333, 1987.

147. **Dell'Orco, R. T., Mertens, J. G., and Kruse, P. F., Jr.,** Doubling potential, calendar time, and senescence of human diploid cells in culture, *Exp. Cell. Res.,* 77, 356, 1973.

148. **Holliday, R., Huschtscha, L. I., Tarrant, G. M., and Kirkwood, T. B. L.,** Testing the commitment theory of cellular aging, *Science,* 198, 366, 1977.

149. **Kaji, K. and Matsuo, M.,** A low-density inoculation method for the serial subcultivation of human diploid fibroblasts: an efficient model system for the study of cellular aging, *Mech. Ageing Dev.,* 13, 219, 1980.

150. **Matsumura, T., Hagashi, M., and Konishi, R.,** Immortalization in culture of rat cells: a genetic study, *J. Natl. Cancer Inst.,* 74, 1223, 1985.

151. **Chen, T. R. and Ruddle, F. H.,** Chromosome changes revealed by the Q-Band staining method during cell senescence of WI-38, *Proc. Soc. Exp. Biol. Med.,* 147, 533, 1974.

152. **Harnden, D. G., Benn, P. A., Oxford, J. M., Taylor, A. M. R., and Webb, T. P.,** Cytogenetically marked clones in human fibroblasts cultured from normal subjects, *Som. Cell Genet.,* 2, 55, 1976.

153. **Salk, D., Bryant, E., Au, K., Hoehn, H., and Martin, G.,** Systematic growth studies, cocultivation and cell hybridization studies of Werner Syndrome cultured skin fibroblasts, *Hum. Genet.,* 58, 310, 1981.

154. **Schneider, E. L. and Gilman, B.,** Sister chromatid exchanges and aging. III. The effect of donor age on mutagen-induced siser chromatid exchange in human diploid fibroblasts, *Hum. Genet.,* 46, 57, 1979.

155. **Beaupain, R., Icard, C., and Macieira-Coelho, A.,** Changes in DNA alkali-sensitive sites during senescence and establishment of fibroblasts *in vitro, Biochim. Biophys. Acta,* 606, 251, 1980.

156. **Yao, M.-C., Choi, J., Yokoyama, S., Austerberry, C. F., and Yao, C.-H.,** DNA elimination in tetrahymena: a developmental process involving extensive breakage and rejoining of DNA at defined sites, *Cell,* 36, 433, 1984.

157. **Macieira-Coelho, A., Bengtsson, A., and Van der Ploeg, M.,** Distribution of DNA between sister cells during serial subcultivation of human fibroblasts, *Histochemistry,* 75, 11, 1982.

158. **Capanna, E.,** *Cytotaxonomy and Vertebrate Evolution,* Academic Press, London, 1973, 783.

159. **Sanford, K. K.,** Malignant transformation of cells *in vitro, Int. Rev. Cytol.,* 18, 249, 1965.

160. **Cooper, G. M.,** Cellular transforming genes, *Science,* 218, 801, 1982.

161. **Bourgeois, C. A., Raynaud, N., Diatlott-Zito, C., and Macieira-Coelho, A.,** Effect of low dose rate ionizing radiation on the division potential of cells *in vitro.* VIII. Cytogenetic analysis of human fibroblasts, *Mech. Ageing Dev.,* 17, 225, 1981.

162. **Schmid, C. W. and Jelinek, W. R.,** The Alu family of dispersed repetitive sequences, *Science,* 216, 1065, 1982.

163. **Macieira-Coelho, A.,** Reorganization of the cell genome as the basis of aging in dividing cells, in *Recent Advances in Gerontology,* Orimo, H., Shimada, M., Iriki, D., and Maeda, J., Eds., Excerpta Medica, Amsterdam, 1979, 111.

164. **Schwartz, A. G. and Moore, C. J.,** Inverse correlation between species life span and capacity of cultured fibroblasts to bind 7,12-dimethylbenzaanthracene to DNA, *Exp. Cell Res.,* 109, 448, 1977.

165. **Hart, R. W. and Setlow, R. B.,** Correlation between deoxyribonucleic acid excision-repair and life span in a number of mammalian species, *Proc. Natl. Acad. Sci. U.S.A.,* 5, 67, 1976.

166. **Mullaart, E. P., van der Lohman, P. H. M., and Vijg, J.,** Differences in pyrimidine dimer removal between rat skin cells *in vitro* and *in vivo, J. Invest, Dermatol.,* 90, 346, 1988.

167. **Yagi, T.,** DNA repair ability of cultured cells derived from mouse embryos in comparison with human cells, *Mutat. Res.,* 96, 89, 1982.

168. **Elliot, G. C. and Johnson, R. J.,** DNA repair in mouse embryo fibroblasts. II. Responses of nontransformed preneoplastic and tumorigenic cells to ultraviolet irradiation, *Mutat. Res.,* 145, 185, 1985.

169. **Diatloff-Zito, C., Deschavanne, P. J., Loria, E., Malaise, E. P., and Macieira-Coelho, A.,** Comparison between the radiosensitivity of human, mouse and chicken fibroblast-like cells using short-term endpoints, *Int. J. Rad. Biol.,* 39, 419, 1981.

170. **Cleaver, J. E.,** Defective repair replication of DNA in Xeroderma Pigmentosum, *Nature,* 218, 652, 1968,

171. **Hanania, N., Diatloff-Zito, C., and Schaool, D.,** An abnormal expression of a tumor-activated multigenic set in cells from cancer prone patients with inherited Fanconi's anemia (FA) and retinoblastoma (Rb), *Cancer Lett.,* 39, 297, 1988.

172. **Brothman, A. R., Cram. L. S., Bartholdi, M. F., and Kraemer, P. M.,** Preneoplastic phenotype and chromosome changes of cultured human Bloom syndrome fibroblasts (strain GM 1492), *Cancer Res.,* 46, 791, 1986.

173. **Mikol, Y. B. and Lipkin, M.,** Methionine dependence in skin fibroblasts of humans affected with familial colon cancer or Gardner's syndrome, *J. Natl. Cancer Inst.,* 72, 19, 1984.

174. **Mayne, L. V., Priestley, A., James, M. R., and Burke, J. F.,** Efficient immortalization of human fibroblasts by transfection with SV40 DNA linked to a dominant marker, *Exp. Cell Res.,* 162, 530, 1986.

175. **Jacobs, P. A., Brown, W. M. C., and Doll, R.,** Distribution of human chromosome counts in relation to age, *Nature,* 191, 1178, 1961.

176. **Puvion-Dutilleul, F. and Macieira-Coelho, A.,** Aging dependent nucleolar and chromatin changes in cultivated fibroblasts, *Cell Biol. Int. Rep.,* 7, 61, 1983.

177. **Puvion-Dutilleul, F., Puvion, E., Icard-Liepkalns, C., and Macieira-Coelho, A.,** Chromatin structure, DNA synthesis and transcription through the lifespan of human embryonic lung fibroblasts, *Exp. Cell Res.,* 151, 283, 1984.

178. **Dell'Orco, R. T., Whittle, W. L., and Macieira-Coelho, A.,** Changes in the higher order organization of DNA during aging of human fibroblast-like cells, *Mech. Ageing Dev.,* 35, 199, 1986.

179. **Icard-Liepkalns, C., Doly, J., and Macieira-Coelho, A.,** Gene reorganization during serial divisions of normal human cells, *Biochem. Biophys. Res. Commun.,* 141, 112, 1986.

180. **Macieira-Coelho, A. and Puvion-Dutilleul, F.,** Evaluation of the reorganization in the high order structure of DNA occurring during cell senescence, *Mutat. Res.,* 219, 165, 1989.

181. **Stein, G. H.,** SV40-transformed human fibroblasts: evidence for cellular aging in precrisis cells, *J. Cell. Phys.,* 125, 36, 1985.

182. **Ide, T. Tsuji, Y., Nakashima, T., and Ishibashi, S.,** Progress of aging in human diploid cells transformed with a tsA mutant of Simian virus 40, *Exp. Cell Res.,* 150, 321, 1984.

183. **Macieira-Coelho, A. and Loria, E.,** Stimulation of ribosome synthesis during retarded aging of human fibroblasts by hydrocortisone, *Nature,* 251, 67, 1974.

184. **Sun, A. S., Alvarez, L. J., Reinach, P. S., and Rubin, E.,** 5'-nucleotidase levels in normal and virus transformed cells, *Lab. Invest.,* 41, 1, 1979.

185. **Raes, M., Houbion, A., and Remacle, J.,** The purification of plasma membranes from WI-38 fibroblasts. Effects of aging on their composition, *Biochim. Biophys. Acta,* 642, 313, 1981.

186. **Muggleton-Harris, A. L. and Desimone, D. W.,** Replicative potentials of various fusion products between WI-38 and SV40 transformed WI-38 cells and their components, *Som. Cell Genet.,* 6, 689, 1980.

187. **Bunn, C. L. and Tarrant, G. M.,** Limited lifespan in somatic cell hybrids and cybrids, *Exp. Cell Res.,* 127, 385, 1980.
188. **Pereira-Smith, O. M. and Smith, J. R.,** Evidence for the recessive nature of cellular immortality, *Science,* 221, 964, 1983.
189. **Martinez, A. O., Norwood, T. H., Prothero, J. W., and Martin, G. M.,** Evidence for clonal attenuation of growth potential in HeLa cells, *In Vitro,* 14, 996, 1978.
190. **Le Borgne de Kaouël, C., Billard, C., and Macieira-Coelho, A.,** Growth characteristics *in vitro* of hybrids between normal and transformed cell lines, *Int. J. Cancer,* 21, 338, 1978.

Chapter 2

AGE-DEPENDENT MODIFICATIONS OF CONNECTIVE TISSUES, POSSIBLE RELATIONSHIPS TO TUMOR GROWTH, AND METASTASIS FORMATION

J. Labat-Robert and L. Robert

TABLE OF CONTENTS

I. INTRODUCTION

Most degenerative diseases exhibit an increasing tendency with age. Most, if not all, of these diseases directly and/or indirectly concern connective tissues. Cancer, or at least some forms of malignancies, exhibit age-dependent modifications in their frequency and also severity. These statistical considerations do not specify any direct causal relationship between the malignant disease and aging. Statistical correlations, as provided by epidemiological studies do, however, justify an in-depth inquiry if such causal relations may exist between the recognized mechanisms of malignant transformations, tumor spreading, and the age-dependent modifications of tissues. This chapter provides a tentative assessment of the possible existence of such relationships based on available experimental and epidemiological evidence.

Epidemiology — A recent health statistic of the World Health Organization (WHO) states that 25.40% of total death causes in 29 countries between 65 and 74 years are malignant tumors. It was also stated that more than 80% of total cancers occur above 50 years of age.[1] Post-mortem studies carried out at the General Hospital of Malmö and reviewed by Ponten[2] suggest a steep increase of several different malignancies, especially of prostate and gastro-intestinal cancers, but also all forms of cancers with age. A more recent critical assessment of these and other figures by Macieira-Coelho[3] led to the conclusion that the increase with age is not a general property of all cancers and even those which do show such a tendency often exhibit a plateau or even a decline above a certain age. It could be argued that a more adequate immune function may be an important selective factor enabling some individuals to pass a certain age limit (70 to 80 years) because of their increased resistance to cancer.

Recent experimental evidence also points to the possibility of an increased resistance of some organisms with age to cancer spread. The team of Weksler[4] showed recently that the growth rate of the B16 melanoma in mice decreases with age. This could be partly attributed to the age-dependent decline of a subset of T-lymphocytes which favors tumor growth, but parabiotic experiments suggested that something in the aging organisms also contributed to the limitation of tumor growth. It could well be a different structure of peritumoral matrix. The tumor-stroma reaction or desmoplastic reaction was considered by some pathologists as a defense reaction of the organism to tumor growth. The changing composition and structure of connective tissues could exert such an action at least at some sites and for some types of tumor cells.

Whatever the evolution of cancers as a function of age, the above cited figures clearly indicate that some correlation might exist between tumor formation, spreading, and the age-dependent modifications of tissues. The formation and spreading of tumors does involve interactions between tumor cells and surrounding tissues. We shall therefore examine some of these interactions, their possible modifications with age, and their possible role in the age-dependent behavior of malignancies. Connective tissues are considered as especially important in this respect. Such tissues differ from others mainly in their higher content of extracellular matrix. Cell-matrix interactions may therefore play an especially important role in these processes. Extracellular matrix is often considered as a barrier to tumor spreading which has to be overcome before tumor cells can enter the circulation and reach other tissues. This question was recently reviewed (Van den Hoff,[5] Tarin[6]). They insist, and rightly so, on the fact that connective tissue remodeling, more than degradation alone, can be considered as a general characteristic of malignant growth. Van den Hoff proposes the upset of the regulation of morphogenetically important genomic entities (homeotic genes given as an example) as underlying malignant growth. The recently acquired knowledge on the informational content and importance of extracellular matrices for contacting cells and their behavior is a more realistic consideration than the merely destructive effects of tumor cells. Such catabolic effects do however exist and have also to be taken into consideration.[6] We shall therefore concentrate on the age-dependent modifications of extracellular matrices and their possible role in tumor spread.

II. COMPOSITION OF EXTRACELLULAR MATRIX AND ITS AGE-DEPENDENT MODIFICATIONS

A. THE MACROMOLECULES OF EXTRACELLULAR MATRICES

Generally speaking, extracellular matrices can be considered as composed of a variety of macromolecules which can be grossly separated in four major classes. It has to be stated also that the delimitation between these classes is not absolute.

1. Collagens

The first major class of extracellular matrix macromolecules is the family of collagens. We actually recognize the existence of at least 14 different collagen types. Their constituent α-chains '3 per molecule', which may be different or identical, are coded by distinct structural genes. By far the most frequent are the so-called fibrous interstitial collagens type I, II, and III with compositions and structures analogous although distinct from one type to the other.[7,8]

The other collagen types, although quantitatively less important, are also quite specifically distributed in a variety of tissues and may well play important and distinct structural and functional roles. This is widely recognized for collagen type IV which is the major constituent of basal lamina in capillaries and between mesenchymal and ectodermal and endodermal tissues.

Although the main structural feature of all these collagens is the presence of a triple helical portion, the importance of this triple helix is quite variable. The fibrillary interstitial collagens contain a very large proportion of these triple helical relatively rigid rod-like structures. For the other collagen types the proportion of the noncollagenous mostly glycoprotein-like portions can be quite important. This is the case for collagen type VI which has approximately a 40% triple helix for 60% of nontriple helical glycoprotein-like constituents (Figure 1).

Recently, it was shown that alternative splicing can occur in some genes coding for collagen α-chains.[8] If such processes would show age-dependent variations, structural (qualitative) alterations could occur in collagenous components with age.

As collagens represent nearly 30% of the total body proteins, they have to be considered important tissue components for the understanding of tumor metastatic spreading. For a more detailed description of these extracellular matrix components, we shall refer to specialized monographies.[7,8]

2. Elastin

Elastin is a major constituent of vessel walls; it also represents about 4% to 5% of lung parenchyma and 2% to 3% of skin. It is present also in cartilage and in smaller amounts in several other connective tissues.

Its main component is a polymeric form of the biosynthetic monomer, tropoelastin, about 70 kDa molecular weight protein rich in lysine residues which are involved in crosslinking through the action of lysyl-oxidase and the formation of heterocyclic crosslinks (desmosine and isodesmosine)[9,10] (Figure 2). Polymeric fibrous elastin is by far the most resistant component of the organism. Its purification can be achieved by heating tissues in 0.1 N sodium hydroxide to 100°C for 45 min.[11] This drastic procedure will result in the solubilization of all other tissue proteins except elastin. This strong resistance is due to the predominance of hydrophobic interactions stabilizing the elastin peptide fold. In the presence of organic solvents, this resistance is lost and elastin is easily depolymerized by alkaline solvents.[10,11] Elastin is also resistant to most proteolytic enzymes except some of them which are therefore classified as elastase-type proteases.[11,12] It has to be stated, however, that these proteases can also degrade other body constituents. As a matter of fact, polymorphonuclear leukocyte elastase, which is one of the most potent elastase-type proteases, can degrade most if not all constituents of extracellular matrices.

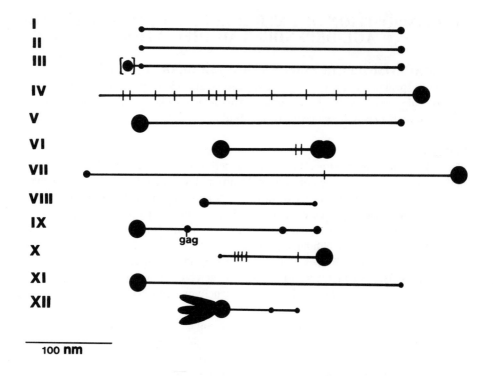

FIGURE 1. Schematic representation of the different types of collagens. The rods represent the triple-helical portion, the bulbs, the nonhelical portions, and the small vertical rods are short interruptions in GLY.X.Y sequences. Types I, II, and III are the interstitial collagens; type IV is the basement membrane collagen; types V and VI are quite widely distributed in tissues; type VII forms anchoring fibrils at dermoepideremal basement membranes; types IX, X, and XI are found in cartilaginous tissues; type XII was detected in several connective tissues (tendon, ligament, cornea, skin). The structure of type XIII is not yet determined. For more details, see Reference 7 and 8. (After P. Kern, Connective Tissue Research Laboratory, Créteil). (Reproduced with permission of author.)

It is for this reason that study of elastase-type proteases is of particular interest in tissue destructions and metastasis formation. Because of its hydrophobic nature, elastin exhibits strong affinity for lipidic components.[9,10] During aging, it is enriched in lipids of all sorts and calcium salts. This will result in the loss of its elasticity and render easier its degradation by elastase-type enzymes.

3. Proteoglycans

Proteoglycans are composed of a protein core onto which glycosaminoglycan chains are attached covalently.[13-15] According to the nature of the protein chain and the number, quality, and length of the glycosaminoglycan chains, they can be very rich, moderately rich, or even poor in carbohydrate constituents. Although their designation is still largely decided by the nature of the glycosaminoglycan chains, it became clear during the last years (especially as a result of the studies of Ruoslahti et al.[15]) that the protein core determines the quality of the proteoglycans as well as the density and the nature of the glycan chains which are attached to it (Figure 3).

Proteoglycans are present on cell membranes, in basement membranes, and in the extracellular matrices. The quality and quantity of these important tissue components varies to a large extent from one tissue to the other. Because of their strong negative charge and their presence on cell membranes, basement membranes and in the matrix, they play an important role in cell-

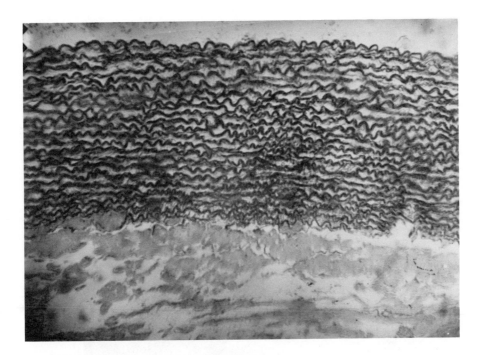

A

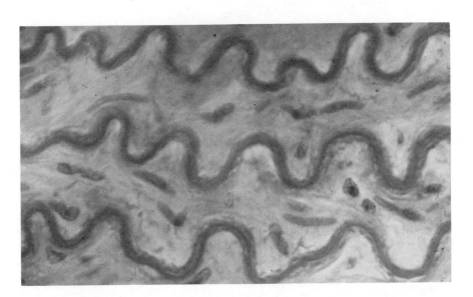

B

FIGURE 2. Elastin and elastic fibers. Optical microscopic picture of elastic fibers in rabbit aorta, A: at low (× 200) and B: at higher (× 800) magnification. C: Electron microscopy of elastic fibers surrounding a smooth muscle cell (× 27,000, photo by G. Godeau). The translucent, amorphous structures represent the crosslinked elastin component; the dark fibrillar structures, in and around elastin, are the microfibrillar structural glycoprotein-components C: collagen fibers. D Elastic fibers in an elastotic breast cancer. Strong perivascular elastosis. (Weigert staining × 200.) (Reproduced with permission of author and editor.)

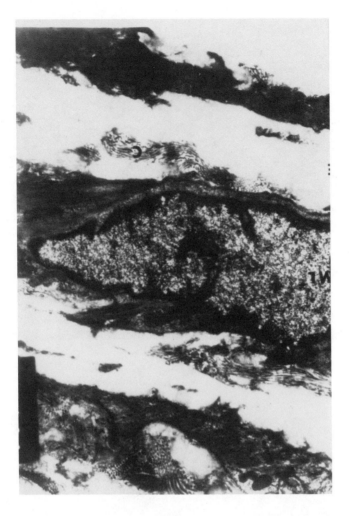

FIGURE 2C.

cell and cell-tissue interactions and were therefore intensively studied in relation to tumor formation and metastatic spreading.

4. Structural Glycoproteins

This heterogenous class of connective tissue components was identified during the early 1960s[16] when it was recognized that besides the above-mentioned three types of macromolecules, extracellular matrices contain glycoproteins with a composition similar to those of circulating blood glycoproteins. As the blood-borne glycoproteins are mostly synthesized in the liver, in order to distinguish the tissue glycoproteins, we proposed to designate them as structural glycoproteins.[16-18] This designation implies that they are synthesized locally by mesenchymal cells and play some structural role in the connective tissues. Other designations such as matrix glycoproteins or connective tissue glycoproteins or nectins are also in use to designate them. As there is no general agreement on their nomenclature, and as their number increases steadily, we will use the original designation we proposed in the early 1960s until such a general agreement can be reached.

Table 1 gives a nonexhaustive list of these structural glycoproteins. It can be recognized from its inspection that their most important biological role concerns the mediation of interactions

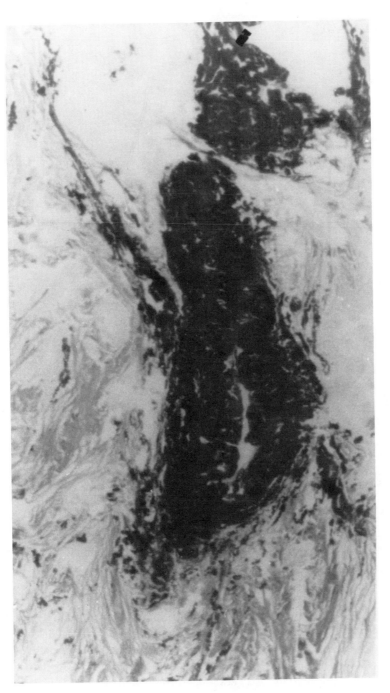

FIGURE 2D.

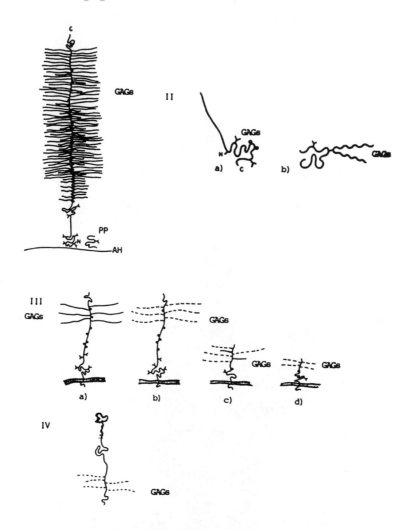

FIGURE 3. Schematic representation of proteoglycans (PG).(I) Cartilage proteoglycans: c: core protein with the laterally anchored glycosaminoglycan (GAG) chains and the *N*-glycosidically linked glycan residues (-<). The GAG-free portions contain the recognition site for hyaluronate (AH), this interaction being further strengthened by the link proteins (PP). (II) Dermatan-sulfate (DS) proteoglycan from skin (a) and keratan-sulfate (KS) proteoglycan from cornea. These proteoglycans contain fewer and shorter GAG-chains than the cartilage PG. (III) Cell membrane proteoglycans: a. Chondroitin-sulfate (CS)-dermatan-sulfate (DS) PG; b. Heparan-sulfate (HS)-CS-DS-PG from mammary epithelium; and c. PGHS from hepatocytes. (IV) PGHS from basement membranes.

between cells and matrix components. As a matter of fact, fibronectin and laminin, which are the best studied components of this matrix glycoprotein family, will be dealt with in more detail because of their important linking function between cells and the extracellular matrix.

Figure 4 shows the way in which fibronectin is considered to mediate interaction of cells and extracellular matrix. It was also recognized that the receptors which mediate interaction of these matrix glycoproteins with the cell itself are mostly transmembrane proteins and many of them are designated as integrins or cytoadhesins. These integrins are composed usually of two peptide chains with a transmembrane domain protruding inside the cell where they contact cytoskeletal components. It was also recognized that as a result of this contact established by the structural glycoproteins and their transmembrane receptors between the inside of the cell and the outside,

TABLE 1
Some Structural Glycoproteins

Fibronectin

Chondronectin

Hyaluronectin

Vitronectin

Osteonectin

Laminin

Entactin/nidogen

Mesonectin

Fibrillin

Tenascin

Elastonectin

Thrombospondin

Von Willebrand factor

Cytotactin

Merosin

messages and instructions can be conveyed through this relay mechanism from the extracellular matrix to the cell. This led us to the proposal of an informational feedback mechanism between cell and extracellular matrix as shown in Figure 5.

This feedback loop starts with the biosynthesis of a specific extracellular matrix which then contacts the cell it surrounds by the intermediary of structural glycoproteins and their receptors and can therefore influence cell behavior. As the matrix composition changes with age, this may well introduce age-dependent modifications in the behavior of the cell.

External factors may also produce a perturbation of this informational feedback loop as, for instance, destruction of some extracellular matrix macromolecules or modifications of the composition, structure, and function of the cell membrane receptors. All these factors appear to play an important role in tumor formation and spreading and are considered in more detail below.

B. AGE-DEPENDENT MODIFICATIONS OF EXTRACELLULAR MATRIX COMPONENTS

As a great deal of information is available on the modifications of the previously mentioned matrix macromolecules, we shall only briefly cite some of these modifications which may be of importance for tumor formation and metastatic spreading. For other details, monographs and reviews can be consulted.[19-21]

1. Aging of Collagens

One of the most important early discoveries in experimental gerontology was made by Verzar in the early 1950s concerning the age-dependent modifications of collagen structure. He observed that the heat-dependent shrinkage of collagen fibers extracted from rat tail tendons and other tissues can be inhibited by an applied contrary force which will keep the tendons in a stretched form. He also observed that this force increases exponentially with the age of the animals. Verzar proposed that this was due to the increasing crosslinking of collagen with aging.[22]

Later studies with refined biochemical procedures could confirm the modification of the quality and quantity of crosslinks, although no general agreement exists for the moment on the nature of the crosslinks which increase with age. As they are mostly nonreducible with tritiated borohydride, it is probable that they can be either of the pyridinoline type or resulting from the Maillard reaction.[23-25] The continuous and long-term interactions of reducing sugars such as

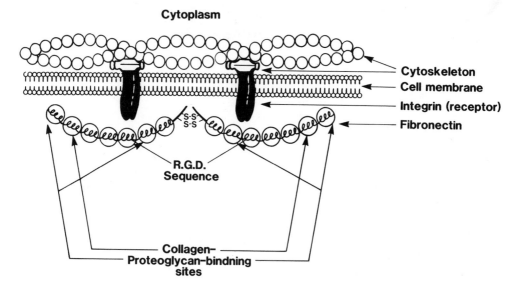

FIGURE 4. Schematic representation of fibronectin with its domain structure, anchored to its cell membrane receptor (integrin) which communicates with the cytoskeleton.

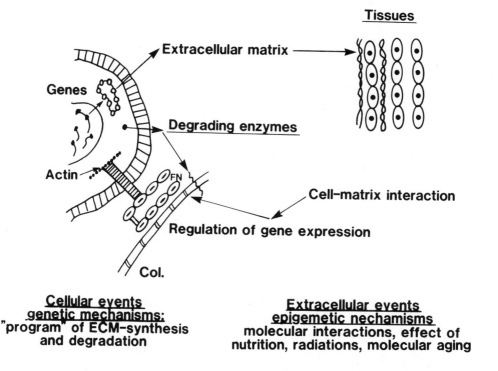

FIGURE 5. Schematic representation of the informational feedback relationship between cells and surrounding extracellular matrix. (a) The cells synthesize the macromolecules of the extracellular matrix according to their genetic "program" of differentiation; their program changes with age. The macromolecules interact with each other and form the tissue specific patterns. (b) The extracellular matrix remains in close contact with the cells it surrounds through the mediation of structural glycoproteins or nectins (fibronectin, FN on the figure). (c) These nectins contact their specific cell membrane receptor (integrin or adhesin) and also other matrix macromolecules (a collagen fiber, col, on the figure). The cytoplasmic end of the integrins contact the cytoskeleton and transmit to the interior of the cell messages coming from the surrounding matrix.

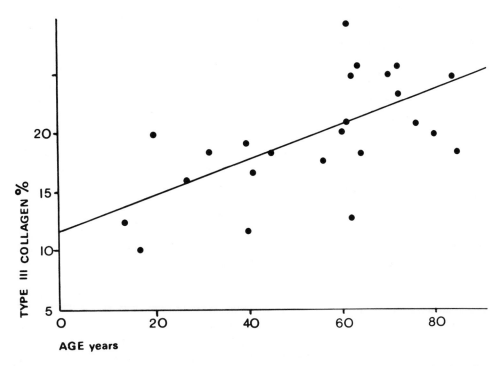

FIGURE 6. Increase with age of the ratio collagen type III to collagen type I in human conjunctival biopsies (From Kern et al.[26]). Abscissa: age in years. Ordinates: collagen type III to collagen type I + III ratio. (Reproduced with permission of author and editor.)

glucose with free amino groups and especially with the ε-amines of lysine can result in covalent crosslink formation between proteins. It is, as a matter of fact, quite plausible to believe that this process leads to the increasing crosslinking of collagen fibers with age.[25]

Another quite general modification of collagens with age was found by Kern et al.[26] and which consists in the steady increase of the ratio of collagen type III to collagen type I in connective tissues. As shown in Figure 6, this ratio is linearly increasing with age in human connective tissues.

It was also proposed on the basis of morphological and ultrastructural studies that the overall density of collagen fibers decreases in some connective tissues at least such as the dermis with age (Bouissou[27]). As our knowledge on the number and diversity of collagen types increased quite fast during the last decade, very little is yet known on their age-dependent modifications. No doubt further research in this area will yield important new insights on the age-dependent modifications of tissues in general and their resistance to tumor invasion in particular.

2. Elastin

The age-dependent modifications of elastin were investigated in detail in our laboratory as well as in several others.[9,10,28,29] We have to distinguish here between elastin itself and the elastic fibers as histological entities, as they occur in the organism. As a matter of fact, the elastic fibers are composed of a microfibrillar structure containing a variety of glycoproteins and the polymer of tropoelastin itself. They are surrounded by other matrix macromolecules and heparan-sulfate proteoglycan appears to be in close apposition to elastic fibers, at least in the major blood vessels.

Age-dependent modifications of elastic fibers involve increasing amounts of lipids which deposit in the protein fold. They potentiate the deposition of calcium salts. The β-turns of the elastic fibers were shown by Urry[30] to be preferential sites for calcium fixation. Adult and aging elastic fibers will also be degraded increasingly by the elastase-type enzymes, liberating elastin peptides in the circulation. Aging of elastin can therefore be characterized by an increasing lipid and calcium content and increasing fragmentation.[9,10]

A sensitive ELISA method which was worked out recently in our laboratory enabled us to determine the circulating serum-elastin peptide concentration which ranges between a fraction of µg/ml to more than 10 to 20 µg/ml.[113] The slightly increasing concentration of circulating elastin peptides with age may well be the reflection of the increasing biosynthesis of elastase-type enzymes by several cell types as shown previously.[10,20,21,29] As these enzymes can degrade most if not all matrix constituents, their increasing synthesis may well result in an increasing degradation with age of extracellular matrix macromolecules in general and of elastin in particular.

These modifications may well be of significance in the increasing tendency of tumor growth and metastasis formation as mentioned in the Introduction.

3. Proteoglycans

Relatively little is known on the age-dependent modifications of the biosynthesis of proteoglycans at different sites of the organism in different tissues. Studies were performed in the articular cartilage where the ratio of proteoglycans with chondroitin-4-sulfate and 6-sulfate varies with age and the total amount of proteoglycans decreases with age.[13]

As far as the cell membrane proteoglycans are concerned, not too much is known on their age-dependent modifications. For basement membranes which represent an important barrier for tumor cell spreading, detailed information is available mainly on the diabetic modifications of basement membrane proteoglycans.[31,32] As type II diabetes imitates in several respects an accelerated aging process, it is probable that similar modifications occur without diabetes in aging basement membranes. Figure 7 shows the increasing thickness of capillary basement membranes as measured by electron microscopy which is due to an increasing synthesis of collagen type IV, fibronectin and laminin.[31,32]

Heparan-sulfate proteoglycan was shown to decrease in diabetic basement membranes.[31] Similar results were reported by Schaeverbeke's team on the nondiabetic aging glomerular basement membranes of rats.[32] It is therefore probable that with increasing thickness of basement membranes with age, an increasing permeability can also be observed with a decreasing selectivity in the regulation of permeability.

4. Structural Glycoproteins and Aging

Detailed information is only available on fibronectin which was intensively studied in our laboratory. It could be shown that plasma fibronectin increases with age exponentially (Figure 8). This increase is strongly attenuated in mammary cancer patients and also in uterine cancers as well as in diabetes.[33-36]

Recently we could show that the biosynthesis of fibronectin increases with age in extracellular matrix.[37] Similar results were reported for *in vitro* aging skin fibroblasts: their fibronectin synthesis increased with passage number at least up to the beginning of phase III, the decline of cell proliferation.[38] It appears therefore that both liver cells and skin fibroblasts exhibit a continuous up-regulation with age of the gene coding for fibronectin. As fibronectin is highly susceptible to degradation by proteases in general and elastases in particular, it is highly probable that this increasing amount of fibronectin, together with the increasing elastase activity synthesized by several cell types, will result in an increased degradation of fibronectin. It was shown some time ago by Barlati et al.[39] that some fragments of fibronectin are able to potentiate the transformation of chick embryo fibroblasts by a Rous sarcoma virus. This observation deserves further study and extension to other models because the previously mentioned increasing concentration and increasing degradation of fibronectin with age may well represent a factor favoring malignant transformation and tumor spreading.

We have mentioned the increasing amounts of fibronectin associated with capillary basement membranes during aging which was studied by immunohistochemical methods in a number of diabetic skin biopsies.[35,36] Diabetic skin biopsies as well as skin biopsies in diseases imitating a highly accelerated aging as in Werner patients showed a strongly increased immunofluores-

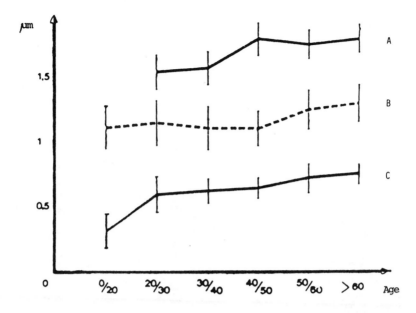

FIGURE 7. Increase of basement membrane thickness in diabetic and non-diabetic conjunctival capillaries. Subpalpebral conjunctival biopsies were taken from nondiabetics (C), diabetics (B), and diabetics exhibiting within the capillary basement membrane fine cross striated collagen fibers (type III intermingled with type IV) (A). Abscissa: age in years. Ordinates: basement membrane diameter evaluated by electron microscopy, in microns. (From information contained in References 31-37 and 107. Reproduced with permission of author and editor.)

cence for fibronectin at the dermoepidermal and capillary basement membranes and diffusely in the dermis.

Other age-dependent modifications of fibronectin and other matrix glycoproteins concern alterations of binding and interacting properties. Several authors provided evidence for a deficiency in fibronectin synthesized by *in vitro* aged (late passage) human skin fibroblasts to form pericellular fibrillar aggregates.[29,40,41] Late passage cells showed an increased tendency to bind plasma fibronectin and an increased rate of accumulation of newly synthesized fibronectin in the extracellular matrix.[41] Nonenzymatic glycation increases with age and concerns most if not all matrix components, especially fibronectin and collagen type IV.[25,42] Glycated forms of these macromolecules exhibit altered interactions with other matrix macromolecules and cells. Glycated fibronectin showed a nearly threefold decrease of its affinity for collagen IV as compared to native fibronectin. Cooperative interactions between fibronectin, collagen IV, and heparin were also severely reduced by nonenzymatic glycation.[42]

Recent data show that during development there is a modification in the isoforms of fibronectin synthesized by the cells through the regulation of alternative splicing.[43,44] Such splicing modifications might be at the origin of the oncofetal forms of fibronectin as shown by monoclonal antibodies.[45] The increased subunit molecular weight found by these authors for fibronectin produced by embryonic (WI 38) fibroblasts and malignant cells (hepatomas, colon carcinomas) appear to be attributable to increased glycosylation of an extradomain (recognized by the FDC-6 monoclonal antibody) situated between the "Hep 2" and "Fib-2" domains in the COOH-terminal region of fibronectin. Little is known of the effects of these alterations on the interactive properties of fibronectin.

Another domain of vital importance for cell-matrix interactions is the cell surface recognition domain of fibronectin. Three amino acids, arginine, glycine, and glutamic acid (R-G-D), and their flanking regions, determine the critical conformation of this site which enables its interaction with the cell surface receptor, the integrin molecule.[46,47]

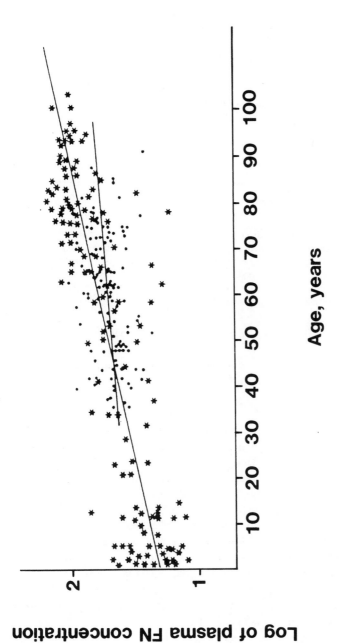

FIGURE 8. Exponential increase of plasma fibronectin with age in clinically "normal" individuals (∗) and strong attenuation of this age-dependent increase in mammary cancer patients (•).[33-37] (Reproduced with permission of author and editor.)

Similar or identical sequences were found in a number of macromolecules, some of them showing age and/or tumor growth dependent modifications.[46,47-52] As fibronectin exhibits major modifications in its relationships to cells during malignant growth,[53-55] these interactions may well be involved in these alterations.

5. The Cell Surface Receptors of Matrix Glycoproteins, the Integrins, or Cytoadhesins

This family of cell membrane receptors recognizing specific cell-binding sequences in matrix glycoproteins is now the focus of attention of a number of laboratories.[46-49] It appears that most are composed of two subunits, α and β. The α subunit is often composed of two disulfide linked (heavy and light) subunits. The β subunit also contains internal disulfide bonded regions. The α subunits appear to regulate binding specificity to the ligand macromolecules, the β subunits may be shared among several cytoadhesins. The selectivity on the ligand site may be imparted by the flanking sequences on both sides of the -R-G-D- recognition signals modifying its steric conformation.[46,47] Other recognition sequences were also proposed.[47-52] For fibronectin, Humphries et al.[56] identified a second and a third recognition sequences, in the alternatively spliced IIICS or V regions and involved in B16 melanoma cell recognition. These sites are C-terminal to the main cell-recognition RGD site. Site directed mutagenesis experiments of the cell binding domain of human fibronectin[51] also suggested the existence of two or more separate synergistic sites for cell fibronectin interactions. The cooperation of these sites appears also to be involved in the interaction of the cytoplasmic portions of integrins with the cytoskeleton and actin microfilament organization. As alternative splicing and fibronectin biosynthesis may vary with age, the adhesive properties, and as a consequence tissue structure, may also be altered. Similar cytoadhesins are also involved in blood cell differentiation and mononuclear cell interactions and function as well as in complement functions.[55-57] As immunological competence declines with age, the role of the above observations in the variations of the host resistance to tumor growth and spreading deserves further attention.

III. MODIFICATIONS OF EXTRACELLULAR MATRIX DURING TUMOR GROWTH AND METASTASIS FORMATION

A. THE STROMA REACTION

An important aspect of the role of extracellular matrix in tumor formation is the progressive modification of the extra cellular matrix during the development and spreading of the tumor. Destructive interactions are mostly emphasized, but some types of tumors lead to increased deposition of extracellular matrix. This so-called stroma reaction is observable especially in mammary tumors of the squirrhus type. This reaction consists in an increased biosynthesis and deposition of extracellular matrix, rich in collagen fibers and sometimes in elastin (in squirrhus type of elastotic breast tumors), as well as in proteoglycans and glycoproteins.[14,60-63] An extensive study was carried out in our laboratory on the behavior of elastin and fibronectin in solid human tumors.[53,54,64-68]

Previous experiments by Gahmberg and Hakomori[69] and Hynes,[70] did show that tumor cells in culture do not express immunohistochemically recognizable fibronectin on their cell membrane. This finding could be confirmed and extended in a variety of solid human tumors which were investigated in our laboratory in collaboration with Adnet and Birembaut and with Szendröi and Lapis.[53,54,65-68,71-73] In all of the investigated tumors, the stroma reaction was characterized by a strong immunofluorescence of fibronectin, surrounding the clusters of tumor cells which were devoid of immunofluorescence (Figure 9). A more detailed investigation of the development of mammary tumors showed that already in the atypical dystrophic modifications which could be suspected as early signs of tumor formation, the continuity of the glandular basement membrane staining by antifibronectin antibodies was disrupted.[53-55] An early sign of malignant transformation was the disappearence of fibronectin from the glandular cell mem-

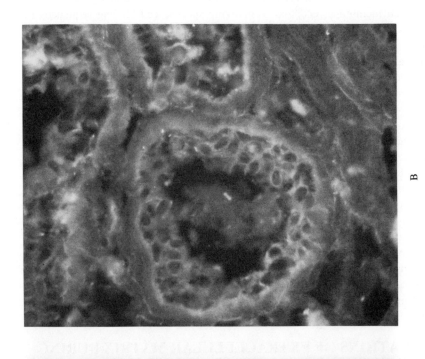

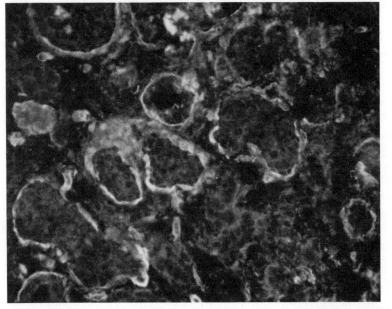

A

B

FIGURE 9. Distribution of fibronectin in tumor-stroma as compared to normal tissues as shown by indirect immunofluorescence.(A): normal mammary gland, fibronectin surrounds the glandular cells, glandular basement membranes and is present in the periglandular stroma. (Magnification 250.) (B): fibronectin immunofluorescence in a atypical hyperplasia of the mammary gland with uneven staining and discontinuities of basement membranes. (Magnification ×100.) (C and D): strong fluorescence of the peritumoral stroma in invasive adenocarcinomas of the breast. (Magnification C: ×100; D: ×150.)[53-55] (Reproduced with permission of author and editor).

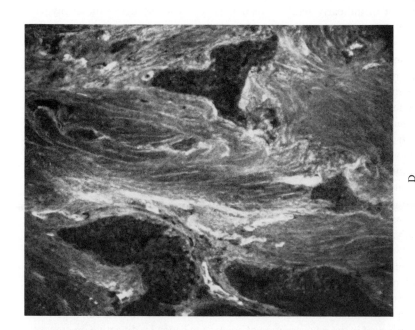

D

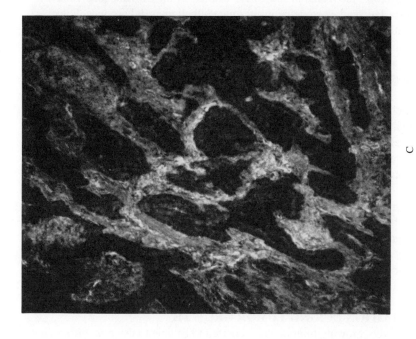

C

FIGURE 9

branes. At a later stage, the complete disorganization of the fibronectin immune histochemical pattern could be observed with completely black areas of tumor cells and a very strong immunofluorescence of the surrounding stroma (Figure 9). This effect may be related to the secretion by tumor cells of stimulating substances (growth factors?) inducing an increased matrix biosynthesis by surrounding stromal cells (see Table 2).

Another matrix glycoprotein which was shown to occur selectively in mammary tumors is tenascin.[74,75] It is present in the early fetal rat mammary gland in the dense mesenchyme surrounding the epithelial rudiment but diseappears from the mature rat mammary gland. It appears again in the stroma of rat mammary adenocarcinoma induced by *N*-methyl-*N*-nitrosourea. It was also shown to appear in virus-induced mammary tumors and malignant human mammary tumors. It could not be detected in benign tumors. This matrix glycoprotein may therefore be considered to be a relatively selective marker of the tumor-stroma reaction.

It was shown to be inducible in chicken fibroblasts by serum and βTGF, as is fibronectin,[76] and also to possess a number of consecutive epidermal growth factor-like sequences. This may be related to its growth promoting activity in serum free media. Nothing is as yet known on its age-dependent behavior. The above properties suggest however a major potential importance for this protein in tumor-tissue interactions.

As in some mammary tumors, a strong elastotic reaction can be observed. The authors also investigated the possible stimulating role of tumor cells on the development of the stroma reaction. When mammary tumor extracts were added to smooth muscle cells maintained in explant cultures (rabbit aorta media explants), a strong increase of matrix biosynthesis could be observed.[77] Using rabbit aorta media explants containing only smooth muscle cells surrounded by their matrix, we could eliminate cell proliferation and observe only the biosynthetic activity of these cells. Smooth muscle cells synthesize a variety of constituents of extracellular matrix such as collagens types I, III, IV, V, and VI, and elastin, proteoglycans, and glycoproteins.[78] When benign or malignant mammary tumor extracts were added to smooth muscle cell explants, an increase could be observed in the incorporation of some of the added radioactive precursors in the matrix macromolecules recovered in successive extracts of the explants (see Table 2).

Only the highly metastatic and elastogenic infiltrating epitheliomas did produce, however, an increased incorporation of the label in polymeric elastin. Therefore, it appears that probably several different stimulating substances are secreted by tumor cells which can induce an increased biosynthetic activity in the surrounding fibroblasts. It appears therefore that the stroma reaction can vary according to the type of the matrix stimulating substances synthesized by the cancer cells.

When elastin and elastase-type enzyme activity was determined in a series of mammary tumors, a close correlation could be observed between the expression of these two types of substances. The more elastin was synthesized by mammary tumor explant cultures, the more it contained of the elastase-type activity as determined on K-elastin agarose gels.[64-68] Both of these parameters (elastin content and elastase-type protease activity) increased with the age of the patients (Figure 10).

As far as the physiopathological importance of the stroma reaction is concerned only speculations are possible. There are arguments pointing to a possible protective role of the surrounding stroma against tumor growth. The experiments of Weksler et al.[4] mentioned in the introduction also suggest that for some tumors at least, the aging matrix may be less favorable than the young one for spreading. No firm statements can be made until more information is available on this topic.

B. MATRIX DESTRUCTION DURING TUMOR GROWTH

Most if not all invasively growing tumors were reported to be able to destroy surrounding connective tissues.[79-80] This can be attributed to the production of lytic enzymes by the tumor cells or the induction of secretion of such enzymes by surrounding nontransformed cells.[64-68]

TABLE 2
Stimulation of Extracellular Matrix Biosynthesis by Mammary Tumor Extracts

Extract of tumor added	Aorta extract (cpm/mg protein)			
	NaCl	Gua	NaOH	El
—	1,648	404	190	283
	±150	±94	±21	±60
Normal breast	910	400	200	240
Benign tumor	730	945	400	285
Cyst	3,810	780	566	109
Dystrophy	2,800	1,226	400	285
Trabecular infiltrating adenoma	5,000	422	826	110
Infiltrating adenoma	11,520	650	676	760

Note: Incorporation of ^{14}C-lysine in rabbit aorta organ cultures in presence and absence of human breast tumor extracts (for details, see Reference 62 to 66 and 108). NaCl: 1 *M* NaCl extract (soluble proteins); Gua: 4 *M* guanidine extract (proteoglycans, glyco-proteins); NaOH: 0. 1 N NaOH extract (at 100°: insoluble collagen); El: elastin (residue of the above extraction containing crosslinked elastin).

Even the most resistant tissues such as bone and cartilage can be degraded by enzymes attacking matrix macromolecules such as collagens, proteoglycans, and glycoproteins. Basement membrane degrading enzymes may play a particularly important role in this respect and especially neutral proteases capable of attacking type IV collagen, laminin, fibronectin, and proteoglycans. Such enzymes were identified in several tumors. Basement membrane thickness increases with age[31-37] due mainly to increased deposition of collagen type IV, fibronectin, and laminin, but decreased heparan-sulfate proteoglycan content. As heparin derived glycosaminoglycans were shown to inhibit PMN elastase,[81] these alterations may well result in an increased age-dependent susceptibility of basement membranes to proteolytic destruction. Fibronectin was shown to be especially susceptible to proteolytic degradation, mainly by elastase-type proteases.

Several of the enzymes were shown to increase with age, *in vivo* and *in vitro*.[20,21,29] Fibronectin, laminin, and some of their proteolytic fragments were shown to induce chemotactic migration of some tumor cells.[82] Inhibitors of such proteases (plasminogen activator, collagenases, serum proteases) could inhibit *in vitro* and *in vivo* basement membrane penetration and metastasis formation.[83] As collagens are the major macromolecular components of connective tissues, the demonstration of collagenases and other collagen destroying enzymes is of importance in regulating tumor invasion. Such enzymes were demonstrated by several authors in a variety of tumors.[79,80,84-86] Sträuli and Baici in the V_2 carcinoma of the rabbit evidenced a cysteine proteinase (cathepsin B) and a collagenase, probably involved in the invasive mechanisms of this tumor, accompanied also by matrix synthesis.[87-89]

Liotta[84] and Tarin[86] also insisted on the importance of collagenase-type enzymes in the progression and metastatic spread of tumors. Vaheri recently documented the production of plasminogen activators by malignant cells and the importance of the membrane localization of such enzymes.[90-94] This membrane localization of activating enzymes and their interaction with fibronectin underlie the proposition of Vaheri concerning membrane directed extracellular proteolysis. Many other similar data could still be cited but as their relevance to age-associated matrix modifications is still a hypothetical one, the above examples should suffice.

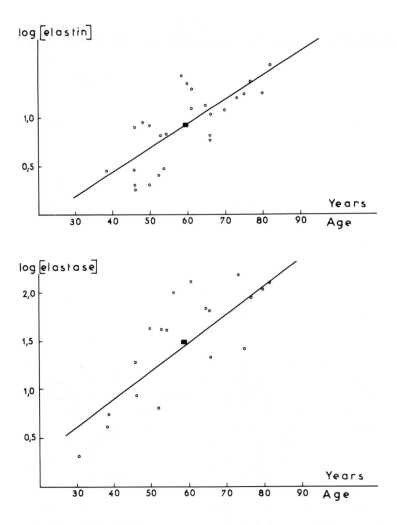

FIGURE 10.   Age-dependent increase of the elastin content (upper graph) and the elastase activity (lower graph) of human mammary carcinomas. Abscissa: age in years. Ordinates: log elastin content in mg/100 mg dry tissue (upper graph, r = 0.80, p <0.001) and log elastase activity, expressed as microgram equivalents of pancreatic elastase activity per milligram dry tissue (lower graph, r = 0.65, p <0.001). For other details, see References 9, 10, and 63 to 66. (Experiments of Hornebeck, Adnet, Robert et al.; reproduced with permission of author and editor.)

IV. AGING AND THE MECHANISMS OF METASTASIS FORMATION

Tumor cell matrix interactions play an important role not only in primary tumor growth as exemplified by the stroma reaction but also in metastasis formation.

Several different steps of this process directly concern the interaction between tumor cells and extracellular matrix macromolecules. One of them is the passage of tumor cells through extracellular matrix containing tissues, followed by the entrance in the blood circulation, then the exit of the cells from the bloodstream through the capillary basement membranes, then further transit through extracellular matrix containing tissues, and finally their fixation at the site of the metastasis formation.[79,80,95]

All of these processes require a variety of interactions between tumor cells and extracellular matrix. For instance, the association of tumor cells with basement membranes is supposed to proceed through the interaction with basement membrane constituents by the mediation of membrane receptors expressed by tumor cells such as integrins or cytoadhesins. The penetration through the basement membrane requires the expression of lytic enzymes by the tumor cells which can degrade one or several of the macromolecules composing the basement membranes. Several of these mechanisms were mentioned above; more details can be found in the cited reviews.

The exit of the tumor cells from the capillary lumen requires interaction with endothelial cells and basement membrane components, the lysis of the basement membrane, and further penetration through the connective tissues necessitating again lytic enzymes.

A crucial step in metastasis formation is the "choice" of the target organ. Although a great deal of detailed observations were published on this topic, the century-old analogy of Paget is still the best way to sum them up,[95] that is, the seed and soil hypothesis. This picture might be helpful for our considerations because the "seed" and also the "soil" do change with age. We ignore how a freshly mutated, transformed cell (the "seed") differs when it originates from "old" or "young" cells. Probably the previous mitotic and interactive history of the cell will turn out to be important. The recent studies cited in the Introduction and many other data of the literature (see other chapters of this volume) clearly show that the susceptibility of the "soil" changes with age. For some tumors it does become more difficult to penetrate, for others maybe easier. In this respect again, the cytoadhesins or integrins expressed on the capillary endothelial cells and on the tumor cells appear to be of primary importance. It is probable that the capillary endothelial cells, besides the general markers of endothelial surfaces, also express organ specific recognition signals (for a review, see Reference 95). Once the endothelial layer is passed, the receptors for basement membrane macromolecules do probably play an important role.

A special role for laminin and the laminin receptor was proposed by Martin, Liotta and their colleagues.[83,84,96,97] The team of Martin[96] showed that melanoma cells can express receptors both for laminin and fibronectin. These receptors appear to be expressed in a reciprocal fashion according to the nature of the matrix components contacting the cells. The phenotype of the malignant cell can therefore be influenced by the surrounding matrix. As with age and in diabetes, laminin and fibronectin were shown to increase in basement membranes, but heparansulfate proteoglycans decrease (see above); these changes may be important for age-dependent modifications of tumor spreading.

The relative density and distribution of surrounding matrix macromolecules will change with age. The exact effect of these changes for the age-dependent variations of metastasis formation has still to be determined. It is however interesting that Martin's team could also show that peptides derived from the laminin receptor recognition sequence (YIGSR) could decrease lung metastasis formation in mice injected with melanoma cells.[97] A similar role was attributed in host-tumor cell interactions to the RGD-sequence by Ruoslahti's team.[98] Such peptides were shown to inhibit the penetration of amniotic basement membranes by human melanoma and glioblastoma cell lines. The GRGDTP-peptide inhibition of attachment to collagen I as well as to fibronectin was more efficient than RGD-peptides acting only on fibronectin- or vitronectin-mediated attachment. Cheresh and Spiro[99] also confirmed the expression of the RGD-specific receptor on human melanoma lines (M21). They could select a variant cell line with defective α-chain synthesis and in β-chain processing and receptor assembly on the surface of the cells. These cells (M21-L) are incapable of attaching to vitronectin, von Willebrandt factor, fibrinogen, or RGD-containing heptapeptide, but do attach to fibronectin. There is also evidence that oncogene activation (src, ras) can lead in virus transformed cells to a modification of expression and assembly of α and β subunits of integrins.[100] Modified receptor expression and surface distribution may well explain modified adhesive (social) behavior of malignant cells and lead to disturbed cell matrix interactions.

Another mechanism was recently elucidated and may play an important role in metastasis formation at least in elastin rich organs such as the lung for instance. We could show that mesenchymal cells, but also highly metastatic tumor cells such as some Lewis lung carcinoma cell lines and human melanoma cell lines, express the capacity to adhere strongly to elastic fibers.[101] Using human skin fibroblasts and porcine aorta smooth muscle cells, this activity could be ascribed to a cell membrane glycoprotein complex. The main component of this adhesive complex was shown to be a 120 kDa macromolecule we designated elastonectin.[102]

This adhesion mechanism of cells to elastin fibers was studied in highly metastatic and low metastatic Lewis lung carcinoma cell lines and in human melanoma cell lines. As shown in Figure 11, the highly metastatic cells exhibit much faster adhesion kinetics to elastic fibers than the normal mesenchymal cells. The low metastatic cell lines did not show any significant adhesion to elastic fibers.[101]

In normal mesenchymal cells, adhesion was preceded by a long lag period which could be accelerated by the addition of soluble elastin peptides. Adhesion could also be inhibited by cyloheximide showing that active protein synthesis is a prior requirement for adhesion.[102] When the adhesive complex was isolated from the adhering elastic fibers besides the 120 kDa glycoprotein, three other protein components could be seen on the polyacrylamide gels with 67, 60, and 45 kDa approximate molecular weights.[102] Similar molecular weight components were found as being parts of the elastin receptor recently evidenced by our team and by Mecham's team.[103-107]

The activation of the elastin receptor was studied in our laboratory by Jacob, Fulöp and co-workers,[105,106] who could show that when this receptor is activated by elastin peptides, a G protein mediated activation of phospholipase C follows with the increase of inositol triphosphate and liberation of diacylglycerol. This leads to the opening of calcium channels and will increase intracellular calcium concentration. This elastin peptide dependent calcium influx documented in mesenchymal cells and mononuclear blood cells[105,106] could also be evidenced with the highly metastatic Lewis lung carcinoma cell line, but not with the low metastatic cell line.[101] It appears that the rapid adhesion to elastic fibers can be due to the constitutive expression of elastonectin on these cell lines which is only inducible in the normal nontransformed mesenchymal cells.

Figure 12 shows the hypothetical mechanism responsible for this rapid adhesion of tumor cells and for the inducible adhesion in mesenchymal cells. In normal mesenchymal cells, interaction of the elastin receptor with elastin peptides triggers among other phenomena the biosynthesis and membrane localization of elastonectin. In tumor cells, elastonectin appears to be expressed constitutively, but its activation is also dependent on the presence of the elastin receptor. However, the coupling of the elastin receptor to the adhesive complex appears to be different from nontransformed cells. Recent experiments also showed that elastonectin expression varies with *in vitro* aging (passage number) of human skin fibroblast;[107] a maximum is reached at about the 10 to 15th passage followed by a decline. Adhesion of normal (and possibly malignant) cells to elastic fibers might therefore be age dependently regulated.

Similar results concerning malignant cell adhesion to elastic fibers were reported recently by Zetter and co-workers[108] studying different highly metastatic tumor cell lines. These authors also arrive at the conclusion that these tumor cells exhibit a high affinity for elastic fibers. We could ascribe this high affinity to the expression of elastonectin and the elastin receptor. It appears therefore that the expression of this elastin adhesive complex and the receptor may well play an important role in tumor formation and metastatic spread in elastic tissue-rich organs such as lung, vessel wall, cartilage, and maybe others. As elastic fibers are degraded and possibly qualitatively modified during aging, probably more than other matrix components, these adhesion phenomena may well be part of the age-dependent alteration of tumor spreading and metastasis formation.

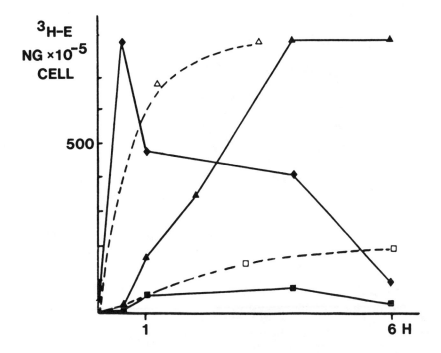

FIGURE 11.   Kinetics of adhesion of human skin fibroblasts and of highly metastatic (HML) and low metastatic (LM) Lewis lung carcinoma cells to elastin fibers. (▲ -▲) Human skin fibroblasts. Notice the long lag period. (Δ-Δ) Human skin fibroblasts in presence of K-elastin (inductive acceleration of adhesion). (❑-❑) Human skin fibroblasts in presence of cycloheximide (inhibition of adhesion). (-) Highly metastatic Lewis lung carcinoma cells. (■-■) Low metastatic Lewis lung carcinoma cells. (Reproduced with permission of author and editor.)

V. AGE-DEPENDENT MODIFICATIONS OF EXTRACELLULAR MATRIX POSSIBLY INFLUENCING TUMOR GROWTH AND SPREADING

Although a great deal remains to be done experimentally on this important aspect of the age dependence of tumor formation and metastatic spreading, some preliminary conclusions can be reached on the basis of what was said before. It appears that cell aging and the age-dependent modifications of extracellular matrix may influence tumor formation and metastatic spreading by several mechanisms.

Let us reiterate Paget's soil and seed allegory. The recent demonstration of genomic rearrangements and loss of DNA during repeated cell division cycles[3,109] could accredit the contention attributing different characteristics to malignant cells according to their previous life history. This important point certainly deserves further attention. So much for the "seed".

As far as the "soil" is concerned, it certainly does change with age. The importance and quality of change will depend on the type of tissue under consideration. The continuous modifications with age of host tissues is a fact: both cells, their membranes, and other organelles, as well as the extracellular matrix, change with age. How these changes may affect tumor growth and metastatic spreading is still largely conjectural. The recently established facts concern the existence of families of cell membrane recognition signals and receptors (integrins, cytoadhesins) mediating cell-cell and cell matrix interactions. Some of these were briefly described as well

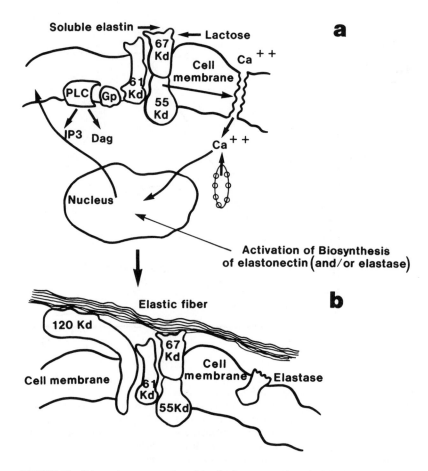

FIGURE 12.   Schematic representation of the elastin receptor (A) and of the induction of the adhesion mechanism (B) of cells to elastin fibers (elastonectin). The reaction of the receptor (three subunits shown) with soluble elastin peptides triggers via a G-protein-phospholipase C-inositolphosphate (IP$_3$) mobilization, the opening of calcium channels, and the synthesis and membrane localization of elastonectin. This mechanism of induced adhesion becomes constitutive in highly metastatic cells (rapid adhesion with no lag period; see Figure 11), although the elastin receptor is present and when occupied can increase the intensity of adhesion. None of these mechanisms (adhesion and receptor function) are present in low metastatic cells. [99,108,109] (Reproduced with permission of author and editor.)

as their modification in transformed cells and their potential role in tumor growth and metastasis formation.

Among the well-characterized age-dependent changes of matrix macromolecules we insisted on the increase of plasma and tissue fibronectin with age and its increase in capillary basement membranes and loose connective tissues, especially in diabetes and Werner's syndrome.[112] The increased proteolytic degradation of fibronectin by elastase type proteases, which are also up-regulated with age, may produce biologically active fragments with some potential in malignant transformation and growth.[39,82] As laminin was also shown to increase in diabetic basement membranes, it is conceivable (although not yet demonstrated) that it also increases with age without the appearance of overt diabetes. These changes might be considered as possibly favoring tumor growth and metastatic spreading. The decrease of heparan-sulfate proteoglycans in aging basement membranes is also a negative factor in this respect.[110]

The fragmentation of elastic fibers producing an increase of circulating elastin peptides may well be another factor, which according to the above-mentioned observations on the elastin receptor[111] may also favor tumor cell migration and increased adhesion to elastic fibers in matrix-rich tissues such as the lung. On the other hand, age-dependent modifications of matrix constituents may also decrease their interactions with tumor cells; increased crosslinking of collagen fibers, their glycation, and the increased lipid and calcium contents of elastic fibers may represent such factors. All these suggestions are, however, mostly speculative. Altered immune function and modifications of postmitotic cells may and probably do play equally important roles in this respect. In order to do more than speculate, we have to accumulate a great deal more experimental results.

REFERENCES

1. Special Programme for Research and Aging, Description of Programme, World Health Organization, July 1987.
2. **Ponten, J.,** Abnormal cell growth, in *Handbook of the Biology of Aging,* Finch C.E. and Hayflick, L., Eds., van Nostrand-Reinhold, New York, 1977, 536.
3. **Macieira-Coelho, A.,** Review article, cancer and aging, *Exp. Gerontol.,* 21, 483, 1986.
4. **Weksler, M. E., Tadaaki Tsuda, Young Tai Kim, and Siskind, G. W.,** Immunobiology of aging and cancer, submitted for publication.
5. **Van den Hooff, A.,** Connective tissue as an active participant in the process of malignant growth, *Anticancer Res.,* 6, 775, 1986.
6. **Tarin, D. and Price, J. E.,** Influence of microenvironment and vascular anatomy on "metastatic" colonization potential of mammary tumors, *Cancer Res.,* 41, 3604, 1981.
7. **Mayne, R. and Burgeson, R. E.,** *Structure and Function of Collagen Types,* Academic Press, New York, 1987.
8. **Fleischmajer, R., Olsen, R. B., and Kühn, K., Eds.,** Structure, Molecular Biology and Pathology of Collagen, *Ann. N.Y. Acad. Sci.,* 1990.
9. **Robert, A. M. and Robert, L.,** Biology and pathology of elastic tissues, in *Frontiers of Matrix Biology,* Vol. 8, Robert, L., Ed., S. Karger, Basel, 1980.
10. **Robert, L. and Hornebeck, W. Eds.,** *Elastin and Elastases,* Vol. I-II, CRC Press, Boca Raton, FL, 1989.
11. **Jacob, M. P. and Hornebeck, W.,** Isolation and characterization of insoluble and kappa-elastins, in *Frontiers of Matrix Biology,* Vol. 10, Robert, L., Ed., S. Karger, Basel, 1985, 92.
12. **Bieth, J.,** Elastases: structure, function and pathological role, in *Frontiers of Matrix Biology,* Vol. 6, Robert, L., Ed, S. Karger, Basel, 1978, 1.
13. **Robert, L. and Moczar, M.,** Age-related changes of proteoglycans and glycosaminoglycans, in *Glycosaminoglycans and Proteoglycans in Physiological and Pathological Processes of Body Systems,* Varma, R.S. and Varma, R., Eds, S. Karger, Basel, 1982, 440.
14. **Iozzo, R. V.,** Biology of disease. Proteoglycans: structure, function and role in neoplasia, *Lab. Invest.,* 53, 373, 1985.
15. **Ruoslahti, E.,** Structure and biology of proteoglycans, *Ann. Rev. Cell Biol.,* 4, 229, 1988.
16. **Robert, L.,** in *Frontiers of Matrix Biology,* Vol. 11, Robert, L., Ed., S. Karger, Basel, 1986, 1.
17. **Robert, L., Junqua, S., and Moczar, M.,** Structural glycoproteins of the intercellular matrix, in *Frontiers of Matrix Biology,* Vol. 3, Robert L., Ed., S. Karger, Basel, 1976, 113.
18. **Robert, L. and Moczar, M.,** Structural glycoproteins, in *Methods in Enzymology,* Vol. 82, Part A, Colowick, S.P. and Kaplan, N.O., Eds., Academic Press, New York, 1981, 839.
19. **Robert, B. and Robert, L.,** Aging of connective tissue-skin, in *Frontiers of Matrix Biology,* Vol. 1, S. Karger, Basel, 1973, 1.
20. **Labat-Robert, J. and Robert, L.,** Aging of the extracellular matrix and its pathology, *Exp. Gerontol.,* 23, 5, 1988.
21. **Robert, L. and Labat-Robert, J.,** Aging of extracellular matrix, its role in the development of age-associated diseases, in *Sandoz Lectures: Crossroads in Aging,* 1988, 105.
22. **Verzar, F.,** The aging of collagen, *Sci. Am.,* 208, 104, 1963.
23. **Bailey, A. J. and Robins, S. P.,** Development and maturation of the crosslinks in the collagen fibres of skin, in *Frontiers of Matrix Biology,* Vol. 1, Robert, L., Ed., S. Karger, Basel, 1973, 130.
24. **Fujimoto, D., Moriguchi, T., Sakamoto, K., Mizuno, A., and Motegi, K.,** Pyridinoline, a new crosslink of collagen and its change in aging, in *Degenerative Diseases of Connective Tissue and Aging,* Robert, L., Murata, K., and Nagai, Y., Eds., Kodansha, Tokyo, 1985, 35.
25. **Cerami, A.,** Aging of proteins and nucleic acids: what is the role of glucose? *TIBS,* 11, 311, 1986.

26. **Kern, P., Sebert, B., and Robert, L.,** Increased type III/type I collagen ratios in diabetic human conjunctival biopsies, *Clin. Physiol. Biochem.,* 4, 113, 1986.

27. **Bouissou, H., Pieraggi, M.T., and Julian, M.,** Aging of elastic tissue in skin and arteries, in *Degenerative Diseases of Connective Tissue and Aging,* Robert, L., Murata, K., and Nagai, Y., Eds., Kodansha, Tokyo, 1985, 203.

28. **Robert, L., Jacob, M. P., Frances, C., Godeau, G., and Hornebeck, W.,** Interaction between elastin and elastases and its role in the aging of the arterial wall, skin and other connective tissues. A review, *Mech. Ageing Dev.,* 28, 155, 1984.

29. **Robert, L., Labat-Robert, J., and Hornebeck, W.,** Aging and atherosclerosis, in *Atherosclerosis Reviews,* Vol.14, Gotto, A.M. and Paoletti, R., Eds., Raven Press, New York, 1986, 143.

30. **Urry, D. W.,** Sequential polypeptides of elastin: structural properties and molecular pathologies, in *Frontiers of Matrix Biology,* Vol. 8, Robert, L., Ed., S. Karger, Basel, 1980, 78.

31. **Rohrbach, D. H., Wagner, C. W., Star, V. L., Martin, G. R., Brown, K. S., and Ji-Won Yoon,** Reduced synthesis of basement membrane heparan sulfate proteoglycan in streptozotocin-induced diabetic mice, *J. Biol. Chem.,* 258, 11672, 1983.

32. **Schaeverbeke, J., Cornet, S., Corman, B., Bakala, H., and Cheignon, M.,** Glomerular basement membrane alterations in ageing rats, in *Progress in Basement Membrane Research,* Gubler, M.C. and Sternberg, M., Eds., John Libbey, London, 1988, 69.

33. **Labat-Robert, J., Potazman, J. P., Derouette, J. C., and Robert, L.,** Age-dependent increase of human plasma fibronectin, *Cell Biol. Int. Rep.,* 5, 969, 1981.

34. **Labat-Robert, J. and Robert, L.,** Modifications of fibronectin in age-related diseases: diabetes and cancer, *Arch. Gerontol. Geriatr.,* 3, 1, 1984.

35. **Potazman, J. P., Le Doussal, V., Pouillard, J., Jallais, L., and Labat-Robert, J.,** Plama fibronectin in mammary and uterine carcinomas, *Clin. Physiol. Biochem.,* 6, 12, 1988.

36. **Labat-Robert, J., Leutenegger, M., Llopis, G., Ricard, Y., and Derouette, J. C.,** Plasma and tissue fibronectin in diabetes, *Clin. Physiol. Biochem.,* 2, 39, 1984.

37. **Boyer, B., Fourtanier, A., and Labat-Robert, J.,** Effect of age on skin fibronectin and collagen biosynthesis, submitted.

38. **Shevitz, J., Jenkins, C. S. P., and Hatcher, V. B.,** Fibronectin synthesis and degradation in human fibroblasts with aging, *Mech. Ageing Dev.,* 35, 221, 1986.

39. **Barlati, S., Adamoli, A., and De Petro, G.,** Presence and role of fibronectin fragments in transformed cells, in *Frontiers of Matrix Biology,* Vol. 11, Robert, L., Ed., S. Karger, Basel, 1986, 174.

40. **Chandrasekhar, S. and Mills, A. J .T.,** Fibronectin from aged fibroblasts is defective in promoting cellular adhesion, *J. Cell. Physiol.,* 103, 47, 1980.

41. **Mann, D. M., McKeown-Longo, P. J., and Mills, A. J. T.,** Binding of soluble fibronectin and its subsequent incorporation into the extracellular matrix by early and late passage human skin fibroblasts, *J. Biol. Chem.,* 263, 2756, 1988.

42. **Tarsio, J. F., Reger, L. A., and Furcht, L. T.,** Decreased interaction of fibronectin, type IV collagen and heparin due to nonenzymatic glycation. Implications for diabetes mellitus, *Biochemistry,* 26, 1014, 1987.

43. **Sekiguchi, K., Klos, A. M., Hirohashi, S., and Hakomori, S.,** Human tissue fibronectin: expression of different isotypes in the adult and fetal tissues, *Biochem. Biophys. Res. Commun.,* 141, 1012, 1986.

44. **Oyama, F., Murata, Y., Suganuma, N., Kimura, T., Titani, K., and Sekiguchi, K.,** Patterns of alternative splicing of fibronectin pre-mRNA in human adult and fetal tissues, *Biochemistry,* 28, 1428, 1989.

45. **Matsuura, H. and Hakomori, S.,** The oncofetal domain of fibronectin defined by monoclonal antibody FDC-6: its presence in fibronectins from fetal and tumor tissues and its absence in those from normal adult tissues and plasma, *Proc. Natl. Acad. Sci. U.S.A.,* 82, 6517, 1985.

46. **Ruoslahti, E.,** Fibronectin and its receptors, *Ann. Rev. Biochem.,* 57, 375, 1988.

47. **Ruoslahti, E. and Pierschbacher, M. D.,** New perspectives in cell adhesion: RGD and integrins, *Science,* 238, 491, 1987.

48. **Buck, C. A. and Horwitz, A. F.,** Cell surface receptors for extracellular matrix molecules, *Ann. Rev. Cell Biol.,* 3, 179, 1987.

49. **Juliano, R. L.,** Membrane receptors for extracellular matrix macromolecules: relationship to cell adhesion and tumor metastasis, *Biochim. Biophys. Acta,* 907, 261, 1987.

50. **Obara, M., Kang, M. S., and Yamada, K. M.,** Site-directed mutagenesis of the cell-binding domain of human fibronectin: separable, synergistic sites mediate adhesive function, *Cell,* 53, 649, 1988.

51. **Zardi, L., Carnemolla, B., Siri, A., Petersen, T. E., Paolella, G., Sebastio, G., and Baralle, F. E.,** Transformed human cells produce a new fibronectin isoform by prefererntial alternative splicing of a previously unobserved exon, *EMBO J.,* 6, 2337, 1987.

52. **Gehlsen, K. R., Dillner, L., Engvall, E., and Ruoslahti, E.,** The human laminin receptor is a member of the integrin family of cell adhesion receptors, *Science,* 241, 1228, 1988.

53. **Labat-Robert, J., Birembaut, P., Adnet, J. J., Mercantini, F., and Robert, L.,** Loss of fibronectin in human breast cancer, *Cell Biol. Int. Rep.,* 4, 609, 1980.

54. **Labat-Robert, J., Birembaut, P., Robert, L., and Adnet, J. J.,** Modification of fibronectin distribution pattern in solid human tumors, *Diag. Histopath.,* 4, 299, 1981.

55. **Ruoslahti, E.,** Fibronectin in cell adhesion and invasion, *Cancer Metastasis Rev.,* 3, 43, 1984.

56. **Humphries, M. J., Olden, K., and Yamada, K. W.,** A synthetic peptide from fibronectin inhibits experimental metastasis of murine melanoma cells, *Science,* 233, 467, 1986.

57. **Ginsberg, M. H., Loftus, J. C., and Plow, E. F.,** Cytoadhesins, integrins and platelets, *Thromb. Haem.,* 59, 1, 1988.

58. **Entwistle, R. A. and Furcht, L. T.,** C1q component of complement binds to fibrinogen and fibrin, *Biochemistry,* 27, 507, 1988.

59. **Leivo, I. and Engvall, E.,** C3d fragment of complement interacts with laminin and binds to basement membranes of glomerulus and trophoblast, *J. Cell Biol.,* 103, 1091, 1986.

60. **Iozzo, R. V. and Müller-Glauser, W.,** Neoplastic modulation of extracellular matrix: proteoglycan changes in the rabbit mesentery induced by V2 carcinoma cells, *Cancer Res.,* 45, 5677, 1985.

61. **Iozzo, R.,** Neoplastic modulation of extracellular matrix, *J. Biol. Chem.,* 260, 7464, 1985.

62. **Martinez-Hernandez, A., Francis, D. J., and Silverberg, S. G.,** Elastosis and other stromal reactions in benign and malignant breast tissue, *Cancer,* 40, 700, 1977.

63. **Tremblay, G.,** Elastosis in tubular carcinoma of the breast, *Arch. Pathol.,* 98, 302, 1974.

64. **Hornebeck, W. and Robert, L.,** Elastase-like enzymes in aortas and human breast carcinomas: quantitative variations with age and pathology, in *Elastin and Elastic Tissue,* Sandberg, L.B., Gray, W.R., and Franzblau, C., Eds., Plenum Press, New York, 1977, 145.

65. **Hornebeck, W., Derouette, J. C., Bréchemier, D., Adnet, J. J., and Robert, L.,** Elastogenesis and elastinolytic activity in human breast cancer, *Biomedicine,* 26, 48, 1977.

66. **Hornebeck, W., Adnet, J.J ., and Robert, L.,** Age-dependent variation of elastin and elastase in aorta and human breast cancers, *Exp. Gerontol.,* 13, 293, 1978.

67. **Hornebeck, W., Bréchemier, D., Bellon, G., Adnet, J. J., and Robert, L.,** Biological significance of elastase-like enzymes in atherosclerosis and human breast cancer, in *Proteinases and Tumor Invasion,* Vol. 6, Straüli, P., Barrett, A.J., and Baici, A., Eds., Raven Press, New York, 1980, 117.

68. **Adnet, J. J., Birembaut, P., Sadrin, R., Gaillard, D., Pastisson, C., Robert, L., Dousset, H., and Bogomoletz, W. V.,** Elastolysis in human breast cancer. I. Morphological studies, in *New Frontiers in Mammary Pathology,* Hollman, de Brux, and Verley, Eds., Plenum Press, New York, 1981, 145.

69. **Gahmberg, C. G. and Hakomori, S.,** Altered growth behaviour of malignant cells associated with changes in externally labeled glycoprotein and glycolipid, *Proc. Natl. Acad. Sci. U.S.A.,* 70, 3329, 1973.

70. **Hynes, R. O.,** Alteration of cell-surface proteins by viral transformation and by proteolysis, *Proc. Natl. Acad. Sci. U.S.A.,* 70, 3170, 1973.

71. **Labat-Robert, J., Potazman, J. P., and Robert, L.,** Modification of the age-dependent increase of plasma fibronectin in cancer patients, *Biochem. Soc. Trans.,* 12, 660, 1984.

72. **Szendroï, M., Lapis, K., Zalatnai, A., Robert, L., and Labat-Robert, J.,** Appearance of fibronectin in putative preneoplastic lesions and in hepato-cellular carcinoma during chemical hepatocarcino-genesis in rats and in human hepatomas, *J. Exp. Pathol.,* 1, 189, 1984.

73. **Labat-Robert, J., Birembaut, P., Potazman, J. P., Adnet, J. J., and Robert, L.,** Modification of plasma and tissue fibronectin in cancer, in *Extracellular Matrix: Structure and Function,* Vol. 25, Reddi, Ed., Alan R. Liss, 1985, 413.

74. **Chiquet-Ehrismann, R., Mackie, E. J., Pearson, C. A., and Sakatura, T.,** Tenascin: an extracellular matrix protein involved in tissue interactions during fetal development and oncogenesis, *Cell,* 47, 131, 1986.

75. **Mackie, E. J., Chiquet-Ehrismann, R., Pearson, C. A., Inaguma, Y., Taya, K., Kawarada, Y., and Sakakura, T.,** Tenascin is a stromal marker for epithelial malignancy in the mammary gland, *Proc. Natl. Acad. Sci. U.S.A.,* 84, 4621, 1987.

76. **Pearson, C. A., Pearson, D., Shibahara, S., Hofsteenge, J., and Chiquet-Ehrisman, R.,** Tenascin: cDNA cloning and induction by TGF-β, *EMBO J.,* 7, 2677, 1988.

77. **Robert, L., Labat-Robert, J., and Davidson, G.,** Interaction between tumor cells and the extracellular matrix. Mechanisms involved in the stromal reaction, in *14th International Cancer Congress,* Abstracts of Lectures, 1, 300, 1986.

78. **Robert, L.,** Cellular and molecular biology of the vessel wall, in *Atherosclerosis, Biology and Clinical Science,* Olsson, A.G., Ed., Churchill Livingstone, New York, 1987, 98.

79. **Tryggvason, K., Höyhtyä M., and Salo, T.,** Proteolytic degradation of extracellular matrix in tumor invasion, *Biochim. Biophys. Acta,* 907, 191, 1987.

80. **Nakajima, M., Welch, D. R., Irimura, T., and Nicolson, G. L.,** Basement membrane degradative enzymes as possible markers of tumor metastasis, in *Cancer Metastasis: Experimental and Clinical Strategies,* Alan R. Liss, New York, 1986, 113.

81. **Redini, F., Tixier, J. M., Petitou, M., Choay, J., Robert, L., and Hornebeck, W.,** Inhibition of leucocyte elastase by heparin and its derivatives, *Biochem. J.,* 252, 515, 1988.

82. **Furcht, R., McCarthy, J. B., Palm, S. L., Basara, M. L., and Enenstein, J.,** Peptide fragments of laminin and fibronectin promote migration (haptotaxis and chemotaxis) of metastatic cells, in *Basement Membranes and Cell Movement,* Ciba Foundation Symposium Pitman, London, 108, 1984, 130.

83. **Reich, R., Thompson, E. W., Iwamoto, Y., Martin, G. R., Deason, J. R., Fuller, G. C., and Miskin, R.,** Effects of inhibitors of plasminogen activator, serine proteinases and collagenase IV on the invasion of basement membranes by metastatic cells, *Cancer Res.,* 48, 3307, 1988.

84. **Liotta, L. A., Rao, N. C., Barsky, S. H., and Bryant, G.,** The laminin receptor and basement membrane dissolution: role in tumour metastasis, in *Basement Membranes and Cell Movement,* Ciba Foundation Symposium 108, Pitman, London, 1984, 146.

85. **Mikuni-Takagaki, Y. and Gross, J.,** Degradation of cartilage matrix by Yoshida sarcoma cells, in *Extracellular Matrix,* Hawkes, S. and Wang, J.L., Eds., Academic Press, New York, 1982, 379.

86. **Tarin, D., Hoyt, B. J., and Evans, D. J.,** Correlation of collagenase secretion with metastatic-colonization potential in naturally occuring murine mammary tumours, *Br. J. Cancer,* 46, 266, 1982.

87. **Graf, M., Baici, A., and Sträuli, P.,** Histochemical localization of cathepsin B at the invasion front of the rabbit V2 carcinoma, *Lab. Invest.,* 45, 587, 1981.

88. **Baici, A., Graf, M., and Gyger-Marazzi, M.,** The V2 carcinoma of the rabbit as a model for tumor invasion: 3. Proteolytic activities, in *Proceedings of the Sixth Meeting of the European Association of Cancer Research,* Kugler Publications, Amsterdam, 1982, 47.

89. **Baici, A., Gyger-Marazzi, M., and Sträuli, P.,** Extracellular cysteine proteinase and collagenase activities as a consequence of tumor-host interaction in the rabbit V2 carcinoma, *Invasion Metastasis,* 4, 13, 1984.

90. **Pöllänen, J., Saksela, O., Salonen, E. M., Andreasen, P., Nielsen, L., Dano, K., and Vaheri, A.,** Distinct localizations of urokinase-type plasminogen activator and its type 1 inhibitor under cultured human fibroblasts and sarcoma cells, *J. Cell Biol.,* 104, 1085, 1987.

91. **Pöllänen, J., Stephens, R., Salonen, E. M., and Vaheri, A.,** Proteolytic mechanisms operating at the surface of invasive cells, *Adv. Exp. Med. Biol.,* 233, 187, 1988.

92. **Pöllänen, J., Hedman, K., Nielsen, L. S., Dano, K., and Vaheri, A.,** Ultrastructural localization of plasma membrane-associated urokinase-type plasminogen activator at focal contacts, *J. Cell Biol.,* 106, 87, 1988.

93. **Stephens, R., Alitalo, R., Tapiovaara, H., and Vaheri, A.,** Production of an active urokinase by leukemia cells: a novel distinction from cell lines of solid tumors, *Leuk. Res.,* 12, 419, 1988.

94. **Vaheri, A. and Salonen, E. M.,** Fibronectin and regulation of proteolysis in cancer and tissue destruction, *Proc. Finn. Dent. Soc.,* 84, 13, 1988.

95. **Nicolson, G.L.,** Cancer metastasis: tumor cell and host organ properties important in metastasis to specific secondary sites, *Biochim. Biophys. Acta,* 948, 175, 1988.

96. **Martin, G. R., Kleinman, H. K., Terranova, V. P., Ledbetter, S., and Hassell, J. R.,** The regulation of basement membrane formation and cell-matrix interactions by defined supramolecular complexes, in *Basement Membranes and Cell Movement,* Ciba Foundation Symposium 108, Pitman, London, 1984, 197.

97. **Iwamoto, Y., Robey, F. A., Graf, J., Sasaki, M., Kleinman, H. K., Yamada, Y., and Martin, G. R.,** YIGSR, a synthetic laminin pentapeptide, inhibits experimental metastasis formation, *Science,* 238, 1132, 1987.

98. **Gehlsen, K. R., Argraves, W. S., Pierschbacher, M .D., and Ruoslahti, E.,** Inhibition of *in vitro* tumor cell invasion by Arg-Gly-Asp-containing synthetic peptides, *J. Cell Biol.,* 106, 925, 1988.

99. **Cheresh, D. A. and Spiro, R. C.,** Biosynthetic and functional properties of an Arg-Gly-Asp-directed receptor involved in human melanoma cell attachment to vitronectin, fibrinogen and von Willebrand factor, *J. Biol. Chem.,* 262, 17703, 1987.

100. **Plantefaber, L. C. and Hynes, R. O.,** Changes in integrin receptors on oncogenically transformed cells, *Cell,* 56, 281, 1989.

101. **Timar, J., Lapis, K., Varga Z., Fulop, T., Tixier, J. M., Robert, L., and Hornebeck, W.,** Interactions between elastin and Lewis lung (3LL) tumor cell lines with different metastatic potential, submitted.

102. **Hornebeck, W., Tixier, J. M., and Robert, L.,** Inducible adhesion of mesenchymal cells to elastic fibers: elastonectin, *Proc. Natl. Acad. Sci. U.S.A.,* 83, 5517, 1986.

103. **Hinek, A., Wrenn, D. S., Mecham, R. P., and Barondes, S. H.,** The elastin receptor: a galactoside-binding protein, *Science,* 239, 1539, 1988.

104. **Wrenn, D. S., Hinek, A., and Mecham, R. P.,** Kinetics of receptor-mediated binding of tropoelastin to ligament fibroblasts, *J. Biol. Chem.,* 263, 2280, 1988.

105. **Fülöp, T., Jacob, M. P., Varga, Z., Foris, G., Leovey, A., and Robert, L.,** Effect of elastin peptides on human monocytes: Ca^{2+} mobilization, stimulation of respiratory burst and enzyme secretion, *Biochem. Biophys. Res. Commun.,* 141, 92, 1986.

106. **Jacob, M. P., Fülöp, T., Foris, G., and Robert, L.,** Effect of elastin peptides on ion fluxes in mononuclear cells, fibroblasts and smooth muscle cells, *Proc. Natl. Acad. Sci., U.S.A.,* 84, 995, 1987.

107. **Hornebeck, W., Ferrari, P., Groult, V., and Robert, L.,** Induction of cell adhesion to elastin fibers (elastonectin) by the activated elastin receptor, submitted.

108. **Blood, C. H., Sasse, J. H., Brodt, P., and Zetter, B. R.,** Indentification of a tumor cell receptor for VGVAPG, an elastin-derived chemotactic peptide, *J. Cell Biol.,* 107, 1987, 1988.

109. **Dell'orco, R. T., Whittle, W. L., and Macieira-Coelho, A.,** Changes in the higher order organization of DNA during aging of human fibroblast-like cells, *Mech. Ageing Dev.,* 35, 199, 1986.
110. Robert, L., *Mecanismes Cellulaires et Moléculaires du Vieillissement,* Masson, Paris, 1983.
111. **Varga, Z., Jacob, M. P., Robert, L., and Fulöp, T.,** Identification and signal transduction mechanism of elastin peptide receptor in human leukocytes, *FEBS Lett.,* 258, 5, 1989.
112. **Robert, L., Jacob, M. P., Fulöp, T., Timar, J., and Hornebeck, W.,** Elastonectin and the elastin receptor, *Pathol. Biol.,* 37, 736, 1989.
113. **Jacob, M. P., Wei, S. M., and Robert, L.,** in preparation.

Chapter 3

DEVELOPMENTAL CHANGES OF THE MAMMARY GLAND IN RELATION TO MAMMARY TUMOR DEVELOPMENT

Hiroshi Nagasawa

TABLE OF CONTENTS

I. INTRODUCTION

Development and growth of normal mammary glands are the prerequisite conditions of mammary tumor development at advanced ages. Hormonal history (altered profoundly by pregnancy, lactation, endocrine therapy, perinatal exposure to hormones, etc.) is as important as chronological age in determining mammary gland growth, a feature that has also recently been demonstrated *in vitro*.[1] There are several reviews and original articles on the growth of normal mammary glands in murine,[2-5] human[6-13] and other species.[14-18] In this chapter, mammary gland growth is discussed only in relation to mammary tumor development and a review of all literature on mammary gland growth completed to date is not attempted. Hormonal control of normal and neoplastic mammary gland growth is also discussed elsewhere[16,19-33] and is beyond the focus of this chapter.

II. METHODS FOR EVALUATING MAMMARY GLAND GROWTH

Methods used extensively for evaluating mammary gland growth are as follows with several modifications:[3,22]

1.   Morphological and morphometrical observations including wholemount preparations employed mainly for the glands developing in two dimensions
2.   Deoxyribonucleic acid (DNA) content assessment
3.   Immunohistochemical observation
4.   DNA synthesis or labeling index estimated by [³H]-thymidine incorporation into mammary DNA

These methods should be regarded as complementary, but not alternative. However, the last method (4) is the most valuable indicator for mammary gland growth when considered in relation to mammary tumor development, since mammary gland proliferative activity around the time when carcinogenic agents attack the gland is a limiting factor for this process.[34-38] There is a close relationship in rats between mammary tumorigenic potential of a carcinogen and mammary DNA synthesis.[39-42] Dietary restriction is generally protective for mammary tumorigenesis. Associated with this, the restriction significantly inhibited mammary gland mitosis in young female rats.[43] It has also been observed in rats that a temporary inhibition of a high mammary DNA synthesis during youth resulted in a marked suppression of spontaneous mammary tumor development at advanced ages.[44,45] Furthermore, the epidemiological studies on the incidence of breast cancer among atomic bomb survivors at Hiroshima and Nagasaki strongly suggest that the earlier the age exposed to radiation, the higher the risk of breast cancer.[46] In this respect, the mitotic rate of mammary gland cells is high during youth and decreases with age in humans,[37,47] and the significance of mitotic activity of the terminal end-buds of the gland (Figure 1) in this process has been stressed by the intensive studies of Russo and his colleagues.[10,37,48-50]

Finally, from the viewpoint of dynamic changes of mammary glands, Anisimov[51] discussed the age related mammary tumorigenic potential in response to carcinogens.

III. MAMMARY GLAND GROWTH AT VIRGINAL STAGE IN RELATION TO MAMMARY TUMOR DEVELOPMENT

In general, the mammary gland, especially the end-bud system, shows better development in mice with high mammary tumorigenic potential than in those with low potential. Mammary tumor virus (MTV) , which is an essential factor for mouse mammary tumor development,[52,53]

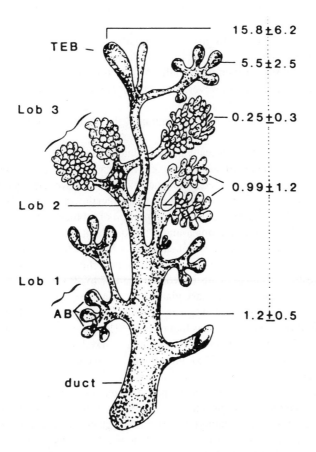

FIGURE 1. Topographic components of human mammary glands. TEB: terminal end-buds, AB: alveolar buds, Lob 1, 2 and 3: lobule types, 1, 2 and 3. DNA-LI: labeling index of DNA (mean ± SD). (From Reference 10 with permission.)

is reported to increase mammary gland susceptibility to mammotropic hormones.[54] The current status of MTV-related sequence in human cellular DNA was also discussed.[52] Mammary gland DNA synthesis in virgin rats is high between 30 to 60 d of age and declines abruptly thereafter.[39] In detail, mammary DNA synthesis in virgin rats at 55 to 60 d of age increases markedly from day 2 of diestrus toward proestrus and shows a peak activity on the afternoon of estrus followed by decrease. On the other hand, the synthesis in 80 to 85-d-old rats shows a high value only at estrus.[55] This cyclic pattern persists throughout fertile life. Thus, in young rats at 50 to 60 d of age, mammary tumorigenic response to 7,12-dimethylbenz(a)anthracene (DMBA)[40] or N-methyl-N-nitrosourea (NMU)[42,56] was higher if the carcinogen was given at proestrus-estrus than at diestrus. In this respect, Ratko et al.[57] examined the difference between estrous stages in mammary gland DNA alkylation by NMU in rats and found the delay in removal of O^6-methylguanine (a primary lesion implicated in alkylation carcinogenesis) from the mammary gland DNA 8 and 24 h after NMU injection at proestrus or estrus.

Anderson et al.[58] examined the effects of age and laterality on the cell multiplication (mitosis) and cell deletion (apoptosis) within the lobules of the "resting" human mammary glands during the menstrual cycle. While all three age groups (15 to 24, 25 to 34, and 35 to 45 years) showed significant cyclic variations for mitosis, there was no significant difference in the variations among groups. On the other hand, for apoptosis, the significant variation was observed among groups with a progressive flattening of the sinusoidal curve with advancing ages as well as laterality difference within each age.

While thymidine labeling index (TLI) in normal human mammary gland was high during the second half of the menstrual cycle, it declined with age.[59] No significant variations in immunohistochemical staining of immunoglobulin A, secretory component, and α-lactoalbumin were seen among cyclic phases, however, the positive staining tended to be associated with high TLI values.[59]

Detailed histologic changes in the human mammary glands during menstrual cycle were reported by Vogel et al.[60]

Hutson et al.[61] examined morphometrically the age related changes (10 to 80 years) of normal mammary glands in human. The relative amount of epithelial and connective tissue varied with age, and the epithelial elements (combined lobular and extralobular) were unevenly distributed within the gland, with the lower quadrants containing more than the upper ones. The upper outer quadrant, however, usually contained the largest proportion of lobular units, which may relate to the higher incidence of lobular carcinoma found in this quadrant. Involution was shown to be a premenopausal rather than postmenopausal phenomenon. Mammary dysplastic changes were uncommon in all age groups. Ferguson[62] also studied ultrastructurally the mitosis and cytokinesis of the normal resting mammary cells of women aged 17 to 40 years.

In contrast to rats and humans, mammary gland DNA synthesis in virgin mice with high mammary tumor potential is little affected by age. In addition, the rate of synthesis at estrus of mice is always two to three times as high as that of rats.[35] Thus, the temporary suppression of mammary DNA synthesis during youth resulted in a marked inhibition of spontaneous mammary tumor development in rats,[44,45] but no influence on the stimulation was observed in mice by the same treatment.[63]

A distinct difference in mammary gland response to mammotropic hormones was also observed between mice and rats. Underneath grafting with anterior pituitaries, from which only prolactin is secreted predominantly, stimulated mammary gland growth morphologically in both mice and rats. However, DNA synthesis of the gland was high only in mice,[64,65] but low in rats,[39] resulting in an enhanced[65] and inhibited[66] mammary tumorigenesis, respectively. These phenomena in mice were seen only in high mammary tumor strains; in low mammary tumor strains the situation was quite the same as observed in rats.[64]

Immunopotentiation by cell wall skeleton of *Nocardia rubra* inhibited spontaneous mammary tumors of mice[67] and carcinogen-induced mammary tumors of rats[68] associated with a decreased DNA synthesis of normal mammary glands.[67] The results suggest that prevention of mammary tumor development by immunopotentiators may partly be due to their inhibition of mammary cell mitosis.

IV. MAMMARY GLAND GROWTH DURING PREGNANCY IN RELATION TO MAMMARY TUMOR DEVELOPMENT

Morphologically, mammary parenchymal growth in rats becomes pronounced with the advance of pregnancy. Meanwhile, mammary DNA synthesis during pregnancy peaks around day 6 and abruptly decreased thereafter (Figure 2). The latter half of pregnancy is the period of proliferative rest, differentiation, hypertrophy, and secretion of cells.[55] The average value for DNA synthesis on days 18 and 22 of pregnancy are less than one third and one fifth of the value at estrus, respectively. Thus, as a whole, the rate of mammary DNA synthesis during the same period is much lower in pregnant rats than in virgins with the similar age (Figure 2). Similarity exists between mammary gland growth pattern during pregnancy in rats and humans.[55,69] Both animals and humans are constantly exposed to carcinogenic agents during their lifetime. It appears that the longer the total period of low mammary DNA synthesis, i.e., proliferative-

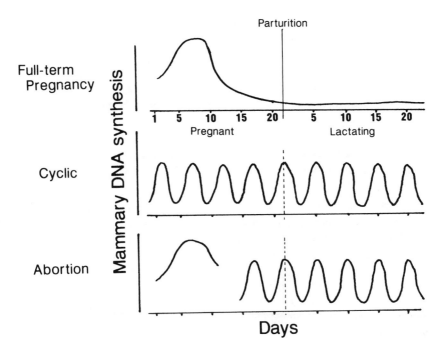

FIGURE 2. Scheme of mammary gland mitosis (DNA synthesis) in pregnant-lactating, virgin, and aborted rats.

mitotic rest, the smaller is the risk of mammary malignancy. Accordingly, the protective role of pregnancy in mammary tumors observed in rats[70,71] and humans[72,73] can be explained by mammary mitotic rest during pregnancy.

Grubbs et al.[74] reported the prevention of NMU-induced mammary tumorigenesis in rats by hormonal prestimulation of the glands to late pregnant state. Associated with this, mammary glands prestimulated were characterized by the absence of terminal end-buds and terminal ducts (Figure 1), which were the most sensitive to carcinogens.[37,48-50] From these results, the authors concluded that the stimulation of the mammary glands to a high differentiated state early in life can provide protection against carcinogen exposure.

Meanwhile, if malignant mammary foci exist before pregnancy, their growth is accelerated during subsequent pregnancy, resulting in an earlier appearance of tumors.[75] This agrees well with the results that in rats the administration of carcinogens followed by pregnancy stimulated mammary tumorigenesis.[70,71] An analogous condition is observed in women with late pregnancy after 35 years of age in whom the risk of mammary tumors and tumor growth are greater than in nulliparous women of the same age groups.[72,73]

According to Russo and Russo,[10] terminal end-buds (TEB) and lobules type 1 (Lob 1) (Figure 1) have the higher mitotic ability and, therefore, show a higher responsiveness to carcinogenic agents than the more differentiated lobules; the ratio of TEB and Lob 1 are greatly decreased by parity. Mammary tissue consisting mostly of Lob 1 was very sensitive to carcinogen exposure *in vitro*, which was independent of age, but was strongly influenced by both the reproduction and clinical history of the donor.[76] These results are in good accord with the results of Moon[71] that the parous rats showed a lower incidence of carcinogen-induced mammary tumors than the virgins irrespective of parous ages. On the contrary, mammary DNA synthesis of high mammary tumor strains of mice is very high even at the end of pregnancy,[77] whereas morphological changes of mammary glands during pregnancy are quite similar to those of rats. This accounts well for the higher and earlier mammary tumor development in breeders than in virgin mice.

Neither mitotic nor apoptosis fluctuation was significantly different between multiparous and nulliparous women even after age adjustment.[58]

It is generally considered that abortion, both induced and spontaneous, increases the risk of breast cancer. This would be well accounted for by mammary gland DNA synthesis; an abortion followed by the menstrual cycle would result in a longer period of a high mammary mitosis compared to normal pregnancy (Figure 2). However, in the study of 3200 cases of breast cancer and 4844 control under 70 years, the risk of breast cancer was not related to the number and the time of induced or spontaneous abortions.[78] Similar results were also obtained for women under 40 years, among whom the frequency of induced abortions was relatively high.[78]

V. MAMMARY GLAND GROWTH DURING LACTATION IN RELATION TO MAMMARY TUMOR DEVELOPMENT

During lactation, mammary DNA synthesis is maintained very low in both rats[55] and mice.[77] Multiparous mice without lactation have a higher and an earlier incidence of mammary tumors than those with lactation.[30] Thus, lactation is generally considered to be protective to mammary tumor development in experimental animal models,[70] while the protective role of lactation in human breast cancer is still far from conclusive.

It is well established that lactational performance closely parallels the amount of mammary parenchyma[79-82] and the importance of mammary cell number in lactation has also been discussed.[83] Meanwhile, experimental results suggesting that a high lactational performance may increase mammary tumor risk have been accumulated. There is a significantly positive correlation in SLN mice between spontaneous mammary tumor incidence and the weight or the growth rate of pups used as the index of lactational performance.[84] The high mammary tumor strains of mice (C3H/He or SHN) have higher lactational performance than the low mammary tumor strains (C57BL/6 or SLN).[85-87] Moreover, a positive relationship was seen between mammary gland DNA synthesis and lactational performance.[88,89] Since mammary DNA synthesis is a limiting factor for mammary tumor development in providing mammary gland conditions favorable for the action of carcinogenic agents,[34,40] the hypothesis presented in Figure 3 is proposed as the cause of the positive relationship between lactational performance and the risk of mammary tumors; both have relations through mammary growth potential and lactational performance itself has no direct role in the risk of mammary tumors. Supporting this hypothesis, Lund et al.[90] reported the breast cancer incidence subsequent to surgical reduction of the breast. Among 1205 women who were treated surgically for breast hypertrophy, a total of 18 breast cancers developed compared to 30.3 expected, yielding a relative risk (RR) of 0.59. The greater risk reduction was observed in women who had 600 g or more of breast tissue removed (RR = 0.27).

As a possible step in evaluating the role of tumor promoters in normal cells, the effects of phorbol and its esters, 12-*O*-tetradecanoyl-phorbol-13-acetate (TPA), on normal mammary cell function was studied.[91] Subcutaneous injection of these promoters between days 12 to 14 of lactation resulted in a significant decline in litter growth and the rate of RNA synthesis/DNA synthesis in the mammary glands. On the contrary, mammary gland DNA synthesis increased by the treatments associated with no alteration in the endocrine system. These findings strongly suggest that tumor promoters can directly shift mammary gland cells from a functional state to a mitotic state, causing an inhibition of lactation and an increase in mammary gland response to carcinogenic agents.

VI. EFFECTS OF PERINATAL MODULATION OF MAMMARY GLAND GROWTH ON MAMMARY TUMOR DEVELOPMENT

An increased risk of cancer in the cervix and vagina in female offspring whose mothers were given diethylstilbestrol (DES) during pregnancy is well known in both laboratory animal[92,93] and

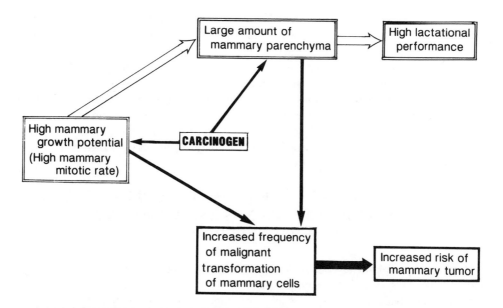

FIGURE 3. Relationship between mammary gland growth potential, lactational performance, and mammary tumor risk. (From Reference 88 with permission.)

human models.[94,95] Such clinical information is not available on the mammary glands, however, the long-term effects of perinatal exposure to hormones and related substances on mammary glands have been extensively studied in laboratory animals,[96,97] since both mammary glands and female reproductive tracts are under the control of similar hormones. While daily injections of sex hormones and their analogs during perinatal life of mice generally induce a stimulation of normal, preneoplastic, and neoplastic mammary gland growth, the sequence varies according to the perinatal stages of exposure to hormones as well as to the animal species.[96,97] Tomooka and Bern[98] found that in female BALB/c mice daily injections of estradiol or DES for the first 5 d of perinatal life inhibited mammary gland growth on day 6, whereas the treatment stimulated the growth after 4 weeks. Testosterone and 5α-dihydrotestosterone (5α-DHT) also enhanced mammary gland growth 4 weeks after treatment, however, they showed no effects at 6 d of age.[98] Similar estradiol treatment between 1 to 5 d of age induced the most mammary abnormalities at 12 months of age, such as dilated ducts, hyperplastic alveolar nodule (HAN)-like lesions, or aberrant secretory state. The incidence of abnormalities declined markedly when treatment was began after day 5.[99] Mammary tumor incidence increased with age in mice receiving single injections of progesterone or the vehicle; at prenatal day 12, however, the treatment with DES significantly retarded mammary tumor development. This difference was not altered by an additional treatment with estradiol benzoate (EB) during 3 months between 2 to 5 months of age. A single injection of progesterone at prenatal day 17 with or without EB after maturity also inhibited mammary tumorigenesis at advanced ages. Mammary tumor development was enhanced by progesterone or DES on the day of birth, however, it was arrested by EB after maturity. All observations indicate that long-term effects of perinatal exposure to hormones on mammary tumor development at advanced ages are largely dependent upon perinatal age of the subjects and that sex hormones given after maturity can modulate the perinatal hormone effects.[100]

Mammary gland growth in rats at 60 d of age was scarcely affected by daily injections of estradiol or prolactin during 20 or 40 d of postnatal life, however, the glands of these animals regressed completely at 180 d of age associated with no appearance of carcinogen-induced mammary tumors.[101]

It has been reported that some agents which have little adverse effects in adults show profound long-term effects on mammary gland growth when treated perinatally. Daily injections during 5 d of postnatal life of Vitamin A, known as well as its synthetic analogs to be effective inhibitors of several types of tumors including mammary tumors,[102-104] enhanced pregnancy-dependent, and autonomous mammary tumors in GR/A mice.[105] Mammary gland growth of mice given single injections of monosodium glutamate(MSG) at birth was markedly retarded after 90 d of age.[106,107] Furthermore, perinatal and neonatal treatments with 5β-DHT, which is biologically inactive and does not bind to receptors in adults, induced a marked stimulation of normal as well as preneoplastic and neoplastic mammary gland growth[108] and the effects were stronger than biologically active 5α-DHT.[109]

VII. RELATIONSHIP BETWEEN THE PRENEOPLASTIC STATE OF MAMMARY GLANDS AND MAMMARY TUMOR DEVELOPMENT

Mammary hyperplastic alveolar nodule (HAN), which is the outgrowth of normal end-bud or lobulo-alveolar system of the mammary glands,[100,111] has a higher susceptibility to hormones than normal end-buds[3] and is a representative preneoplastic state of mammary tumors of mice. Modulation of HAN by some treatments, however, does not always reflect mammary tumorigenesis. Whereas a single injection of MSG on the day of birth induced a marked inhibition of HAN formation between 4 to 11 months of age, mammary tumorigenesis in the MSG-treated mice was not much different from that in the control.[107] Despite the pellet implantation of medroxyprogesterone acetate, megestrol acetate, or melengestrol acetate significantly inhibited the HAN formation,[112-114] mammary tumorigenesis was apparently enhanced by any treatment.[113,114] Some possibilities are plausible as the causes of this phenomenon:

1. The suppression of HAN formation by these agents was not complete and some HAN might remain unresponsive and/or might become tolerant to the agents
2. Mammary tumor incidence is a qualitative criterion and HAN formation a quantitative one and, therefore, they may not parallel each other

Even if there is a large difference in the number of HAN between mice, each animal is counted as bearing a cancer if a HAN in these mice transformed malignantly to develop to a palpable tumor.

HAN-like lesions have been found in the mammary glands of rats (both intact and carcinogen-treated), dogs, and nonhuman primates.[111] However, their potential to malignant transformation is much lower than that of mice or has not been determined. Wellings et al.[110] reported that atypical lobules, type A, which are abnormal terminal ductal lobular units consisting of ductules (acini) together with intralobular and extralobular terminal units, are somewhat similar to HAN. They increase in number with age and appear more frequently in the breast of women at high risk. No direct evidence that this lesion transforms to malignancy has been obtained.

Pregnancy-dependent mammary tumor (PDMT)[111] is another preneoplastic state of mammary tumors in GR/A and some other mouse strains of European origin. PDMT appears after the middle of pregnancy, reaches maximal size at the end of pregnancy, regressed completely immediately after parturition regardless of lactation, and appears again during the next pregnancy. According to Yanai and Nagasawa,[115] 30% of PDMT reappeared as autonomous tumors, which corresponded to 37% of all tumors developing after retirement. In other words, about 63% of tumors appeared after retirement, mostly originating from HAN. The recurrent tumors appeared significantly earlier than newly developing tumors.

It has also been observed that about 30% of PDMT transplanted into female nude mice became palpable by 20 weeks after transplantation and all were completely autonomous in growth and diagnosed as adenocarcinoma.[116] These may be attributable to the fact that PDMT consists of several types of tumor cells. PDMT was found to disturb the growth of normal mammary glands during pregnancy, which resulted in suppressed lactation.[117]

In humans, the risk of benign breast lesions to evolve toward malignancy is an important problem. Wellings et al.[110] discussed the early lesions of the human breast and reported hyperplastic fibrocystic disease (mammary dysplasia complex) as one type of the preneoplastic state of human breast cancer. The lesion has a correlation to past, present, and future development of breast cancer. During 4 to 15 years of follow-up, 11 out of 365 patients with 7 types of biopsy-proven breast diseases developed breast cancers, which corresponded to a 2.6–fold risk over the reference populations.[118] No association was observed between patients who developed cancer and those who did not with respect to the initial histologic features, the age at entry by decades, menopause, the presence of cysts or calcification in the biopsy specimen, a family history of breast cancer, or the number of observation years.[118]

Mansel[119] pointed out that the predictive power of a previous personal histology of benign breast disease is weak and is of no practical value to the clinician, while some histologic changes such as changes of fibroadenoma, duct ectasia, etc., have been shown to carry no increased risk. Thus, the simple clinical diagnosis of the disease is not very helpful in the assessment of future cancer risk. Mansel pointed out the following:

1. The subjective nature of histologic reports and the lack of agreement on precise terminology between pathologists
2. The retrospective nature of nearly all histologic risk prediction
3. The need for a high level of experience and accuracy for histologic assessment of benign biopsy specimen

Mansel stressed the significance of the use of monochlonal antibody, immunohistochemistry, and other markers.

VIII. MALE CONTRIBUTION TO FEMALE MAMMARY GLAND GROWTH IN RELATION TO MAMMARY TUMOR DEVELOPMENT

As described previously, mammary gland growth and lactation are some of the essential factors for mammary tumorigenesis at advanced ages, and numerous studies have been done on mammary gland growth in several species.[2-18] However, almost all of these studies were on females with little attention to males, despite the genetical contribution of males to mammary gland growth potential of the offspring. In this regard, Nagasawa et al. examined mammary gland growth of four strains (SHN, SLN, GR/A, and C3H/He) of male mice in comparison with females and found a marked difference in the growth pattern[120] and susceptibility to hormones[121] of the mammary glands, not only among strains but also between sexes within a strain. They also observed the heterogenesis in normal and neoplastic mammary gland growth of F1 females between SHN and GR/A, both having the highest mammary gland growth potential in the female and the male, respectively.[122] These results directly demonstrated the male contribution to normal and neoplastic mammary gland growth of the female offspring. It is impossible to estimate directly mammary gland growth potential of males even in most experimental animals. Thus, these mouse models would be valuable in studying the genetic mechanism(s) of normal and neoplastic mammary gland growth, especially the male contribution to this process.

IX. MESENCHYME AND MAMMARY GLAND GROWTH IN RELATION TO MAMMARY TUMOR DEVELOPMENT

Like many other organs, mammary glands are composed of two different tissues, epithelium and mesenchyme. Cell to cell interactions of these two tissues are essential for growth, morphogenesis, and cytodifferentiation.[5,123-126] Indeed, several studies have stressed the role of mesenchyme or stroma during mammary tumor development, although the clear conclusion has yet to be solved.[126]

The interaction between mammary epithelium and mesenchyme during mammary gland growth is mediated by the extracellular matrix,[127] including proteins produced by either or both of these tissues, such as fibronectin, laminin, and proteoheparan sulfate. Recently, a new protein named tenascin was found in mammary mesenchyme closely surrounding the budding epithelial rudiments in the embryo.[128] It is not detected in the adult mammary gland even during pregnancy, however, it reappears in mammary tumors at the site of tumor growth and in the fibroblast in contact with the neoplastic epithelium.[5,128] The importance of the paracrine-acting or stroma-released substances, which might positively or negatively influence mammary gland growth in some way, has been postulated.[129]

ACKNOWLEDGMENTS

I thank T. Naito for his help in preparation of the manuscript. My thanks are also due to the Editorial Board of *Medical Hypothesis*, Plenum Press, and Drs. J. Russo and H. Russo for their permission to cite figures.

REFERENCES

1. **Choongkittaworn, N., Hosick, H. L., and Jones, W.,** *In vitro* replication potential of serially passaged mammary parenchyma from mice with different reproductive histories, *Mech. Ageing Dev.,* 35, 147, 1987.
2. **Hoshino, K.,** Mammary transplantation and its histogenesis in mice, in *Physiology of Mammary Glands,* Yokoyama, A., Mizuno,H., and Nagasawa, H., Eds., Japan Scientific Societies Press/University Park Press, Tokyo, Baltimore, 1978, 163.
3. **Nagasawa, H. and Yanai, R.,** Normal and abnormal growth of the mammary glands, in *Physiology of Mammary Glands,* Yokoyama, A., Mizuno, H., and Nagasawa, H., Eds., Japan Scientific Societies Press/University Park Press., Tokyo, Baltimore, 1978, 121.
4. **Daniel, C. W. and Silberstein, G. B.,** Postnatal development of the rodent mammary gland, in *The Mammary Gland Development, Regulation, and Function,* Neville, M. C. and Daniel, C. W., Eds., Plenum Press, New York, 1987, 3.
5. **Sakakura, T.,** Mammary embryogenesis, in *The Mammary Gland, Development, Regulation, and Function,* Neville, M. C. and Daniel, C. W. Eds., Plenum Press, New York, 1987, 37.
6. **Raynaud, A.,** Morphogenesis of the mammary glands, in *Milk: The Mammary Glands and Its Function,* Vol. 1, Kon, S. K. and Cowie, A. T., Eds., Academic Press, New York, 1961, 3.
7. **Bässler, R.,** The morphology of hormone induced structural changes in the female breast, *Curr. Top. Pathol.,* 53, 1, 1970.
8. **Vorherr, H.,** *The Breast, Morphology, Physiology and Lactation,* Academic Press, New York, 1974, 1.
9. **Drife, J. O.,** Breast development in puberty, *Ann. N.Y. Acad. Sci.,* 464, 58, 1986.
10. **Russo, J. and Russo, H.,** Development of the human mammary gland, in *The Mammary Gland, Development, Regulation, and Function,* Neville, M. C. and Daniel, C. W., Plenum Press, New York, 1987, 67.
11. **Yang, J., Balakrishnan, A., Hamamoto, S., Elias, J. J., Rosenau, W., Beattie, C. W., Das Gupta, T. K., Wellings, S. R., and Nandi, S.,** Human breast epithelial cells in serum-free collagen gel primary culture: growth morphological, and immunohistochemical analysis, *J. Cell. Physiol.,* 133, 228, 1987.
12. **McKiernan, J., Coyne, J., and Cahalane, S.,** Histology of breast development in early life, *Arch. Dis. Child.,* 63, 136, 1988.

13. **Whitworth, N. S.,** Lactation in humans, *Psychoneuroendocrinology,* 13, 171, 1988.

14. **Smith, V. R.,** *Physiology of Lactation,* 5th ed., Iowa State University Press, Ames, 1959, 1.

15. **Anderson, R. R.,** Embryonic and fetal development of the mammary apparatus, in *Lactation, A Comprehensive Treatise,* Vol. 4, Larson, B. L., Ed., Academic Press, New York, 1978, 3.

16. **Cowie, A. T., Forsyth, I. A., and Hart, I. C.,** *Hormonal Control of Lactation,* Springer-Verlag, New York, 1980, 58.

17. **Anderson, R. R.,** Mammary gland, in *Lactation,* Larson, B. L., Ed., Iowa State University Press, Ames, 1985, 3.

18. **Tucker, A. H.,** Quantitative estimates of mammary growth during various physiological states: a review, *J. Dairy Sci.,* 70: 1958, 1987.

19. **Smith, V. R.,** *Physiology of Lactation,* 5th ed., Iowa State University Press, Ames, 1959, 50.

20. **Jacobsohn, D.,** Hormonal regulation of mammary gland growth, in *Milk: The Mammary Gland and Its Secretion,* Vol. 1, Kon, S. K. and Cowie, A. T., Eds. Academic Press, New York, 1961, 127.

21. **Meites, J.,** Control of mammary growth and lactation, in *Neuroendocrinology,* Vol. 1, Martini, L. and Ganong, W. F., Eds., Academic Press, New York, 1966, 669.

22. **Ceriani, R. L., and Hilgers, J.,** Growth of the mouse mammary gland *in vivo,* in *Mammary Tumors in the Mouse,* Hilgers, J. and Sluyser, M., Eds., Elsevier/North-Holland, Amsterdam, 1981, 302.

23. **Nagasawa, H.,** Human prolactin and normal and abnormal breast tissue, in *Hormones and Normal and Abnormal Human Tissues,* Vol. 1, Fotherby, K. and Pal, S. B., Eds., Walter de Gruyter, New York, 1981, 115.

24. **Welsch, C. W., McManus, M. J., Haviland, T. J., Dombroske, S. E., Swim, E. L., Sharpe, S., and Conley, E.,** Hormonal regulation of DNA Synthesis of normal and hyperplastic human breast tissues *in vitro* and *in vivo,* in *Endocrinology of Cystic Breast Disease,* Angeli, A., Bradlow, H. L., and Dogliotti, L., Eds., Raven Press, New York, 1983, 47.

25. **Tucker, H. A.,** Endocrine and neural control of the mammary gland, in *Lactation,* Larson, B. L., Ed., Iowa State University Press, Ames, 1985, 29.

26. **Kleinberg, D. L., and Newman, C. B.,** The pituitary gland in primate mammary development: evidence that prolactin is not essential, *Ann. N.Y. Acad. Sci.,* 464, 37, 1986.

27. **Nagasawa, H., Ohta, K., Nakajima, K., Noguchi, Y., Miura, K., Niki, K., and Namiki, H.,** Interrelationship between pituitary and ovarian hormones in normal and neoplastic growth of mammary glands of mice, *Ann. N.Y. Acad. Sci.,* 464, 301, 1986.

28. **Dembinski, T. C. and Shiu, R. P.,** Growth factors in mammary gland development and function, in *The Mammary Gland, Development, Regulation, and Function,* Neville, M. C. and Daniel, C. W., Eds., Plenum Press, New York, 1987, 355.

29. **Haslam, S. Z.,** Role of sex steroid hormones in normal mammary gland function, in *The Mammary Gland, Development, Regulation, and Function,* Neville, M. C. and Daniel, C. W., Eds., Plenum Press, New York, 1987, 499.

30. **Shyamala, G.,** Endocrine and other influences in the normal development of the breast, in *Fundamental Problems in Breast Cancer,* Paterson, A. H. G. and Lees, A. W., Eds., Martinus Nijhoff, Boston, 1987, 127.

31. **Thordarson, G. and Talamantes, F.,** Role of the placenta in mammary gland development and function, in *The Mammary Gland, Development, Regulation, and Function,* Neville, M. C. and Daniel, C. W., Eds., Plenum Press, New York, 1987, 459.

32. **Vonderhaar, B. K.,** Prolactin: transport, function, and receptors in mammary gland development and differentiation, in *The Mammary Gland, Development, Regulation, and Function,* Neville, M. C. and Daniel, C. W., Eds., Plenum Press, New York, 1987, 383.

33. **Sheffield, L. G., and Welsch, C. W.,** Transplantation of human breast epithelia to mammary-gland-free fat-pads of athymic nude mice: influence of mammotrophic hormones on growth of breast epithelia, *Int. J. Cancer,* 41, 713, 1988.

34. **Nagasawa, H.,** Mammary gland DNA synthesis as a limiting factor for mammary tumorigenesis, *IRCS J. Med. Sci.,* 5, 405, 1977.

35. **Nagasawa, H.,** The cause of species differences in mammary tumorigenesis: significance of mammary gland DNA synthesis, *Med., Hypoth.,* 5, 499, 1979.

36. **Nagasawa, H.,** Causes of age-dependency of mammary tumour induction by carcinogens in rats, *Biomedicine,* 34, 9, 1981.

37. **Russo, J. and Russo, I. H.,** Is differentiation the answer in breast cancer prevention?, *IRCS J. Med. Sci.,* 10, 935, 1982.

38. **Nagasawa, H.,** Age-related changes in mammary gland DNA synthesis as a limiting factor for mammary tumorigenesis in rats and its implication for human breast cancer, in *Age-Related Factors in Carcinogenesis,* Likachev, A., Anisimov, V., and Montesano, R., Eds., International Agency for Research Cancer (IARC), Lyon, 1986, 105.

39. **Nagasawa, H. and Yanai, R.,** Frequency of mammary cell division in relation to age; its significance in the induction of mammary tumors by carcinogen in rats, *J. Natl. Cancer Inst.,* 52, 609, 1974.

40. **Nagasawa, H., Yanai, R., and Taniguchi, H.,** Importance of mammary gland DNA synthesis on carcinogen-induced mammary tumorigenesis in rats, *Cancer Res.,* 36, 2223, 1976.

41. **Mhatre, M. C., Shah, P. N., and Juneja, H. S.,** Effect of varying photoperiods on mammary morphology, DNA synthesis, and hormone profile in female rats, *JNCI,* 72, 1411, 1984.

42. **Ratko, T. A. and Beattie, C. W.,** Estrous cycle modification of rat mammary tumor induction by a single dose of N-methyl-N-nitrosourea, *Cancer Res.,* 45, 3042, 1985.

43. **Lok, E., Nera, E. A., Iverson, F., Scott, F., So, Y., and Clayson, D .B.,** Dietary restriction, cell proliferation and carcinogenesis: a preliminary study, *Cancer Lett.,* 38, 249, 1988.

44. **Nagasawa, H. and Morii, S.,** Prophylaxis of spontaneous mammary tumorigenesis by temporal inhibition of prolactin secretion in rats at young ages, *Cancer Res.,* 41, 1935, 1981.

45. **Nagasawa, H. and Morii, S.,** Inhibition by early treatment with bromocriptine of spontaneous mammary tumour development in rats with no side-effects, *Acta Endocrinol.,* 101, 51, 1982.

46. **Tokunaga, M., Land, C. E., Yamamoto, T., Asano, M., Tokuoka, S., Ezaki, H., and Nishimori, I.,** Incidence of female breast cancer among atomic bomb survivors, Hiroshima and Nagasaki, 1950-1980, *Rad. Res.,* 112, 243, 1987.

47. **Meyer S. J.,** Cell proliferation in normal human breast ducts, fibroadenomas, and other ductal hyperplasias as measured by tritiated thymidine, effects of menstrual phase, age and oral contraceptive hormones, *Human Pathol.,* 8, 67, 1977.

48. **Russo, J., Wilgus, G., Tait, L,. and Russo, I. H.,** Influence of age and parity on the susceptibility of rat mammary gland epithelial cells in primary cultures to 7,12-dimethylbenz(a)anthracene, *In Vitro,* 17, 877, 1981.

49. **Russo J. and Russo, I. H.,** Differentiation of the mammary gland susceptibility to carcinogenesis, *Breast Cancer Res. Treat.,* 2, 5, 1982.

50. **Russo, J., and Tait, L. and Russo, I. H.,** Susceptibility of the mammary gland to carcinogenesis. III. The cell of origin of rat mammary carcinoma, *Am. J. Pathol.,* 113, 50, 1983.

51. **Anisimov, V.,** *Carcinogenesis and Aging,* Vol. 1, CRC Press, Boca Raton, FL, 1987, 54.

52. **Callahan, R.,** Retrovirus and proto-oncogene involvement in the etiology of breast neoplasia, in *The Mammary Gland, Development, Regulation, and Function,* Neville, M. C. and Daniel, C. W., Eds., Plenum Press, New York, 1987, 323.

53. **Salmons, B. and Gunzburg, W. H.,** Current perspectives in the biology of mouse mammary tumor virus, *Virus Res.,* 8, 81, 1987.

54. **Nagasawa, H., Yanai, R., and Miyamoto, M.,** Participation of mammary tumor tumor virus in mammary gland sensitivity to prolactin in mice, *Jpn. J. Zootech. Sci.,* 43, 519, 1972.

55. **Nagasawa, H. and Vorherr, H.,** Rat mammary deoxyribonucleic acid synthesis during the estrous cycle, pregnancy, and lactation in relation to mammary tumorigenesis. Its implication for human breast cancer, *Am. J. Obst. Gynecol.,* 127, 590, 1977.

56. **Lindsey, W. F., Das Gupter, T. K., and Beattie, C. W.,** Influence of estrous cycle during carcinogen exposure on nitrosomethylurea-induced rat mammary carcinoma, *Cancer Res.,* 41, 3857, 1981.

57. **Ratko, T. A., Braun, R.J., Pezzuto, J. M., and Beattie, C. W.,** Estrous cycle modulation of rat mammary gland DNA alkylation by N-methyl-N-nitrosourea, *Cancer Res.,* 48, 3090, 1988.

58. **Anderson, T. J., Ferguson, D. J. P., and Raab, G. M.,** Cell turnover in the "resting" human breast: influence of parity, contraceptive pill, age and laterality, *Br. J. Cancer,* 46, 376, 1982.

59. **Going, J. J., Anderson, T.J., Battersby, S., and MacIntyre, C. C. A.,** Proliferative and secretory activity in human breast during natural and artificial menstrual cycles, *Am. J. Pathol.,* 130, 193, 1988.

60. **Vogel, P. M., Georgiade, N. G., Fetter, B. F., Vogel F. S., and McCarty, K. S., Jr.,** The correlation of histologic changes in the human breast with the menstrual cycle, *Am. J. Pathol.,* 104, 23, 1981.

61. **Hutson, S. W., Cowen, P. N., and Bird, C. C.,** Morphometric studies of age related changes in normal human breast and their significance for evolution of mammary cancer, *J. Clin. Pathol.,* 38, 281, 1985.

62. **Ferguson, D. J. P.,** An ultrastructural study of mitosis and cytokinesis in normal 'resting' human breast, *Cell Tissue Res.,* 252, 581, 1988.

63. **Nagasawa, H. and Mori T.,** Stimulation of mammary tumorigenesis and suppression of uterine adenomyosis by temporary inhibition of pituitary prolactin secretion during youth in mice, *Proc. Soc. Exp. Biol. Med.,* 171, 164, 1982.

64. **Nagasawa, H. and Yanai, R.,** Some discrepancies between the use of DNA synthesis and wholemount preparations as indices of mammary gland response to pituitary mammotrophin, *J. Endocrinol.,* 67, 303, 1975.

65. **Nagasawa, H., Yanai, R., and Taniguchi H.,** Reduction by pituitary grafts of mammary tumor age. Its variability in a high mammary tumor strain of mice. Effects of mammary DNA synthesis, *Eur. J. Cancer,* 12, 1017, 1976.

66. **Welsch, C. W., Clemens, J.A., and Meites, J.,** Effects of multiple pituitary isografts or progesterone on 7,12-dimethylbenzanthracene-induced mammary tumors in rats, *J. Natl. Cancer Inst.,* 41, 465, 1968.

67. **Nagasawa, H., Yanai, R., and Azuma I.,** Suppression by *Nocardia* cell wall skeleton of mammary DNA synthesis, plasma prolactin level, and spontaneous mammary tumorigenesis in mice, *Cancer Res.,* 38, 2160, 1978.

68. **Nagasawa, H., Yanai, R., and Azuma, I.,** Inhibitory effect of *Nocardia rubra* cell wall skeleton on carcinogen-induced mammary tumorigenesis in rats, *Eur. J. Cancer,* 16, 389, 1980.

69. **Battersby, S. and Anderson, T.J .,** Proliferative and secretory activity in the pregnant and lactating human breast, *Virchows Arch. Pathol. Anat. Physiol.,* 413, 189, 1988.

70. **Dao, T. L.,** Inhibition of tumor induction in chemical carcinogenesis in the mammary gland, *Prog. Exp. Tumor Res.,* 14, 59, 1971.

71. **Moon, R. C.,** Influence of pregnancy and lactation on experimental mammary carcinogenesis, in *Bambury Report 8, Hormones and Breast Cancer,* Pike, M.C., Siiteri, P.K., and Welsch, C.W., Eds., Cold Spring Harbor Laboratory, Cold Spring Harbor, NY, 1981, 353.

72. **MacMahon, B. and Cole P.,** Etiology of human breast cancer: a review, *J. Natl. Cancer Inst.,* 50, 21, 1973.

73. **Cole, P.,** Epidemiology of human breast cancer, *J. Invest. Dermatol.,* 63, 133, 1974.

74. **Grubbs, C. J., Farnell, D. R., Hill, D. L., and McDonough, K. C.,** Chemoprevention of N-nitroso-N-methylurea-induced mammary cancers by pretreatment with 17β–estrdiol and progesterone, *JNCI,* 74, 927, 1985.

75. **Juret, P., Couetle, J. E., and Brune, D.,** Age at first birth: an equivocal factor in human mammary carcinogenesis, *Eur. J. Cancer,* 10, 591, 1974.

76. **Russo, J., Reina, D., Frederick, J., and Russo, I. H.,** Expression of phenotypical changes by human breast epithelial cells treated with carcinogens *in vitro, Cancer Res.,* 48, 2837, 1988.

77. **Nagasawa, H., and Yanai, R.,** Mammary nucleic acids and pituitary prolactin secretion during prolonged lactation in mice, *J. Endocrinol.,* 70, 389, 1976.

78. **Rosenberg, L., Palmer, J. R., Kaufman, D. W., Strom, B. L., Schottenfeld, D., and Shapiro S.,** Breast cancer in relation to the occurrence and time of induced and spontaneous abortion, *Am. J. Epidemiol.,* 127, 981, 1988.

79. **Moon, R. C.,** Mammary gland cell content during various phases of lactation, *Am. J. Physiol.,* 203, 939, 1962.

80. **Tucker, H. A.,** Regulation of mammary nucleic acid content by various suckling intensities, *Am. J. Physiol.,* 210, 1209, 1966.

81. **Nagasawa, H., Yanai, R., Kosugiyama, M., and Fujimoto, M.,** *Jpn. J. Zootech Sci.,* 40, 61, 1969.

82. **Nagai, J. and Sarkar, N. K.,** Relationship between milk yield and mammary gland development in mice., *J. Dairy Sci.,* 61, 733, 1978.

83. **Knight, C. H. and Wilde, C. J.,** Mammary growth during lactation: implications for increasing milk yield, *J. Dairy Sci.,* 70, 1991, 1987.

84. **Nagasawa, H. and Nakajima, Y.,** Relationship between incidence and onset age of mammary tumors and reproductive characteristics in mice, *Eur. J. Cancer,* 16, 1111, 1980.

85. **Nagasawa, H., Kanzawa, F., and Kuretani, K.,** Lactational performance of the high and low mammary tumor strains of mice, *GANN (Jpn. J. Cancer Res.),* 58, 331, 1967.

86. **Nagasawa, H., Yanai, R., Kosugiyama, M., Fujimoto, M., and Kuretani, K.,** Lactational performance of high (C3H/He) and low (C57BL/6) mammary tumor strains of mice (II), *Exp. Anim.,* 18, 21, 1969.

87. **Nagasawa, H., Yanai, R., Taniguchi, H., Tokuzen, R., and Nakahara, W.,** Two-way selection of a stock of Swiss albino mice for mammary tumorigenesis: establishment of two new strains (SHN and SLN), *J. Natl. Cancer Inst.,* 57, 425, 1976.

88. **Nagasawa, H. and Yamaki, K.,** High lactation potential may increase the risk of mammary tumor?: role of mammary gland growth potential, *Med. Hypoth.,* 9, 259, 1982.

89. **Nagasawa, H.,** Relationship between the rate of mammary gland DNA synthesis and lactational performance in the 1st and the 2nd lactations in GR/A mice, *Bull. Fac. Agr. Meiji Univ.,* 62, 5, 1983.

90. **Lund, K., Ewertz, M., and Schou, G.,** Breast cancer incidence subsequent to surgical reduction of the female breast, *Scand. J. Plast, Reconstr. Surg.,* 21, 209, 1987.

91. **Nagasawa, H., Yanai, R., and Nakajima, Y.,** Suppression of lactation by tumor promoters in mice, *Proc. Soc. Exp. Biol. Med.,* 165, 394, 1980.

92. **Mori, T. and Iguchi T.,** Long-term effects of perinatal treatment with sex steroids and related substance on reproductive organs of female mice, in *Toxicity of Hormones in Perinatal Life,* Mori, T. and Nagasawa, H., Eds., CRC Press, Boca Raton, FL, 1988, 63.

93. **Forsberg, J.-G.,** Histogenesis of irreversible changes in the female genital tract after perinatal exposure to hormones and related substances, in *Toxicity of Hormones in Perinatal Life,* Mori, T. and Nagasawa, H., Eds., CRC Press, Boca Raton, FL, 1988, 39.

94. **Herbst, A. L., Scully, E. E. R., and Robby, S.J.,** Prenatal diethylstilbestrol exposure and human genital tract abnormalities, *J. Natl. Cancer Inst. Monogr.,* 51, 25, 1979.

95. **Rotmensch, J., Frey, K., and Herbst, A. L.,** Effects of female offspring and mothers after exposure to diethylstilbestrol.in *Toxicity of Hormones in Perinatal Life,* Mori, T. and Nagasawa, H., Eds., CRC Press, Boca Raton, FL, 1988, 143.

96. **Mori, T., Nagasawa, H., and Bern H. A.,** Long-term effects of perinatal exposure to hormones on normal and neoplastic mammary growth in rodents: a review, *J. Environ. Pathol. Toxicol.,* 3, 191, 1980.

97. **Nagasawa, H. and Mori, T.,** Longer-term effects of perinatal exposure to hormones and related substances on normal and neoplastic growth of murine mammary glands, in *Toxicity of Hormones in Perinatal Life,* Mori, T. and Nagasawa, H., Eds., CRC Press, Boca Raton, FL, 1988, 82.

98. **Tomooka Y. and Bern, H. A.,** Growth of mouse mammary glands after neonatal sex hormone treatments, *J. Natl. Cancer Inst.,* 69, 1347, 1982.

99. **Bern, H. A., Mills, K. T., and Jones, L. A.,** Critical period for neonatal estrogen exposure in occurrence of mammary gland abnormalities in adult mice, *Proc. Soc. Exp. Biol. Med.,* 172, 239, 1983.

100. **Nagasawa, H., Mori, T., and Nakajima, Y.,** Long-term effects of progesterone or diethylstilbestrol with or without estrogen after maturity on mammary tumorigenesis in mice, *Eur. J. Cancer,* 16, 1583, 1980.

101. **Nagasawa, H., Yanai, R., Shodono, M., Nakamura, T., and Tanabe, Y.,** Effect of neonatally administered estrogen or prolactin on normal and neoplastic mammary growth and serum estradiol-17 level in rats, *Cancer Res.,* 34, 2643, 1974.

102. **Nettesheim, P.,** Inhibition of carcinogenesis by retinoids, *Can. Med. Assoc.,* 122, 757, 1980.

103. **Hill, D. L. and Grubbs, C. J.,** Retinoids as chemopreventive and anticancer agents in intact animals (review), *Anticancer Res.,* 2, 111, 1982.

104. **Moon, R. C. and Mehta, R. G.,** Anticarcinogenic effects of retinoids in animals, in *Essential Nutrients in Carcinogenesis,* Poirier, L. A., Newberne, P. M., and Pariza, M. W., Eds., Plenum Press, New York, 1986, 399.

105. **Nagasawa, H.,** Stimulation by neonatal treatment with vitamin A of spontaneous mammary tumor development in GR/A mice, *Breast Cancer Res. Treat.,* 4, 205, 1984.

106. **Nagasawa, H., Yanai, R., and Kikuyama, S.,** Irreversible inhibition of pituitary prolactin and growth hormone secretion and of mammary gland development in mice by monosodium glutamate administered neonatally, *Acta Endocrinol.,* 75, 249, 1974.

107. **Nagasawa, H., Noguchi, Y., Mori, T., Niki K., and Namiki, H.,** Suppression of normal and preneoplastic mammary growth and uterine adenomyosis with reduced growth hormone level in SHN mice given monosodium glutamate neonatally, *Eur. J. Cancer Clin. Oncol.,* 21, 1547, 1985.

108. **Yanai, R., Mori, T., and Nagasawa, H.,** Long-term effects of prenatal and neonatal administration of 5β-dihydrotestosterone on normal and neoplastic mammary development in mice, *Cancer Res.,* 37, 4456, 1977.

109. **Yanai, R., Nagasawa, H., Mori, T., and Nakajima Y.,** Long-term effects of perinatal exposure to 5α-dihydrotestosterone on normal and neoplastic mammary development in mice, *Endocrinol. Jpn.,* 28, 231, 1981.

110. **Wellings, S. R., DeVault, M., Jenfoft, V., Richards, J., Yang, J., Nandi, S., Guzman, R., and Faulkin, L J.,** Early lesions of the human mammary gland and their relationship to precancerous lesions of other species, in *New Frontiers in Mammary Pathology,* Hollmann, K. H., deBrux, J., and Verbey, J. M., Eds., Plenum Press, New York, 1981, 27.

111. **Squartini, F. and Hart I.,** New concepts and approaches in the analysis of mammary preneoplasia and tumor progression, in *Breast Cancer: Origins, Detection, Treatment,* Rich, M. A., Hager, J. C., and Taylor-Papadimitriou, J., Eds., Martinus Nijhoff, Boston, 1986, 69.

112. **Nagasawa, H., Fujii, M., and Hagiwara, K.,** Inhibition by medroxyprogesterone acetate of precancerous mammary hyperplastic alveolar nodules in mice, *Breast Cancer Res. Treat.,* 5, 31, 1985.

113. **Nagasawa, H., Aoki, M., Sakagami, N., and Ishida, M.,** Medroxyprogesterone acetate enhances spontaneous mammary tumorigenesis and uterine adenomyosis in mice, *Breast Cancer Res. Treat.,* 12, 59, 1988.

114. **Nagasawa, H., Sakagami, N., Ohbayasgi, R., Yamamoto, K., and Petrow, V.,** Effect of megestrol acetate or melengestrol acetate on preneoplastic and neoplastic mammary growth in mice, *Anticancer Res.,* 8, 1399, 1988.

115. **Yanai, R. and Nagasawa, H.,** Development and growth of pregnancy-dependent and -independent mammary tumors in GR/A strain of mice and their relationships, *GANN (Jpn. J. Cancer Res.),* 69, 25, 1978.

116. **Nagasawa, H. and Morii, S.,** Hormone dependency of pregnancy-dependent mammary tumors in mice. II., *Bull. Fac. Agric., Meiji Univ.,* 57, 7, 1982.

117. **Nagasawa, H., Suzuki, M., Yamamuro, Y., Sensui, N., Inaba, T., and Mori, J.,** Suppressed lactation by pregnancy-dependent mammary tumors in GR/A mice, *Proc Soc. Exp. Biol. Med.,* in press.

118. **Ris, H. -B., Niederer, U., Stirnemann, H., Doran, J. E., and Zimmerman, A.,** Long-term follow-up of patients with biopsy-proven benign breast disease, *Ann. Surg.,* 207, 404, 1988.

119. **Mansel, R. E.,** Benign breast disease and cancer risk: new prospectives, *Ann. N.Y. Acad. Sci.,* 464, 364, 1986.

120. **Nagasawa, H., Naito, M., and Namiki H.,** Mammary gland growth and serum levels of prolactin and growth hormone in four strains of male mice in comparison with females, *Life Sci.,* 40, 1473, 1987.

121. **Nagasawa, H., Naito, T., and Mori, T.,** Difference in response to mammotropic hormones of mammary growth and uterine adenomyosis among four strains of mice, *In Vivo,* 2, 171, 1988.

122. **Nagasawa, H., Koshimizu, U., and Yamamoto, K.,** Enhancement of normal and neoplastic mammary growth by crossbreeding between strains of female and male mice with high mammary growth potentials, *Asia-Aust. J. Anim. Sci.,* 1, 43, 1988.

123. **Sheffield, L. G. and Welsch, C. W.,** Influence of submandibular salivary glands on hormone responsiveness of mouse mammary glands, *Proc. Soc. Exp. Biol. Med.,* 186, 368, 1987.

124. **Haslam, S. Z.,** Cell to cell interactions and normal mammary gland function, *J. Dairy Sci.,* 71, 2843, 1988.

125. **Topper, Y. J., Sankaran, L., Chomczynski, P., Prosser, C., and Qasba, P.,** Three stages of responsiveness to hormones in the mammary cells, *Ann. N.Y. Acad. Sci.,* 464, 1, 1986.

126. **Sakakura, T.,** Epithelial-mesenchymal interactions in mammary gland development and its perturbation in relation to tumorigenesis, in *Understanding Breast Cancer. Clinical and Laboratory Concepts,* Rich, M. A., Hager, J. C., and Furmanski, P., Eds., Marcel Dekker, New York, 1983, 261.

127. **Bissell, M. J. and Hall, H. G.,** Form and function in the mammary gland: the role of extracellular matrix, in *The Mammary Gland, Development, Regulation, and Function,* Neville, M.C. and Daniel, C.W., Eds., Plenum Press, New York, 1987, 97.

128. **Chiquet-Ehrismann, R., Mackie, E. J., Pearson, C. A., and Sakakura, T.,** Tenascin: a extracellular matrix protein involved in tissue interactions during fetal development and oncogenesis, *Cell,* 47, 131, 1986.

129. **McGuire, W. L., Dickson, R. B., Osborne, C. K., and Salomon, D.,** The role of growth factors in breast cancer, *Breast Cancer Res. Treat.,* 12, 159, 1988.

Chapter 4

AGE AND IMMUNITY

Bengt Björkstén and Catharina Svanborg

TABLE OF CONTENTS

I. INTRODUCTION

Aging is associated with a general deterioration of many physiological processes including a reduction in immunological vigor. This has been offered as an explanation of the increased susceptibility to infection, autoimmune diseases, and cancer in the elderly. A waning immune surveillance has also been proposed as a mechanism for physical aging. These assumptions are mainly based on studies of aging mice. Less is known about the situation in humans mainly for two reasons. First, studies of elderly individuals have been performed in hospitalized popula- tions where healthy old people usually are underrepresented. For this reason it is not clear if the observed changes in immunological function are due to old age or to disease or poor health conditions associated with old age. The second reason for the limited knowledge about the relation between aging and immunity is methodological.

Like the elderly, infants and children have an increased susceptibility to infections. In both age groups, the infections present obscurely and they are common causes of high morbidity and mortality. Examples are urinary tract infections, pneumonias, and nosocomial infections. The mechanisms explaining the increased susceptibility to infection may, thus, be sought by comparing the age groups at the two extremes of life.

In this chapter, immune functions in old age are discussed. Initially, a brief summary of the immune system is given for the benefit of those who are not immunologists.

II. THE NORMAL IMMUNE RESPONSE

The immune system is able to identify self from nonself. It permits modulation of resistance to infections and other diseases by its hypervariable structure and thus saves man from the need to undergo germ-line evolution to counteract the attack of plagues and other illnesses.

The term "immune system" is mostly used to denote the highly specific components, which respond to antigens, i.e., antibodies, B-, and T-lymphocytes. Lymphocytes with specificity for different antigens are continuously produced in the bone marrow, and circulate in the blood, lymph, and lymph nodes. When lymphocytes meet the antigen, only the ones with specificity for this antigen are stimulated to divide, mature, and produce their effector molecules. Antigen recognition is, thus, required for activation.

The accessory immune system in contrast is continuously active and it does not need specific antigen stimulation. Examples of components in this defense system are phagocytes, comple- ment, proteins, interleukins, and acute phase reactants. This less specific response against foreign invaders is phylogenetically older than the specific immunity and is found in most multicellular organisms.

The generation of a specific immune response requires that the antigen is taken up and processed by antigen presenting cells, e.g., macrophages, dendritic cells, phagocytes, or B- lymphocytes. The antigen is fragmented and expressed on the surface of the antigen-presenting cell together with transplantation antigens (class II). Antigen fragments bound to class II molecules are recognized by T-cells as altered self and they are therefore a legitimate target for the immune attack.

The majority of antigens activate primarily T-lymphocytes and they are therefore called T- dependent. Subsequent to the activation of the T-helper cell, lymphokines are produced which direct the maturation of B-lymphocytes, T-cytotoxic, and T-suppressor cells. The B-lympho- cytes may also be directly activated by antigen in the absence of T-helper cells, in which case the antigen is designated as T-independent.

The effector functions of the specific immune system may be divided into two main categories: B-cell products and T-cell products. The B-cells exert their functions mainly through maturation to antibody producing plasma cells. The T-cell effector systems involves both the production of cytotoxic T-cells, which recognize antigen in the context of transplantation antigens (class I) and the production of lymphokines. Lymphokines from an activated T-helper cell, especially γ-interferon, can also activate macrophages and enhance their ability to kill, for example, intracellular microorganisms, or give rise to the delayed hypersensitivity reactions.

The accessory immune system provides a first line of defense against microorganisms and macromolecules. It is mobilized locally at the site of tissue damage and often leads to the elimination of the harmful agent before the specific immunity is activated. The complement system is composed of proteins, which lyse the membrane of target cells. The reaction products of the complement cascade have many biologic activities and they participate, e.g., in the coagulation system, in the immune response, and in inflammation. The complement components C3b and C5b interact with antibodies and also with granulocytes, which are the second major group of effectors of the accessory immune system. Particles covered by complement components are easily phagocytosed by the neutrophils. This process includes several separate steps, i.e., chemotaxis, adhesion, ingestion, and intracellular microbial killing of the foreign microorganisms (Figure 1). The specific and accessory immune systems cooperate in microbial killing. Thus, both granulocytes and complement factors are required for the antibody molecules to exert their functions.

III. AGE-RELATED CHANGES IN LYMPHOID ORGANS AND CELLS

A. STEM CELLS

Stem cells contain the genetic information required for the production of lymphocytes and certain accessory cell populations. In humans, the density of stem cells in the bone marrow decreases with age.[1] The ability of the stem cell to develop functionally does not, however, appear to deteriorate with age. The relative influence of age on the stem cell and the environment into which the stem cell is placed has been analyzed by adoptive transfer experiments in mice with graft rejection as the end-point. The poor graft rejection of the old mice could not be compensated by transfer of syngeneic stem cells from younger donors. Stem cells from old mice could, however, repopulate the lymphoid system of young recipients. This suggested that the impairment of stem cell function with age is a result of the aging of the environment, e.g., nonimmune components of the body, rather than of the stem cells per se.[2]

B. THE THYMUS AND T-LYMPHOCYTES

Immature lymphocytes from the bone marrow enter the cortex of the thymus gland, where they receive the signals necessary to differentiate into mature T-cell populations. The thymus undergoes marked changes with age. Involution begins already during adolescence. By 45 to 50 years of age, the thymus retains only 5 to 10% of its maximal mass.[3] As a consequence, the transit of immature lymphocytes from bone marrow to thymus decreases.[4] The involved thymus produces less of the polypeptide hormones which are important for the differentiation of pre-and post-thymic lymphocytes. In man, the levels of thymic hormones in serum decline after 30 years of age, to become undetectable after about 60 years of age. The aging thymus, thus, loses its capacity to differentiate immature lymphocytes and such cells are therefore found in increased numbers in the bloodstream of elderly humans.[5]

It has been reported that with age there is a slight drop in the number of circulating lymphocytes and that they show abnormalities of the cytoplasma membrane and of the organelles.[6] The change in numbers of circulating T-lymphocytes with age was initially studied by the E-rosette technique and a slight drop in numbers was only observed in mice and in selected human populations. Recent studies of representative samples of elderly individuals did not support the hypothesis of a general decrease in circulating T-lymphocytes with age.[7]

These observations were recently confirmed with more modern techniques (Table 1). Using monoclonal antibodies and fluorescence activated cell sorters, the peripheral blood lymphocyte

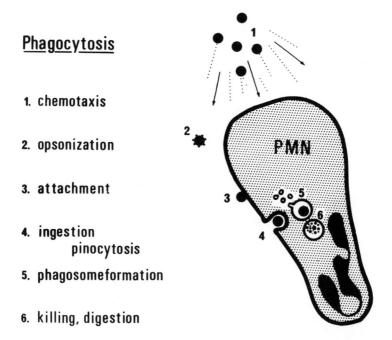

Phagocytosis

1. chemotaxis

2. opsonization

3. attachment

4. ingestion
       pinocytosis

5. phagosomeformation

6. killing, digestion

FIGURE 1. DNA repair pathways. (From Laval, F. and Huet, J., in Monitoring Human Exposure to Carcinogenic and Mutagenic Agents, IARC Sci. Publ. No. 59, Berlin, A., Draper, M., Hemminki, K., and Vainio, H., Eds., IARC, Lyon, 371. With permission.)

distribution in a representative sample of 85-year-old individuals fell within the range of the normal values established for middle-aged healthy blood donors. This is contrary to other studies claiming an increase in the percentage in number of cells with suppressor or cytotoxic characteristics (CD 8) but not of the CD 4 positive helper cell population.[8]

C. B-LYMPHOCYTES

The studies of changes in B-cell population with age have mainly focused on functional aspects, i.e., immunoglobulin production (see below). Studies analyzing the differentiation of pre-B-cells to B-cells in aging animals or in man are largely lacking. The number of circulating immunoglobulin bearing cells has not been found to decrease with age.[9]

D. ACCESSORY CELL FUNCTION

Lymphocytes are dependent on accessory cells for differentiation as well as for exerting their effector functions. In view of the effect of the environment on stem cell differentiation, it may be expected that accessory cells such as macrophages and dendritic cells would impair their function with age. Although morphological studies indicated that the number of macrophages was not impaired by age, the frequency of regulatory macrophages involved in the production of interleukin-1, which is needed by helper T-cells for normal antigen recognition, is reduced.[10]

IV. FUNCTIONAL ASPECTS OF CELL-MEDIATED IMMUNITY

Several studies have demonstrated reduced cell mediated immunity with increasing age. Delayed type hypersensitivity (DTH) reactions in the skin are often reduced in the aged. This includes responsiveness to antigens such as Candida and mumps, as well as model antigens such as dinitrochlorobenzene (DNCB). In a study of responses to the latter antigen, it was shown that 30% of healthy individuals above 70 years of age had a reduced responsiveness, as compared to 5% in younger individuals, according to Waldorf et al.[11]

TABLE 1
Lymphoid Cells in Peripheral Blood in 76-Year-Old Individuals

Markers	Cell type	No.	Mean	SD
okt 3	Total T cells	23	68.4	6.3
okt 4	Helper/inducer	23	43.1	8.1
okt 8	Suppressor/cytox	23	30.1	8.9
Leu 16	B lymphocytes	23	10.3	4.4
Hla-Dr	Lymphoid cells	23	17.3	5.3
Quote 4/8		23	1.6	0.8

Subclasses of IgG in Relation to Age

Age	No.	IgG_1	Mean S.D. (g/l)		
			IgG_2	IgG_3	IgG_4
38	7	6.78	4.76	0.85	0.24
50	8	8.05	3.77	0.86	0.32
62	15	7.05	3.32	0.66	0.28
70	67	7.83	3.81	0.79	0.44

Data from Anderson, B. et al., in preparation.

Marrie et al.[12] recently studied the DTH reactions of 149 healthy adults ranging in age from 25 to 82 years in senior citizens in a nursing home and in an acute care hospital. They found that DTH responses decreased with increasing age and with increasing dependency in a nursing home (Table 2). Anergy, as defined by negative test results to seven different antigens, was not only different in those who were self-sufficient as compared to those living in a nursing home, but it was also influenced by age and sex.

Several studies have demonstrated that *in vitro* response to antigens and plant lectins declines with age. T-lymphocyte preparations from old humans contain only 20 to 30% as many mitogen-responsive cells as similar preparations from young humans.[13] Not only are there fewer T-lymphocytes responsive to mitogen in the blood of elderly humans, but the capacity to divide in culture is impaired.[14]

The results from several previous studies were recently confirmed by a carefully performed study in 260 elderly subjects.[15] They included healthy elderly subjects between the ages of 70 and 106 (mean age 84.6), living independently and not taking any immunosuppressive agents, corticosteroids, or other medication known to decrease immune responsiveness. The control population consisted of 39 young healthy adults between the ages of 23 and 35. The proliferative responses to Concanavalin-A (Con-A) and phytohemaglutinin (PHA) were reduced. In contrast, the proliferative responses to pokeweed mitogen (PWM) were not significantly affected. The oldest group, i.e., those over 90 years, showed less reduction of the proliferative responses than the other elderly group. No response at all to the three mitogens was observed in 13% of the group aged 70 to 89, but in none of the group aged 90 to 106 or in the young controls. These observations suggest that the decreased immune response of the elderly is not directly related to age over the age of 70 and that there may be a selection process in which subjects who live to the age of 90 are those in whom there is less decrease in immune response.

Also in the study natural killer cell activity was investigated. No significant differences between the young controls and any of the elderly groups were recorded, although there was a nonsignificant trend toward a slight increase in percent cytotoxicity in the groups 70 to 79 and 80 to 84 and a slight decrease in the oldest group.

The observation that responsiveness to PWM was not decreased is interesting and supports a previous study by Powell and Fernandez[16] in which responses to PWM even increased in old

TABLE 2
Delayed Type Hypersensitivity (DTH) Responses
in Relation to Age and Health

	Healthy at home			Senior citizens		
Age	25—40	41—65	66+	S	N	H
n	68	42	39	79	25	15
No. of positive DTH (%)						
>3	76.5	50.0	28.2	15.2	4.0	20.0
1—2	22.0	40.5	53.9	43.0	46.0	40.0
0	1.5	9.5	17.9	41.8	60.0	40.0
Mean diameter for positive DTH (mm)						
	3.5	3.6	3.6	3.2	2.4	2.8

Note: The table gives the number of positive (>2 mm diameter) and mean diameter of positive tests in different age groups of healthy and self-sufficient adults (S) and not self-sufficient (N) seniors citizens living in nursing homes and subjects who were hospitalized in an acute care hospital (H). Seven skin tests antigens were employed.

Modified from Marrie et al., 1988.

age. This mitogen induces T-dependent B-cell responses. Although the reasons for difference in mitogen responses is not clear, it could be related to loss of suppressor cells with age.

V. HUMORAL IMMUNITY

The information on changes in immunoglobulin levels and antibody activity with age is inconsistent. This probably reflects the fact that several different mechanisms regulate the changes in B-cells with age.

A. CIRCULATING IMMUNOGLOBULINS

The overall serum immunoglobulin levels increase with age.[17] Some of this rise in circulating immunoglobulin levels can be accounted for by the higher incidence of benign monoclonal gammopathies found in the aged.[18] Whereas the levels of IgG_2 have been proposed to decline with age, the IgA levels increase. This is interesting in view of the hypothesis that IgA producing plasma cells represent the most mature step in the B-cell differentiation.

B. THYMUS DEPENDENT ANTIGENS

The age-related decline in antibody responses to foreign antigens is most pronounced during primary T-cell dependent responses.[19] This may both be a function of the reduced T-helper cell activity and of the decreased production of cytokines required for the T-dependent antigen responses. A consequence of the antibody response after vaccination, e.g., with tetanus and hepatitis B, declines with age. The latter study indicated that the lack of antibody production was due to dysfunction of T-cells.

Concomitant with the reduced response to foreign antigens, there is an increased level of autoantibodies.[21] This has been attributed to the decreased immune surveillance function, which permits expansion of clones which would otherwise be regulated to lower levels of antibody production. Recently it was also shown that autoimmunity could arise from a shift of antibody specificity of an aging B-cell clone. This occurred for B-cells specifically recognizing phosphorylcholine (pc), which through a minor change in the VH region altered the specificity to DNA recognizing antibodies. Other possible explanations for the increase in autoimmunity include a loss of ability to maintain self tolerance, declining T-cell suppression of B-cell proliferation,[23] or alterations in B-cell responsiveness.

C. T-CELL INDEPENDENT ANTIGENS

Carbohydrate antigens give rise to immunity largely through a direction action on B-lymphocytes. Carbohydrate structures are ubiquitous in nature and anticarbohydrate antibodies make up a significant portion of immunoglobulins made by B-cells. For example, a naturally occurring antigalactosyl antibody was reported to comprise 1% of the human immunoglobulin mass.[24]

A decline in anti-carbohydrate antibody levels with advancing age was first reported for the ABO(H) blood group system as referenced in Thomsen et al.[25] The A, B, and H antigens are all carbohydrate determinants on the surface of human cells. In a subsequent study, Furuhata and Eguchi[26] demonstrated a similar decline of B antibody levels with age in the Japanese population.

Phosphorylcholine is an antigen determinant present on the cell wall of *Streptococcus pneumoniae* and in multicellular parasites, as referenced in Thomaz[27] and Clafin.[28] Antibodies to pc are naturally occurring in man and the levels decline with age. Thus, 36% of individuals over 60 years of age had levels below 10 μg/ml of these antibodies. In studies of consecutive samples from individuals at 38 and 50, 50 and 62, or 70, 75, 79, and 81 years of age, it was found that on a population basis the anti-pc antibody levels declined between 38 to 70 years of age but remained stable after that age.[29] This suggested that the B-cell aging occurs in late middle age rather than during old age exclusively.

Several mechanisms may explain the observed decline with age of the levels of anti-pc antibodies:

1. The longevity of the T-cell independent B-cell clones may be shorter than that of other clones. In addition these clones have been proposed to mature later than other B-cells in the young individuals.
2. The local immune responses, which are well developed in young and middle-aged individuals, may reduce the exposure to antigen at systemic sites and thus decrease the B-cell exposure to antigen.
3. The antigen specificity of the B-cell may be altered (see above).

VI. MUCOSAL IMMUNITY

Mucosal membranes are the first line of defense against particles, complex antigens, and microorganisms. Nonspecific components and specific immunity are both essential for the barrier function of the mucosal membranes (Table 3). The gut associated lymphoid tissue contains the majority of all lymphocytes in the body, a higher number than the bone marrow, spleen, thymus, and lymph nodes together. The effect of aging on mucosal immunity has received limited attention. The available information was recently reviewed by Schmucker and Daniels.[30]

Elderly individuals have an increased susceptibility to several mucosal infections. In the gut, age-related changes in microbial flora have been reported.

Pneumococcal pneumonia is more frequent and has a particularly high fatality rate in the elderly. Risk factors for pneumonia include chronic lung disease, alcoholism, smoking, etc., but these factors are insufficient to predict who will attract pneumonia and who will die from the infection. The association between specific immune responses and pneumococcal pneumonia have been extensively studied. Antibodies against the capsular polysaccharides are protective in man.[32] We recently investigated the relationship between anti-pc antibody levels at 70 years

TABLE 3
Components of the Mucosal Host Defense

Nonspecific components	Affected by old age
Anatomically intact barrier	Yes
Motility	Yes
Mucosal secretions	Yes
Ciliary function (in some compartments)	?
Microbial flora	Yes
Phagocytes	No?
Specific immunity	
IgA	No?
Cell mediated immunity	?

of age and subsequent death associated with pneumonia. The hypothesis was that individuals with the lowest anticarbohydrate antibody levels would be the most susceptible to lethal pneumonia. In contrast, we found that the individuals with the highest anti-pc antibody levels at 70 years of age were most likely to die with pneumonia during the follow-up years. This illustrates that the commonly proposed relationship between specific immunity and susceptibility to infection is an oversimplification.

The frequency of bacteriuria increases with age, from about 1% in infants to about 2% in pregnant women, 4% of women around 50-years-old and 9% of women at the age of 60. From the age of 70 and onwards the estimated frequencies of bacteriuria range from 2% among 70-year-old men to 50% among women over 80 years of age. Still higher estimates were reported among elderly people living in institutions. The variation in frequency probably reflects the variable selection of patients for study as well as the criteria used to define bacteriuria. In a recent screening study of bacteriuria in 70 to 79-year-old individuals representative of the general population in Gothenburg, growth of at least 10^5 of a single species was found among 6% of men and 15% of women in this age group.[33] Although these frequencies are in the lower range of those previously reported for the age group, they are consistent with the notion that the susceptibility to bacteriuria increases in old age.

Specific immunity is less important for the natural resistance to bacteriuria than nonspecific defense mechanisms. The hormonal changes in connection with menopause increase the susceptibility of the urogenital mucosal surfaces to infection. This may be counteracted by supplementation with estrogen. Furthermore, there is decreased production of urine and impediment of urine flow through neurogenic changes, prostatic enlargement, etc. Residual urine may provide a good medium for bacterial growth.

The elderly also have a decreased gastrointestinal motility and secretion. Esophageal peristalsis is diminished and there is less production of hydrochloric acid in the stomach. In the respiratory tract, weakened respiratory muscles and decreased elasticity of the lung tissues as well as reduction in the secretion, affect cough and other unspecific defenses against infection.

VII. NUTRITION AND IMMUNITY

Clinical observations in malnourished children, reviewed by Chandra and Chandra,[34] and in old people reviewed by Thompson et al.,[35] as well as an abundance of animal studies, all clearly indicate that malnutrition is associated with immune deficiency, which in turn results in increased susceptibility to infection. Since inadequate nutrition is common among the elderly, the potential role of malnutrition on host defense in old age should be considered. The relative importance of various nutrients is, however, difficult to assess in the clinical situation since in severe clinical malnutrition there is almost always not only a lack of proteins and calories, but also in vitamins and trace elements.

Studies in malnourished children in developing countries, have, in addition to increased susceptibility to infections, shown a number of immunological abnormalities. There are reduced antibody responses to vaccination, depressed cell mediated immunity *in vitro*, and in skin tests and reduced phagocyte function.[34]

In elderly patients undergoing surgery it has been shown that there is an association between cutaneous anergy preoperatively and postoperative wound infections, septicemia, and death.[36] Preoperative parental nutrition to old patients not only normalized cutaneous reactivity but also significantly reduced the rate of postoperative infections.

Less is known about the immunological consequences of lack of trace elements. Studies, both in animals and human patients, have, however, revealed that zinc deficiency results in lowered lymphocyte numbers, reduced proliferative responses of T-lymphocytes, decreased T-cell dependent antibody production, decreased tempo of allograph rejection, decreased natural killer cell activity, and decreased functional activity of thymic hormones. In children who have the hereditary disease acrodermatitis enteropatica, zinc levels in the blood and urine are low and they have a defective cell mediated and humoral immunity as well as abnormal neutrophil chemotactic responsiveness. These children can be completely cured of disease symptoms by zinc supplementation.

In Down Syndrome, abnormally low zinc levels have been reported in addition to various immune deficiencies, and supplementation of zinc to these individuals improved cell mediated reactivity in the skin, increased lymphocyte proliferative responses, as well as neutrophil chemotactic responsiveness.[39]

The relation between nutrition and immunity is, however, not a simple one. Overnutrition may also impair immunity. Thus, it has been long known that the lifespan of experimental animals can be significantly prolonged by a diet restricted in calories.

VIII. IMMUNITY AND SUSCEPTIBILITY TO DISEASE

An intact immune system is obviously of vital importance for the individual's defense against infections. Much has been learned from studies of what types of infections are encountered in individuals with defined immune deficiencies. By such analysis and subsequent confirmation in vitro and in animal experiments the role of cell mediated immunity for defense against viral and fungal infections has been clearly established. Similarly, the role of IgG antibodies in the defense against many common pathogens, such as *pneumococci staphylococci*, and enteroviruses.

The importance of complement in the defense against *meningococci* and *gonococci* has been learned from the observation of increased frequency and severity of such infections in individuals deficient in components of the complement system. Proof of the role of circulatory phagocytes in the defense against infections in the skin and respiratory tract has been obtained from analysis of individuals with abnormal neutrophil chemotaxis.

The role of immunity for the defense against malignancy has been summarized by the term immune surveillance. Immunity, especially that effectuated by T-cells and natural killer cells, limits the growth of tumors with antigens which can be recognized as foreign, e.g., those induced by viral infections. Malignancies in the lymphoid system are especially frequent in immunodeficient individuals as well as in those undergoing immunosuppressive therapy.

Trisomy 21 is characterized by premature aging and multiple abnormalities of the immune system, including inflammatory responses, cell mediated, and humoral immunity.[39-41] These patients also have an increased rate of malignant disease, but this is limited to leukemia and lymphomas.

In contrast to malignancies of the lymphatic system, appearing in various immune deficiency states, the tumors appearing in old age more rarely originate in the lymphoid system but are spontaneous tumors in the gastrointestinal tract, prostata, female genitalia, and in the breast. The immune surveillance theory does not appear to be equally relevant for the development and growth of noninduced spontaneous tumors. The frequency of such tumors is for example, not increased in T-cell defective animals, as compared to immunocompetent controls. As opposed to the virally induced tumors, these cancers do not appear to have foreign surface antigens, but rather are characterized by changes in the proportion of natural antigens. They are, therefore, not recognized as nonself in the immune system. The role of the immunity for the age-related increase in tumor frequency thus remains poorly understood.

Although it is tempting to suggest a relation between immune function and susceptibility to cancer there is probably no clear-cut association for spontaneously occurring tumors, i.e., for the great majority of cancers encountered in the elderly. From an evolutionary point of view the immune system has probably been geared to focus on host defense against the myriad of foreign antigens and potential pathogens encountered throughout life rather than toward protection against spontaneously occurring tumors that appear with age long after the reproduction period. Susceptibility to infections kill the young individual, tumors usually the old.

IX. PROSPECTS FOR THE FUTURE AND CONCLUDING REMARKS

The immune system provides man with an exquisite tool to cope with the exposure to a changing and complex environment. With increasing longevity, the multitude of challenges is augmented, and probably also the likelihood of unsuccessful immune recognition. Superimposed on changes in the immune system are the various disease conditions, which also increase in frequency with age. Chronologic age is, however, a poor description of the functional age of the individual. Criteria applicable to the definition of functional rather than chronologic age remain to be identified. It is possible that immune function will be found to vary more clearly with the functional age of the individual and assessment of them may even be useful to define functional age. This would, however, require more extensive studies in clearly defined groups of elderly individuals at various functional ages and with clearly defined diseases.

REFERENCES

1. **Kay, M. B.,** Aging and the decline of immune responsiveness, in *Basic and Clinical Immunology*, Fudenberg, H. H., Stites, D. P., Celdwell, J. R., and Wells, J. V., Eds., Lange, Los Altos, CA , 1976, 267.
2. **Makinodan, T., James, S. J., Inamizu, T., and Chang, M. P.,** Immunologic basis for susceptibility to infection in the aged, *Gerontology*, 30, 279, 1984.
3. **Weksler, M. E.,** Senescence of the immune system, *Med. Clin. North Am.*, 67, 263, 1983.
4. **Pahwa, R. N., Modak, J. J., McMorrow, T., et al.,** Terminal deoxynucleotidyl transference (TdT) enzyme in thymus and bone marrow, *Cell Immunol.*, 58, 39, 1981.
5. **Moody, C. E., Innes, J. B., Staino-Coico, L., et al.,** Lymphocyte transformation induced by autologous cells. XI. The effect of age on the autologous mixed lymphocyte reaction, *Immunology*, 44, 31, 1981.
6. **Fox, R. A.,** The effect of aging on the immune system, in *Immunology and Infection in the Elderly*, Churchill Livingstone, Edinburgh, 289, 1984.
7. **Bjursten, L. M., Nilsson, L., Hanson, L. Å., and Svanborg, A.,** The immune system in aged humans as judged by *in vitro* tests in 70 year and 75 year old people, unpublished manuscript.
8. **Nagel, J. E., Chest, F. J., and Adler, W. H.,** Enumeration of T-lymphocyte subsets by monoclonal antibodies in young and aged humans, *J. Immunol.* 127, 2086, 1981.
9. **Becker, M. J., Farkas, R., Schneider, M., Drucker, J., and Klajman, A.,** Cell-mediated cytotoxicity in humans: age-related decline as measured by a xenogeneic assay, *Clin. Immunol.. Immunopathol.* 14, 204, 1979.
10. **Inamizu, T., Chang, M. P., and Makinodan, T.,** Decline in Interleukin (IL)-1 production with age, *Gerontologist*, 23, 249, 1983.

1 1. **Waldorf, D. S., Wilkens, R. R., and Decker, J. L.,** Impaired delayed hypersensitivity in an aged population. Association with antinuclear reactivity and rheumatoid factor, *JAMA,* 203, 831, 1968.

12. **Marrie, T. J., Johnson, S., and Duran, H.,** Cell-mediated immunity of healthy adult Nova Scotians in various age groups compared with nursing home and hospitalized senior citizens, *J. Allergy Clin. Immunol.,* 81, 36, 1988.

13. **Inkeles, B., Innes, J. B., Kuntz, M. M., Kadish, A .S., and Weksler, M. E.,** Immunological studies of aging, III. Cytokinetic barrier for the impaired response of lymphocytes from aged persons to plant lecitins, *J. Exp. Med.,* 145, 1176, 1977.

14. **Hefton, J. M., Darlington, G. J., Casazza, B. A., and Weksler, M. E.,** Immunologic studies of aging. V. Impaired proliferation of PHA responsive human lymphocytes in culture, *J. Immunol.,* 125, 1007, 1980.

15. **Murasko, D. M., Nelson, B. J., Silver, R., Matour, D., and Kaye, D.,** Immunologic response in an elderly population with a mean age of 85, *Am. J. Med.,* 81, 612, 1986.

16. **Powell, R. and Fernandez, L. A.,** Proliferative responses of peripheral blood lymphocytes to activation: a comparison of young and elderly individuals, *Mech. Ageing Dev.* 13, 241, 1980.

17. **Walford, R. L.,** The immunologic theory of aging, *Adv. Gerontol. Res.* 2, 159, 1967.

18. **Buckley, C. E., Buckley, E. G., and Dolsey, F. C.,** Longitudinal changes in serum immunoglobulin levels in older humans, *Fed. Proc.,* 33, 2036, 1974.

19. **Makinodan, T., and Peterson, W. J.,** Relative antibody-forming capacity of spleen cells as a function of age, *Proc. Natl. Acad. Sci. U.S.A.,* 78, 234, 1962.

20. **Kishimoto, S., Tomino, S., Mitsuya, H., Fijiwaa, H., and Tsuda, H.,** Age related decline in the *in vitro* and *in vivo* synthesis of antitetanus toxoid antibody in humans, *J. Immunol.,* 125, 2347, 1980.

21. **Goodwin, J. S., Searles, R. P., and Tsing, K. S. K.,** Immunological responses of a healthy elderly population, *Clin. Exp. Immunol.,* 48, 403, 1982.

22. **Sharf, M. D., Aguila, H. L., Behar, S. M., et al.,** Studies on the somatic instability of immunoglobulin genes *in vitro* and in cultured cells, *Immunol. Rev.,* 96, 75, 1987.

23. **Fernandez, L. A. and MacSween, M.,** Decreased autologous mixed lymphocyte reaction with aging, *Mech. Ageing Dev.,* 12, 245, 1980.

24. **Galili, U., Rachmilewitz, E. A., Peleg, A., and Flechner, I.,** A unique natural human IgG antibody with anti-galactosyl specificity, *J. Exp., Med.,* 160, 1519, 1984.

25. **Thomsen, O. and Kettel, K.,** Die Stärke der menschlichen Isoagglutinine und entsprechenden Blutkörperchenrezeptoren in verschiedenen Lebensaltern, *A. Immun. Exp. Ther.,* 63, 67, 1929.

26. **Furuhata, T. and Eguchi, M.,** The change of the agglutinin titer with age, *Proc. Jpn. Acad., Sci.,* 31, 555, 1955.

27. **Thomaz, A.,** Choline in the cell wall of a bacterium: novel type of polymer-linked choline in Pneumococcus, *Science,* 157, 694, 1967.

28. **Clafin, J. L.,** Uniformity of the clonal repertoire for the immune response to phospholcholine in mice, *Eur J. Immunol.,* 6, 66, 1976.

29. **Nordenstam, G., Andersson, B., Bengtsson, C., Briles, D., Scott, G., Svanborg, A., and Svanborg Edén, C.,** Age-related change in anticarbohydrate antibody levels, *Am. J. Epidemiol.,* 129, 89, 1989.

30. **Schmucker, D. L. and Daniels, C. K.,** Aging, gastrointestinal infections and mucosal immunity, *J. Am. Geriatr. Soc.,* 34, 377, 1986.

31. **Briles, D. E., Scott, G., Gray, B., Crain, M. J., Blaese, M., Nahm, N., Scott, V., and Haber, P.,** Naturally occurring antibodies to phosphocholine as a potential index of antibody responsiveness to polysaccharides, *J. Infect. Dis.,* 155, 1307, 1987.

32. **Amman, A.J ., Schiffman, G., and Austrian, R.,** The antibody responses to pneumococcal capsular polysaccharides in aged individuals, *Proc. Soc. Exp. Biol. Med.,* 164, 312, 1980.

33. **Nordenstam, G. R., Odén, A., Svanborg Edén, C., Brandberg, A., and Svanborg, A.,** Bacteriuria and mortality in an elderly population, in *Host-parasite Interactions in Urinary Tract Infections,* Kass, E. H. and Svanborg Edén, C., Eds., University of Chicago Press, 1989, 49.

34. **Chandra, S. and Chandra, R. K.,** Nutrition, immune response and outcome, *Prog. Food Nutr. Sci.,* 10, 150, 1986.

35. **Thompson, J. S., Robbins, J. and Cooper, J. K.,** Nutrition and immune function in the geriatric population, *Clin. Geriatr. Med.,* 3, 309, 1987.

36. **Meakins, J. L., Pietsch, J. B., Bubenick, O., Kelly, R., Rode, H., Gordon, J., and Maclean, L. D.,** Delayed hypersensitivity: indicator of acquired failure of host defenses in sepsis and trauma, *Ann. Surg.,* 186, 241, 1977.

37. **Pietsch, J. B., Meakins, J. L., and Maclean, L. D.,** The delayed hypersensitivity response: application in clinical surgery, *Surgery,* 82, 349, 1977.

38. **Hambidge, K. M., Walravens, P. A., and Neldner, K.,** The role of zinc in the pathogenesis and treatment of acrodermatitis enteropathica, in *Zinc Metabolism: Current Aspects in Health and Disease,* Brewer, G. J. and Prasad A. S., Eds., Alan R. Liss, New York, 1977, 329.

39. **Björkstén, B., Bäck, O., Hägglöf, B., and Tärnvik, A.,** Immune function in Down Syndrome, in *Inborn Errors of Immunity and Phagocytosis,* Güttler, Seakins and Harkness, Eds., MTP Press, Lancaster, England, 1978, 189.

40. **Björkstén, B., Bäck, O., Gustavson, H., Hallmans, B., Hägglöf, B., and Tärnvik, A.,** Zinc and immune function in Down Syndrome, *Acta Paediatr. Scand.,* 69, 183, 1980.

41. **Björkstén, B., Marklund, S., and Hägglöf, B.,** Enzymes of leukocyte oxidative metabolism in Down Syndrome, *Acta Paediatr. Scand.,* 73, 97, 1984.

Chapter 5

EFFECTS OF AGE ON DNA REPAIR IN RELATION TO CARCINOGENESIS

Alexei J. Likhachev

TABLE OF CONTENTS

I. INTRODUCTION

It is well known that in elderly individuals, the overall incidence of cancers is considerably higher than in young ones. This fact may depend, on the one hand, on a cumulative effect of different carcinogenic agents, which answers the concept of summation of their effects.[1] On the other hand, the age-dependent increase in tumor incidence may result from a higher susceptibility of tissues to malignization following exposure to carcinogenic agents. This problem is discussed in many reviews and monographs, and scientists often come to contradictory conclusions.[2,3]

The susceptibility of tissue to the initiating effect of carcinogenic agents depends predominantly on the extent and specificity of alterations of the cellular genome induced by them and the efficiency of a subsequent DNA replication and repair.[4,5] Assuming this, the analysis of age-related changes in repair of DNA damages caused by carcinogenic agents must be regarded as a necessary element in understanding the cause of the different susceptibility to carcinogenic stimuli at different stages of ontogenesis.

Before reviewing the age-related characteristics of DNA repair, it is worthwhile to present a general outlook of this phenomenon.

II. MECHANISMS AND TYPES OF DNA REPAIR

Of all structural and functional elements of the cell, only DNA can be repaired in regard to alterations caused by exposures to various agents including carcinogens. This phenomenon, which is as important for the cellular functioning and reproduction as replication and transcription, was discovered comparatively recently,[4,6] when the consequences of damage to DNA of ultraviolet (UV) irradiation were studied. Since that time, a comprehensive investigation of pathways and molecular mechanisms of DNA repair has been conducted.

It should be stressed that a loss of purines and pyrimidines from DNA occurs also under physiological conditions. Such a loss is estimated to be around several thousand bases per genome per day.[6] However, the cell retains the capacity for reproduction and can function without any disorders, demonstrating the high reliability of the DNA repair system.

Mechanisms of DNA repair have been thoroughly described in many contemporary reviews and monographs.[4-10] They propose several different systems of classification of different types of DNA repair. The most convenient and simple classification seems to be that given by Laval and Huet,[11] who subdivide the types of DNA repair in several classes depending on the type of DNA damage (Figure 1).

The principal feature of the first of these classes is that damage is removed from DNA without rupture of the phosphodiester chain. This class consists of the following types of DNA repair:

1. Repair of UV-induced DNA damage (photoreactivation): an elimination of pyrimidine dimers by specific enzymes which are activated by light with a wavelength above 300 nm. These enzymes require a cofactor of low molecular weight.

2. Repair of "promutagenic" DNA damages induced by monofunctional alkylating agents, i.e., O^6-alkylguanine (O^6-AG), and O^4-alkylthymine (O^4-AT). Both adducts are repaired by a specific protein which accepts their alkyl groups on one of its cysteine residues.[6,7] The protein which repairs O^6-AG, O^6-alkylguanine-DNA alkyltransferase (AT) is not regenerated after transfer of the alkyl group, hence, it is not a true enzyme. Its highest affinity is to O^6-methylguanine (O^6-MG). The bacterial AT transfers the alkyl group of O^4-AT, as well; however, AT of eukaryotes apparently does not repair O^4-AT. It is noteworthy that AT also repairs alkyl groups in the phosphate chain of DNA through a similar mechanism, but does not repair alkylated RNA.[4-7]

3. DNA repair by a direct reinsertion of purine at apurinic sites of DNA. It should be noted, however, that no reliable evidence is yet available favoring the existence of this reaction.[6,11]

The second class refers to those types of DNA repair in which the removal of DNA damage is accompanied by incision of the phosphodiester chain and by the synthesis of a "patch" which replaces a defect in DNA (excision repair). Depending on the pattern of DNA damage, the repair can proceed through two different pathways:

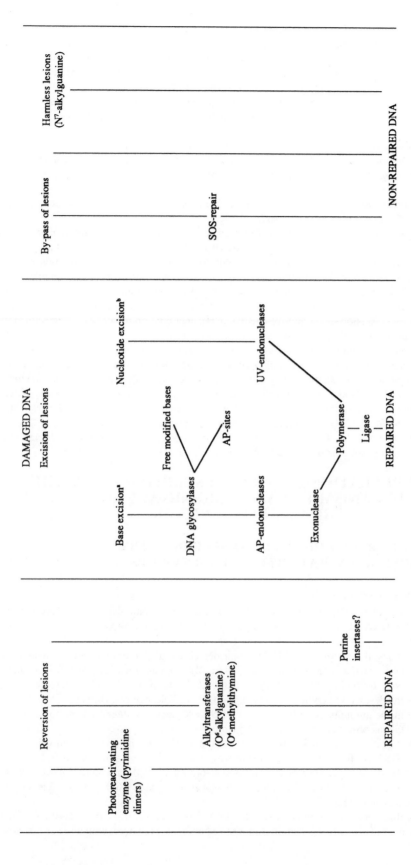

FIGURE 1. Steps in phagocytic process include migration of cells toward invading microorganisms in response to chemical stimuli, opsonization by antibodies, complement, or unspecific opsonins-like fibronectin and phagocytosis.

ª Occurs for small lesions: 3-methyladenine, 7-methylguanine, 3-methylguanine, rom⁷-guanine, hypoxanthine, etc.
ᵇ Occurs for bulky lesions: ultraviolet-induced lesions, psoralen adducts, aflatoxin adducts.

1.   With the excision of a damaged base, if DNA is damaged due to reaction with agents of a comparatively simple structure, i.e., *N*-nitroso and some other related compounds. A specific DNA glycosilase recognizes and excises a damaged base by cleavage of its bond with the deoxyribose; this is followed by formation of a corresponding apurinic or apyrimidinic site (AP) site. This site is recognized, in turn, by an AP endonuclease which nicks the DNA. Then an exonuclease excises the AP site, yielding a gap, and a DNA polymerase fills the gap with the corresponding base. Finally, a polynucleotide ligase restores the continuity of the phosphodiester chain (Figure 1).

2.   With the excision of a site of DNA consisting of some tens of nucleotides, i.e., by a "big patch" mechanism. Specific enzymes "recognize" structural distortions formed by the presence of the adduct in the DNA helix rather than the adduct itself.[4,11]

Postreplication repair concerns the third class. The cell repairs DNA damage which is restored after its replication through a recombination exchange.[8,11]

All above-mentioned types of DNA repair are followed, as a rule, by restoration of its damage (error-free repair), because the double-stranded complementary structure of DNA guarantees that genetic information which is lost by one chain is repaired due to the availability of information on the complementary chain. However, the existence of error-prone repair was postulated.[8,11] Such repair may take place if the DNA damages are situated in proximity of each other on either side of the strand. In this type of DNA repair, a genetic alteration may appear due to the absence of a nondamaged matrix.

As seen below, only excision repair and AT-mediated transmethylation repair have been studied in the investigations concerning the age-related aspects of carcinogenesis.

Since excision repair is a multistage process, it can be measured by means of various approaches, allowing the characterization of a given stage of DNA repair. The following approaches are commonly used: ultracentrifugation in an alkaline sucrose gradient, detection of activity of repair enzymes, sedimentation of nucleoids, and estimation of unscheduled DNA synthesis (UDS) by means of ^{3}H-thymidine incorporation. AT activity is measured either by the levels of accepted methyl groups due to *in vitro* incubation with O^6-MG-containing DNA, or by the decrease in concentration of O^6-MG in this DNA substrate. Besides, the efficiency of DNA repair of each type can be assessed indirectly, by the rate of removal of a given damage from DNA. For detail, see References 8 and 11.

III. INTERRELATION BETWEEN SUSCEPTIBILITY OF THE ORGANISM TO CARCINOGENIC AGENTS, AGING, AND DNA REPAIR

A. EFFICIENCY OF REPAIR OF DNA DAMAGES INDUCED BY CARCINOGENIC AGENTS AT DIFFERENT AGE PERIODS

1. UV-, γ-, and X-Ray Irradiation

As indicated in Section II, DNA damage induced by these agents is repaired by means of an excision mechanism. Besides, DNA damage induced due to exposure to UV can be repaired by a photoreactivation mechanism.

In a series of studies, it was found that DNA repair decreases in aged animals and humans after exposure to irradiation. Thus, an age-dependent decrease in DNA repair, measured by UDS, occurred in human lymphocytes following UV-[12,13] or γ-irradiation.[12] Nette et al.[14] found a decrease in the efficiency of UDS in UV-exposed epidermocytes of 60 to 79 year-old women. However, they did not find any decrease in the amounts of cells in which UDS took place. In other studies, however, no decrease in the UDS was observed in UV-irradiated fibroblasts of aged persons.[15-17]

In similar animal studies conflicting results were also obtained. Thus, in several communications, a decrease in the UDS level following UV exposure was observed in aged animals. Such data were obtained with fibroblasts of 2-year-old mice[18] and 3-year-old rats.[19] In the rat study[19] it was found, however, that only the rate of DNA repair in old animals was decreased, whereas its final level was similar in both young and old rats.

It is interesting that following a comparatively high UV dose the level of UDS in basal epidermal cells of 18-month-old mice was lower than in 2-month-old animals. However, with a lower UV dose there was no difference in the UDS level in mice of different age groups.[20] An age-dependent decrease in the level of UDS also occurred in spleen lymphocytes of two strains of mice following both UV- and γ-irradiation. It was found, however that following γ-irradiation, DNA repair proceeded only in proliferating lymphocytes, whereas UV-induced DNA repair proceeded in both proliferating and resting lymphocytes.[21]

In *in vitro* UV-irradiated hepatocytes isolated from 6-month-old rats, the level of UDS was considerably lower than in the hepatocytes taken from 14-month-old rats. However, in 32-month-old animals, the level of UDS decreased and became similar to that in the 6-month-old group. The rate of total RNA synthesis had a similar age-dependent pattern.[22] Other investigations did not reveal any difference in the rate of UDS in the hepatocytes of 2 to 3 month-old and 28 to 30-month-old rats, following *in vitro* UV irradiation.[23]

In several studies, no distinct age-associated difference in DNA repair was revealed following an exposure to carcinogenic agents of a physical nature. Thus, an essentially similar level of UDS was found in the retinal ganglion cells of rats of different ages following exposure to UV. However, the maximal age of the rats in this study did not exceed 2 years; actually these were adult rats and so DNA repair in old animals was not studied.[24] A similar rate of DNA repair, as measured by detection of the molecular mass of its fragments, occurred in the neurons of dogs of different ages following an X-ray irradiation. However, they found a progressive decline with age in the molecular mass of the DNA species.[10]

Several attempts were undertaken to measure the rate of DNA repair depending on the animal age by means of physical methods. Thus, the rate of DNA repair in young and old rats was measured by detection of the spectrum of the circular dichroism of DNA which reflects changes in the conformation of the DNA double helix. It was revealed that in the liver and brain DNA of old (38-month-old) rats, the amplitude of circular dichroism was lower than in the same tissues of young rats, indicating some distortions in the DNA helical structure in old animals. However, in young rats, exposed to γ-irradiation, the difference with old rats disappeared.[25] Thus, the distortion of DNA conformation may be associated with the efficiency of DNA repair. This association is supported by the observation that the rate of incision of γ-irradiation damaged bases of liver DNA of 20-month-old mice was lower than that in 2-month-old animals. Assuming that DNA-repairing enzymes, i.e., AP endonuclease and DNA polymerase, had a similar activity in the animals of both groups, it was suggested that the difference in DNA repair efficiency in young and old mice could be attributed to the alteration in the accessibility of damaged bases for these enzymes in the old animals, i.e., to distortions of conformation.[26] It should be mentioned that in the rats exposed to the carcinogen *N*-methyl-acetoxymethylnitrosamine (DMN-OAc), highly organized subnuclear structures (nucleoids) in the hepatocytes of 14-month-old rats were damaged to a higher extent than in 3-month-old rats, thus indicating age-associated distortions in DNA spiralization. However, in nontreated rats of the same age groups nucleoid sedimentation had a similar pattern.[27]

2. Carcinogenic Substances

As mentioned in Section II, DNA damage induced by these agents is repaired either by means of excision repair, or by transmethylation with a specific alkyltransferase.

Kanagalingam and Balis[28] were the first to study the role of age in the repair of DNA damage due to the action of carcinogenic compounds. Having measured the rate of DNA sedimentation by centrifugation in the gradient of alkaline sucrose, they found that adult, i.e., 13 to 15-month-old rats exposed to 1,2-dimethylhydrazine, which induced predominantly colonic tumors in these species, showed a lower efficacy of DNA repair in the crypts as well as in superficial cells as compared to young rats (the age was not specified). Another study revealed an increased rate of UDS in liver cells of 2-month-old rats, as compared to newborns, after administration of *N*-methylnitrosourea (NMU). However, no detectable level of UDS was registered in the kidney and brain DNA of the same rats.[29]

Using an alkaline elution technique, Fort and Cerutti[30] found that following *in vitro* exposure to *N*-ethylnitrosourea (ENU) of rat fibroblasts, DNA fragmentation in 2-year-old animals was less pronounced than in those 3 weeks-old. The authors assumed that their findings indicate an age-associated lowering of excision repair. Niedermüller[31] reported an age-dependent decrease in the rate of UDS in several rat tissues in response to carcinogens. Thus, a decreased UDS of the skin, lungs, brain, and heart was observed in 2-year-old animals following exposure to NMU as compared to that in young rats, i.e., 6-month-old, while following the exposure to methylmethane sulfonate (MMS). It was decreased in the heart and liver, and following the exposure to *N*-nitrosodimethylamine, in the kidney, duodenum, lung, and liver. Following the exposure to these three carcinogens, aged rats manifested a decreased DNA repair in the spleen and testes. In another study, the same author[32] compared age-related efficiency of different steps of DNA excision repair after administration of several chemical carcinogens. It was found that in 28-month-old rats exposed to NMU, UDS in the spleen lungs, heart, testes, muscle, and brain was reduced as compared to 9- or 18-month-old animals. However, following MMS treatment, the pattern of nucleoid sedimentation, which reveals the appearance of single-stranded DNA, was altered only in the testes and brain. However, there was no age-associated difference in the rejoining of double-stranded breaks which appeared due to exposure to 4-nitroquinoline-oxide (NQO), measured by neutral elution technique.

In two other studies, no distinct age-dependent differences in the efficiency of DNA repair was revealed. In one of these studies, UDS was measured in basal epidermal cells of 2- and 18-month-old mice exposed to different doses of NQO.[20] In the other study, after administration of *N*-hydroxy-2-acetylaminofluorene or NMU, the level of UDS was similar in the hepatocytes of 2- to 3-month-old and 28- to 30-month-old rats, although in these animals an age-associated decrease of DNA replication occurred.[23]

As we mentioned in Section II, the repair of some biologically significant adducts, such as O^6-AG and O^4-AT, which are formed in DNA after exposure to monofunctional alkylating agents, i.e., simple *N*-nitroso-, azo-, azoxy-, hydrazo-, and triazo compounds, proceeds with the participation of a specific alkyltransferase.

The activity of this enzyme in fetal and newborn tissues is comparatively low.[5-7] However, the data concerned with its activity at various periods of postnatal development are fragmentary and, in some observations, nonuniform.

Thus, Waldstein et al.[33] did not find any difference in the AT activity in the lymphocytes of males and females ranging from 20 to 60 years old, although individual levels of AT differed appreciably. Other researchers found a similar activity of AT isolated from the liver tissue of both men and women ranging from 19 to 65 years old and individual differences were negligible.[34]

The age-associated efficiency of O^6-AG repair in the DNA and O^6-AG-repairing enzyme, i.e., AT, was also studied in several animal experiments. A similar AT activity was found in the livers of 6-week old and 12-month old rats. However, the latter, as compared to young rats, showed a higher level of AT in the liver in response to administration of a liver carcinogen 2-acetylaminofluorene.[35] In another study it was found that following exposure to DMN-OAc, 3-month-old rats displayed a more efficient repair of O^6-MG from the DNA of different parts of the intestine than adult (14-month-old) rats. However, from the liver DNA, this adduct was repaired more efficiently in adult rats.[27] This observation is in agreement with another experiment which demonstrated an age-associated difference in the susceptibility of rats to the carcinogenic effect of DMN-OAc.[36]

AT activity was also compared in the livers of nontreated rats of several age groups. It was found that in 3-month-old male rats, AT was less efficient than in 1-month-old animals, the second rise in the AT activity was observed at the age of 12 months. Later, after the age of 22 months, there was a decrease in AT activity.[37]

However, Woodhead et al.[38] did not find any significant age-associated difference in the AT activity of the tissues studied, i.e., liver, spleen, brain, and kidney, in rats aged from 1 to 24 months(males) or to 37 months (females); however, some nonsignificant age-related deviations in the level of this DNA-repairing protein were observed. In the animals of all age groups, AT was most active in the liver and somewhat lower in the spleen. It is interesting that dietary restrictions did not alter AT activity in any rat tissue in any age group.

Recently, we measured in detail AT levels in the liver, kidney, and peripheral blood leukocytes of male rats aged from 1 month to 3 years. As in previous investigations,[37] we found a wave-like age-related difference in AT activity in the liver, i.e., it was lower in the rats aged 3 months than in 1-month-old animals. Later on, an increase in AT activity occurred, which reached its highest value between 1 and 2 years of age; by the age of 3 years, it went down again. However, the AT levels in the kidney and leukocytes did not differ significantly with age, and they were lower than those observed in the liver extracts, with the kidney extracts having a higher AT activity than the leukocyte extracts. In the rats of all age groups, we observed considerable individual variations in the AT activity in all the tissues studied, but no correlation could be found between the individual levels of AT in different tissues.

The discrepancies in the age-associated pattern of AT found in the above-mentioned studies could probably result from the strain-dependent peculiarities of the rats used in these experiments. In the other species, i.e., in mice, the AT activity at different ages strongly depended on the strain of animals.[39]

B. CELLULAR AGING *IN VITRO* AND DNA REPAIR

It is well known that *in vitro* normal human and animal cells have a limited number of cell divisions, after which they cease to divide, senesce, and die. Therefore, the number of cellular divisions serves as a measure of age in culture. This depends both on species longevity and donor's age[2,10,12] and allows the study of senescence under *in vitro* conditions.

Numerous experiments demonstrate that the efficiency of repair of DNA damages caused by carcinogenic agents of a physical nature weakens considerably during the period of cellular senescence, i.e., predominantly with the last one to two divisions, in parallel with the alteration of many other cellular functions.[10,12]

Thus, Goldstein[15] found a similar activity of UDS in young (20th passage) and old (56th passage) human fibroblasts following a UV irradiation. However, in the terminal stage of the all-population life span, i.e., at the 57th passage, the level of UDS was considerably decreased. A reduction of UDS occurred together with a reduction of the proliferative activity only at the last stage of cellular senescence in primary embryonal hamster UV- or γ-irradiated cultures. The efficiency of DNA repair in human skin fibroblasts evaluated by the rejoining of DNA strand breaks induced by γ-irradiation was sharply reduced as the cells approached senescence, i.e., at the final one or two population doublings.[10]

Several studies, though, suggest age-associated differences in the efficiency of DNA repair before the cells reach the end of their life span. Thus, it was found that UV-induced DNA repair in fibroblast-like human cells, measured by the calculation of the number of nuclease-sensitive sites in the DNA, was more efficient in cells at a high population doubling level than in younger cells. In nonexposed cells, DNA damages accumulated with aging.[40] However, no difference was revealed in the repair efficiency of X-ray induced single-strand breaks in the culture of young and old human lung fibroblasts,[41] whereas the repair of modified thymine from γ-irradiated exogenous DNA by nuclei from old cells was reduced.[42]

C. RELATIONSHIP BETWEEN THE EFFICIENCY OF DNA REPAIR AND SPECIES LONGEVITY

Many studies show a correlation between species longevity and the efficiency of DNA repair. The first report was published in 1974[43] and showed that the level of UDS in the UV-irradiated DNA of primary fibroblastic cultures taken from seven different species was proportional to species longevity. A similar correlation was found in a study involving 30 different species.[44] In response to UV irradiation, the UDS in primary cultures of hepatocytes proceeded more efficiently in longer living animals, i.e., guinea pigs and rabbits vs. mice and rats.[45] A direct correlation between life span and excision-repair efficiency of spontaneous and irradiation-induced DNA damage was also found in different species of mice[46,47] and of primates.[48] Both mice and primate species studied had considerable differences in their longevity.

Other studies revealed no correlation between the maximal life span and the efficiency of excision repair. Kate et al.[49] did not find any correlation between longevity and DNA repair efficiency in 34 mammalian species. A similar conclusion was made by Woodhead et al.,[50] who studied the interrelation between species longevity and the efficiency of DNA repair in some cold-blooded vertebrates. The discrepancies were suggested to have resulted from the inadequacy of methods used by these two authors.[2]

Some studies demonstrate that it is not only excision-repair that is more efficient in long-living species. As mentioned above, human liver AT has a considerably higher activity than rat liver AT[34] and the liver of another long-living species, the monkey, has an AT activity comparable to that of human liver.[51] Some studies demonstrate that cell cultures from individuals with Werner's and Cockayne's syndromes, as well as with Falkoni's anemia, have a reduced life span.

D. DNA REPAIR IN PREMATURE AGING SYNDROMES

Progeroid syndromes are rare genetic diseases. The data concerning DNA repair in progeria syndrome patients are scarce and do not suggest a deficiency.[2,12] However, deficient excision repair was found in the cells of patients with another progeroid syndrome. Thus, significant reduction of UDS was found in patients with Cockayne's syndrome,[52] as well as in individuals with ataxia telangiectasia.[52] A very high sensitivity to UV is characteristic of both Cockayne's syndrome and ataxia telangiectasia. The incidence of various tumors in patients with ataxia telangiectasia considerably exceeds that in healthy humans. No appropriate data on Cockayne's syndrome are available.[2,12]

Patients with xeroderma pigmentosum, which is characterized by a high sensitivity to sunlight, also show a high probability of tumor development, mainly skin cancer. These patients are also deficient in excision repair.[52] Both hypersensitivity to UV and increased cancer incidence are apparently the consequence of the deficiency in DNA excision repair in this syndrome.

Another type of DNA repair, i.e., AT-mediated transmethylation, is not deficient in the fibroblasts of both ataxia telangiectasia and xeroderma pigmentosum patients.[53,54] The latter study also demonstrated that the activity of the excision repair enzyme, DNA glycoyslase, is reduced in these patients.

IV. CONCLUSION

A survey of the data available concerning repair of DNA damages caused by carcinogenic agents of different natures demonstrates that this problem is poorly studied.

These data give the following general trend. Toward the end of the perinatal period there is an increase in the competence of DNA repair systems.[2,5] Subsequently, the efficiency of repair, with the exception of AT-mediated transmethylation repair, does not change appreciably, and becomes reduced only in the terminal period of the life span.

In the majority of studies, the age-dependent dynamics of DNA repair were not properly studied. For instance, the level of UDS in the hepatocytes of both young and old rats following their *in vitro* UV irradiation was essentially similar.[23] Thus, it can be concluded that aging did not change the efficiency of DNA repair. However, another study[22] indicated a considerable increase in UDS in the hepatocytes of adult rats, as compared to young ones, which was followed by its reduction toward the older age, and hence, led to the loss of differences between young and old animals.

Many investigations revealed no age-related changes in the functioning of different types of DNA repair (Table 1). Such conflicting results could, evidently, be obtained due to the different methods used. For instance, excision repair is often characterized by only one of its steps, which may not reflect the whole process. Another source of conflict results from the fact that it is mainly the rate of repair that has been studied, but not the final result. Besides, in many studies, adult animals are considered as old subjects. In a considerable portion of experiments, the effect of aging on DNA repair was studied on models which corresponded to an artificial situation, e.g., detection of UDS in fibroblasts, leukocytes, or hepatocytes exposed to UV. Furthermore, DNA repair is often analyzed in tissues where a given carcinogen never induces tumors. On the other hand, studies of excision repair following the exposure to monofunctional alkylating agents characterize a restoration of DNA damages which apparently are not related to carcinogenesis. Only in a few experiments has the relationship between carcinogen dose effect and the age characteristics of DNA repair been studied. Moreover, it is evident that the effect of cellular aging on DNA repair in cell cultures cannot be completely identical to an *in vivo* situation.

In some experiments, the age-dependent characteristics of DNA repair were detected by physical methods. Such an approach seems to be quite promising because it allows the study of the primary structure of DNA and the restoration of its conformation, which is necessary for normal DNA functioning.

Experiments on animals with a different life span showed that their longevity usually correlates with the efficiency of different types of DNA repair.

Finally, the studies on the individuals with progeroid syndromes depicted, in general, deficiencies in excision-repair and a reduced life span of their cells. However, these studies often show no correlation between deficient repair and aging. Thus, patients with a true progeria, i.e., Hutchinson-Gilford syndrome, revealed no deficiency in DNA repair, whereas the latter was considerably reduced in the cells of xeroderma pigmentosum patients whose life span was not reduced.[2,52] The data available show that AT activity is not decreased in these syndromes.

The variation in DNA repair efficiency with age could play a role in the different susceptibility to carcinogens during senescence. However, DNA repair alone cannot be responsible since other factors, such as proliferative activity, competence of drug-metabolizing enzymes, adduct formation, and immune status, are also important determinants of the susceptibility to carcinogens.

TABLE 1
Effect of Aging on DNA Repair Efficacy in Carcinogen-Damaged Tissues

Carcinogen	Tissue	Species	Age groups, months/years	Effect of aging
Pyrimidine Dimers				
UV light	Lymphocytes	Human	13-94 years	Decreases
			22 and 54 years	Decreases
			17-69 years	No effect
	Epidermis	Human	0-70 years	No effect
			17-77 years	Decreases
	Kidney	Human	30-82 years	No effect
	Liver	Rat	6 and 14	Increases
			14 and 32	Decreases
	Lens epithelium	Rat	14 and 40	No effect
	Retinal ganglion	Rat	1-6 and 23	No effect
	Kidney, lung	Hamster	1 and 17	No effect
	Brain, liver	Hamster	1.2 and 18	No effect
DNA Strand Breaks				
X-rays	Lymphocytes	Human	0-70 years	Decreases
			7-60 and 60-69 years	Decreases
	Cerebellum	Dog	1.5 months and 13 years	No effect
		Mouse	2 and 22	No effect
γ-Rays	Lymphocytes	Human	0-70 years	Decreases
	Liver	Mouse	1.5-2 and 18-22 mos	Decreases
	Thymus	Mouse	1 and 18 mos	No effect
Electrons	Skin	Rat	1-6 and 13 months	Decreases
Apurinic Sites				
N-OH-2-AFF	Lymphocytes	Human	0-10 and 51-60 years	Decreases
			51-60 and 71-80 years	No effect
NQO, ENU	Retinal ganglion	Rat	1-6 and 23 months	No effect
ENU	Fibroblasts	Rat	3 weeks and 24 months	Decreases
MNU	Skin, lung, brain, heart, spleen, gonads	Rat	6, 24-26 months	Decreases
	Liver, kidney, duodenum, muscle	Rat	6, 24-26 months	No effect
NDMA	Kidney, lung duodenum, heart, gonads, spleen	Rat	6, 24-26 months	Decreases
	Skin, brain, heart, muscle	Rat	6, 24-26 months	No effect
DMH	Colon	Rat	3-4, 13-15 months	Decreases
DMN-OAc	Colon, ileum, lung, liver, uterus	Rat	3,14 months	Decreases
DMBA	Mammary epithelium	Rat	1.5, 5 mos	Increases

TABLE 1 (continued)
Effect of Aging on DNA Repair Efficacy in Carcinogen-Damaged Tissues

Carcinogen	Tissue	Species	Age groups, Months/years	Effect of aging
		Alkylation of Guanine at O⁶ Position		
DENA	Liver	Rat	3 and 14 mos	Decreases
	Kidney	Rat	3 and 14 mos	Increases
DMN-OAc	Liver	Rat	3 and 14 mos	Increases
	Colon, ileum	Rat	3 and 14 mos	Decreases
	Lung	Rat	3 and 14 mos	No effect

Abbreviations: N-OH-2-AAF = N-hydroxy-2-acetylaminofluorene; ENU = N-ethylnitrosourea; NDMA = N-nitrosodimethylamine; DMH = 1,2-dimethylhydrazine; DMBA = 7,12-dimethylbenz(a)anthracene; DENA = N-nitrosodiethylamine.

From Anisimov, V. N., *Carcinogenesis and Aging,* Vol. 1, CRC Press, Boca Raton, FL 1987, 130. With permission

ACKNOWLEDGMENTS

I would like to thank Professor N.P. Napalkov for his continuous interest in this work, Dr. V. N. Anisimov, Dr. L. M. Berstein, Dr. E. H. von Hofe, and Dr. M. A. Zabezhinsky for their valuable suggestions and Mrs. O. N. Mikhailova for her editorial help and typing of the manuscript. Some experiments surveyed in this review were performed in collaboration with Drs. V. N. Anisimov, N. V. Zhukovskaya, and J. Hall.

REFERENCES

1. **Druckrey, H.,** Quantitative aspects in chemical carcinogenesis, in *Potential Carcinogenic Hazards from Drugs,* UICC Monogr. Series No. 7, Truhaut, R., Ed., Springer-Verlag, New York, 1967, 60.
2. **Anisimov, V. N.,** *Carcinogenesis and Aging,* Vols. 1 and 2, CRC Press, Boca Raton, FL, 1987.
3. **Likhachev, A., Anisimov, V., and Montesano, R., Eds.,** *Age-Related Factors in Carcinogenesis,* IARC Sci. Publ. No. 58, International Agency for Research on Cancer, Lyon, 1985.
4. **Singer B. and Grunberger, D.,** *Molecular Biology of Mutagens and Carcinogens,* Plenum Press, New York, 1983.
5. **Napalkov, N. P., Anisimov, V. N., Knyazev, P. G., and Likhachev, A. J.,** *Modern Concepts of Carcinogenesis Mechanisms, Monogr. Rev.,* Vol. 5, All-Union Institute of Medical Information, Moscow, 1987.
6. **Lindahl, T.,** DNA repair enzymes, *Ann. Rev. Biochem.,* 51, 61, 1982.
7. **Karran, P. and Lindahl, T.,** Cellular defense mechanisms against alkylating agents, *Cancer Surv.,* 4, 583, 1985.
8. **Mehlman, M. A., Ser. Ed.,** *Advances in Modern Environmental Toxicology, Vol. XII, Mechanisms and Toxicity of Chemical Carcinogens and Mutagens,* Flamm, W. G. and Lorentzen, R. J., Eds., Princeton Scientific, Princeton, NJ, 1985.
9. **Loeb, L. A. and Preston, B. D.,** Mutagenesis by apurinic/apyrimidinic sites, *Ann. Rev. Genet.,* 20, 201, 1986.
10. **Little, G. B.,** Relationship between DNA repair capacity and cellular aging, *Gerontology,* 22, 28, 1976.
11. **Laval, F. and Huet, J.,** DNA repair in relation to biological monitoring of exposure to mutagens and carcinogens, in *Monitoring Human Exposure to Carcinogenic and Mutagenic Agents,* IARC Sci. Publ. No. 59, Berling, A., Draper, M., Hemminki, K., and Vainio, H., Eds., International Agency for Research on Cancer, Lyon, 1984, 371.
12. **Lehmann, A. R.,** Ageing, DNA repair of radiation damage and carcinogenesis: fact and fiction, in *Age-Related Factors in Carcinogenesis,* IARC Sci. Publ. No. 58, Likhachev, A., Anisimov, V., and Montesano, R., Eds., International Agency for Research on Cancer, Lyon, 1985, 203.
13. **Dilman, V. M. and Revskoy, S. Y.,** Study on correlation between DNA repair and level of cholesterol in serum and lymphocytes, *Hum. Physiol.,* 7, 125, 1981.
14. **Nette, E. G., Xi, Yu-Ping, Sun, Yu-Kay, Andrews, A. D., and King, D. W.,** A correlation between aging and DNA repair in human epidermal cells, *Mech. Ageing Dev.,* 24, 283, 1984.

15. **Goldstein, S.,** The role of DNA repair in aging of cultured fibroblasts from xeroderma pigmentosum and normals, *Proc. Soc. Exp. Biol. Med.,* 137, 730, 1971.

16. **Hennis, H. L., Draid, H. L., and Vincent, R. A.,** Unscheduled DNA synthesis in cells of different shape in fibroblast cultures from donors of various ages, *Mech. Ageing Dev.,* 16, 355, 1981.

17. **Hall, J. D., Almy, R. E., and Scherer, K. L.,** DNA repair in cultured fibroblasts does not decline with donor age, *Exp. Cell Res.,* 139, 351, 1982.

18. **Kempf, C., Schmitt, M., Danse, J.-M, and Kemp. J.,** Correlation of DNA repair synthesis with aging in mice evidenced by quantitative autoradius actoradiography, *Mech. Ageing Dev.,* 26, 183, 1984.

19. **Vijg, J., Mullaart, E., Lohman, P. H. M., and Knook, D. L.,** UV-induced unscheduled DNA synthesis in fibroblasts of aging inbred rats, *Mutat. Res.,* 146, 197, 1985.

20. **Ishikawa, T., and Sakura, J.,** *In vivo* studies on age dependency of DNA repair with age in mouse skin, *Cancer Res.,* 46, 1344, 1986.

21. **Licastro, F. and Walford, R. L.,** Proliferative potential and DNA repair in lymphocytes from short-lived and long-lived strains of mice, relation to ageing, *Mech. Ageing Dev.,* 31, 171, 1985.

22. **Richardson, A., Birchenall-Sparks, M. C., and Plesko, M. M.,** Age-related changes in translation and transcription in isolated hepatocytes, in *Pharmacological, Morphological and Physiological Aspects of Liver Aging,* Bezooijen, C. F. A., Ed., Eurage, Rijswijk, The Netherlands, 1984, 3.

23. **Sawada, N. and Takatoshi, I.,** Reduction of potential for replicative but not unscheduled DNA synthesis in hepatocytes isolated from aged as compared to young rats, *Cancer Res.,* 48, 1618, 1988

24. **Ishikawa, T., Takayama, S., and Kitagawa, T.,** DNA repair synthesis in rat retinal ganglion cells treated with chemical carcinogens or ultraviolet light *in vitro,* with special reference to aging and repair level, *J. Natl. Cancer Inst.,* 61, 1101, 1978.

25. **Vilenchik, M. M., Tretjak, T. M., Lobachev, V. M., and Kuzin, A. M.,** DNA of old rat tissues is characterized by a spectrum of circular dichroism similar to the spectrum of gamma-irradiated DNA, *Dokl. Akad. Nauk SSSR,* 259, 1488, 1981.

26. **Malakhova, L. V. and Fomenko, L. A.,** A slow elimination of altered bases in liver DNA of gamma-irradiated aged mice, *Dokl. Adad. Nauk SSSR,* 257, 725, 1981.

27. **Likhachev, A. J., Oshima, H., Anisimov, V. N., Ovsyannikov, A. I., Revskoy, S. Yu., Keefer, L. K., and Reist, E. J.,** Carcinogenesis and aging. II. Modifying effect of aging on metabolism of methyl(acetoxymethyl)nitrosamine and its interaction with DNA of various tissues in rats, *Carcinogenesis,* 4, 967, 1983.

28. **Kanagalingam, K. and Balis, M. E.,** *In vivo* repair of rat intestinal DNA damage by alkylating agents, *Cancer,* 36, 2364, 1975.

29. **Arfellini, G., Grilli, S., and Prodi, G.,** *In vivo* DNA repair after N-methyl-N-nitrosourea administration to rats of different ages, *Z. Krebsforsch.,* 91, 157, 1978

30. **Fort, F. L. and Cerutti, P. A.,** Altered DNA repair in fibroblasts from aged rats, *Gerontology,* 27, 306, 1981.

31. **Niedermüller, H.,** Age dependency of DNA repair in rats after DNA damage by carcinogens, *Mech. Ageing Dev.,* 19, 259, 1982.

32. **Niedermüller, H., Hofecker, G., and Skalicky, M.,** Changes of DNA repair mechanisms during the aging of the rat, *Mech. Ageing Dev.,* 29, 221, 1985.

33. **Waldstein, E. A., Cao, En-Hua, Bender, M. A., and Setlow, R. B.,** Abilities of extracts of human lymphocytes to remove O^6-methylguanine from DNA, *Mutat. Res.,* 95, 405, 1982.

34. **Pegg, A. E., Roberfroid, M., von Bahr, C., Foote, R. S., Mitra, S., Bresil, H., Likhachev, A., and Montesano, R.,** Removal of O^6-methylguanine from DNA by human liver fractions, *Proc. Natl. Acad. Sci. U.S.A.,* 79, 5162, 1982.

35. **Margison, G. P.,** The effect of age on the metabolism of chemical carcinogens and inducibility of O^6-methylguanine methyltransferase, in *Age-Related Factors in Carcinogenesis,* IARC, Sci., Publ. No. 58, Likhachev, A., Anisimov, B., and Montesano, R., Eds., International Agency for Research on Cancer, Lyon, 1985, 225.

36. **Likhachev, A. J., Anisimov, V. M., and Ovsyannikov, A. I.,** Some peculiarities of carcinogenic effect of methyl (acetoxymethyl)nitrosamine and DNA repair in rats of different age, *Exp. Oncol.,* 8, 18, 1986.

37. **Likhachev, A. J.,** Effect of age on DNA repair in carcinogenesis due to alkylating agents, in *Age-related Factors in Carcinogenesis,* IARC Sc. Publ. No. 58, Likhachev, A., Anisimov, V., and Montesano, R., Eds., International Agency for Research on Cancer, Lyon, 1985, 239.

38. **Woodhead, A. D., Merry, B. J., Cao, En-Hua, Holehan, A. M., Grist, E., and Carlson, C.,** Levels of O^6-methylguanine acceptor protein in tissues of rats and their relationship to carcinogenicity and aging, *J. Natl. Cancer Inst.,* 75, 1141, 1985.

39. **Nakatsuru, Y., Aoki, K., and Ishikawa, T.,** Age and strain dependence of O^6-methylguanine-DNA methyltransferase activity in mice, *Mutat.Res.,* 219, 51, 1989.

40. **Dell'orco, R. T. and Whittle, W. L.,** Evidence for an increased level of DNA damage in high doubling level human diploid cells in culture, *Mech. Ageing Dev.,* 15, 141, 1981.

41. **Clarkson, J. M. and Painter, R. B.,** Repair of X-ray damage in aging WI-38 cells, *Mutat. Res.,* 23, 107, 1974.

42. **Mattern, M. R. and Cerutti, P. A.,** Age dependence of excision repair of gamma-ray-damaged thymine by isolated nuclei from diploid human lung fibroblasts WI 38, *Nature,* 254, 450, 1975.

43. **Hart, R. W. and Setlow, R. B.,** Correlation between deoxyribonucleic acid excision repair and lifespan in a number of mammalian species, *Proc. Natl. Acad. Sci. U.S.A.,* 71, 2169, 1974.

44. **Francis, A. A., Lee, W. H., and Regan, J. D.,** The relationship of DNA excision repair of ultraviolet-induced lesions to the maximum lifespan of mammals, *Mech. Ageing Dev.,* 16, 181, 1981.

45. **Maslansky, C. J. and Williams, G. M.,** Ultraviolet light-induced DNA repair synthesis in hepatocytes from species of differing longevities, *Mech. Ageing Dev.,* 29, 191, 1985.

46. **Hart, R. W., Sacher, G. A. and Hoskins, T. L.,** DNA repair in a short- and long-lived rodent species, *J. Gerontol.,* 34, 808, 1979.

47. **Su, C. M., Brash, D. E., Turturro, A., and Hart, R. W.,** Longevity-dependent organ-specific accumulation of DNA damage in two closely related murine species, *Mech. Ageing Dev.,* 27, 239, 1984.

48. **Hall, K. Y., Hart, R. W., Benirschke, A. K., and Walford, R. L.,** Correlation between ultraviolet-induced DNA repair in primate lymphocytes and fibroblasts and species maximum achievable life span, *Mech. Ageing Dev.,* 24, 163, 1984.

49. **Kato, H., Harafa, M., Tsuchiya, K., and Moriwaki, K.,** Absence of correlation between DNA repair in ultraviolet-irradiated mammalian cells and life span of the donor species, *Jpn. J. Genet.,* 55, 99, 1980.

50. **Woodhead, A. D., Setlow, R. B., and Grist, E.,** DNA repair and longevity in three species of cold-blooded vertebrates, *Exp. Gerontol.,* 15, 301, 1980.

51. **Hall, J., Brésil, H., and Montesano, R.,** O^6-alkylguanine DNA transferase activity in monkey, human and rat liver, *Carcinogenesis,* 6, 209, 1985.

52. **Lehman, A. R.,** Cancer-associated human genetic diseases with defects in DNA repair, *J. Cancer Res. Clin. Oncol.,* 100, 117, 1981.

53. **Medcalf, A. S. C. and Lawley, P. D.,** Time course of O^6-methylguanine removal from DNA of *N*-methyl-*N*-nitrosourea-treated human fibroblasts, *Nature,* 289, 796, 1981.

54. **Harris, A. L., Karran, P., and Lindahl, T.,** O^6-methylguanine-DNA methyltransferase of human lymphoid cells: structural and kinetic properties and absence in repair-deficient cells, *Cancer Res.,* 43, 3247, 1983.

55. **Thompson, K. V. A. and Holliday, R.,** Genetic effects on the longevity of cultured human fibroblasts. II. DNA repair deficient syndromes, *Gerontology,* 29, 73, 1983.

Chapter 6

REPRODUCTIVE AND HORMONAL FACTORS IN RELATION TO CANCER OCCURRENCE IN THE BREAST, PROSTATE, TESTIS, UTERINE CORPUS, OVARY, UTERINE CERVIX, AND THYROID GLAND

H. Olsson

TABLE OF CONTENTS

The incidence of most malignant tumors, in general, increases steadily with age. Mathematically the increase could be represented by the equation[1,2]

$$I(t) = at^k$$

where I = incidence of the malignant tumor, t = age, k = the exponent (often between 4 and 5), and a = a constant.

Examples of tumors demonstrating the above age dependence are cancer of the lung and stomach. The incidence of tumors affecting the reproductive organs is modified by reproductive factors in various modes and in this chapter the occurrence of malignant tumors of the breast, gynecological organs, testis, prostate, and the thyroid are discussed in relation to the age dependency of various risk factors, tumor biology, and latency times. Comprehensive reviews of the incidence and risk factors of tumors originating in reproductive organs have earlier been presented in References 2 through 6.

I. BREAST CANCER

A. AGE AND INCIDENCE

As the most common malignant tumor in women, cancer of the breast comprises one fourth of all malignancies among women.[7] In men, malignant tumors of the breast are rare; only about 1% of all breast tumors occurs in men.[8] The mean age at presentation in industrialized countries is 10 years later for men; approximately 71 years compared with 61 years for women.[7] The incidence of breast cancer increases sharply with age (see Figure 1). Perimenopausally, the increase in incidence of breast cancer in women is slowing down, indicating an important effect of menopause on incidence. This was first described by Clemmesen[9] and later reproduced by others. For men, no such change in incidence is seen,[10] supporting the hypothesis that the reproductive factors affect only the incidence of breast cancer in females. By 45 years of age, the cumulative incidence of breast cancer in women is somewhat less than 1% to reach around 8% by 75 years of age. During a lifetime, approximately 1 woman in 13 develops breast cancer. Premenopausal incidence of breast cancer does not show great geographic differences, while postmenopausal incidence varies extensively between high risk areas (such as the U.S. and Western Europe) and low risk areas (such as Japan).[11-12]

Mammographic screening in postmenopausal women increases cancer incidence in screened age groups, especially during the first screening phase.

B. AGE AND RISK FACTORS

The commonness of malignant tumors of the female breast in relation to the size of the organ is somewhat surprising and most probably is explained by the dynamics of the breast epithelium rather than its cell quantity. The uniqueness of the female breast in propensity to cancer (25% of all malignant tumors in women) is further substantiated by a comparison with some domestic animals. Breast cancer constitutes in dogs approximatively 13%, in cats 5%, and in cattle and horses 1% of all cancers.[13] Both in animals and in man cell proliferation and the number of proliferating cells probably are important for carcinogenesis.[14] Reproductive and hormonal factors, while themselves not carcinogenic, could promote carcinogenesis at the time of initiation by increasing the number of proliferating cells. For the female breast, the susceptibility of the breast to tumor development is augmented during early reproductive years, especially prior to the first pregnancy and between 10 to 25 years of age.[2,6,15,16] This coincides with the time of highest cell proliferation in the normal breast epithelia and with the large increase in breast volume due to development of the ductal epithelium.[17] A full-term pregnancy reduces the proliferation of the breast as does an increasing age of the woman.[18]

1. Latency Time

Knowledge from breast cancer development after ionizing irradiation, extrapolation of growth curves from mammographically diagnosed tumors, and mathematical models extrapolating information from growth rates (labeling indices or S-phases) points to latency times between 10 and 30 years for breast cancer development.[19-22]

2. Ionizing Irradiation

Survivors of the atomic bomb blasts in Hiroshima and Nagasaki experienced a higher risk of breast cancer.[19,20] The increased risk was first and foremost shown for women between 10 to 25 years of age at irradiation.[20] Similar findings have been made among groups of women being exposed to therapeutic ionizing irradiation for benign disorders such as mastitis.[23] However, women irradiated for breast cancer pre-, peri-, or postoperatively have not displayed an increased risk for breast cancer development of the contralateral breast compared with unirradiated patients.[24,25] The latter could at least partially be explained by the fact that the radiation treatment was given at older ages when the breast epithelium was less sensitive for carcinogenesis.

3. Reproductive Factors

An early age at menarche (AM), a late age at first full-term pregnancy (AFFP), a low parity, and a late menopause, all increase the risk for breast cancer.[6,26] These findings strongly suggest that menstrual and reproductive events are related to breast cancer risk. However, all investigations have not confirmed the importance of individual factors. For example, in some Scandinavian investigations the risk association with a late AFFP has been weak.[27-30] These authors suggest that the above factors are only indirectly related to breast cancer risk.

A propensity for short, regular cycles in breast cancer patients and a lack of long cycles made us suggest in 1983 that the cumulative number of menstrual cycles could be of importance for the risk of breast cancer.[31] The hypothesis was further generalized to other gynecological tumors by Johansson[32] and further developed for breast cancer by Henderson et al.[33] incorporating other risk factors for breast cancer. While retrospectively counting the number of cycles prior to the first full-term pregnancy, we recently found that the number of cycles was the most important risk factor for breast cancer, while age at menarche and age at first full-term pregnancy lost their importance as risk factors.[34] Recent investigations of age at menarche, age at first full term

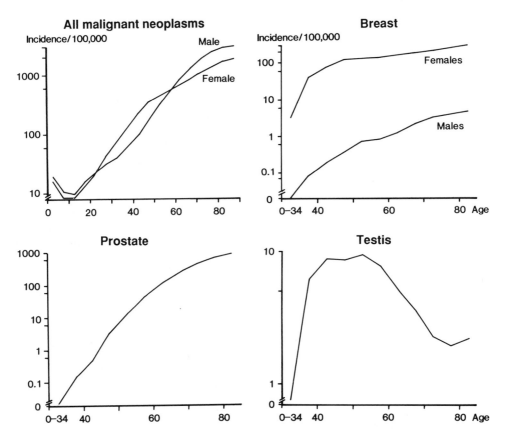

FIGURE 1.   Incidence of all malignant neoplasms, breast cancer, cancer of the prostate, testis, ovary, uterine corpus, uterine cervix, and thyroid in relation to age and sex in the Nordic countries, 1970-1982.[8]

pregnancy, parity, lactation, and menstrual cycle length give further support to the theory that the number of regular cycles is of great importance for the breast cancer risk.[35-39] From the above discussion it could be hypothesized that the effect from the cycles would be expected to be particularly strong in early reproductive life. A number of theories regarding breast cancer development converging on the importance of events in early reproductive life has been published.[2,3,33,40-44] The effect of parity on breast cancer risk may be dual; initially close to the first full-term pregnancy, the risk may be augmented while later reducing the risk.[45]

4. Lactation

Early investigation of lactation and risk for breast cancer did not demonstrate in a convincing way that breast cancer was related to lactation.[46] However, recent investigations have challenged this by showing a protective effect.[39,47,48] The investigation from China[39] describing only a 30% risk of breast cancer in women lactating for very long periods is especially interesting and again gives support to the cumulative menstrual cycle hypothesis as lactation tends to inhibit menstrual cycling.

5. Early Abortions

Some studies have indicated that early abortions may increase the risk of breast cancer.[49,51] This has not been seen for abortions after the first full-term pregnancy.[49-51] It is possible that interrupted pregnancies prior to the first full-term pregnancy, contrary to a full-term pregnancy, increase proliferation of the breast epithelium and thus increase the cancer risk.

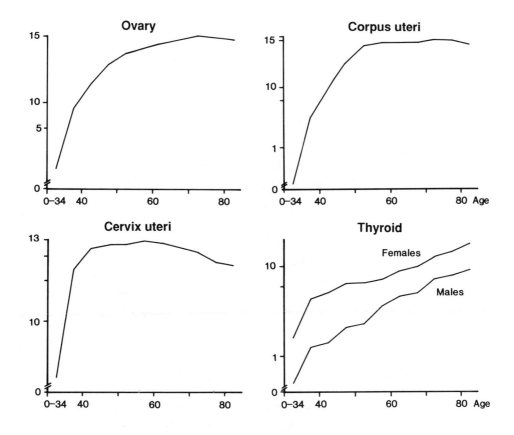

FIGURE 1 (continued).

6. Combined Oral Contraceptives (OCs)

Early studies on OC use did not find an adverse effect on the risk of breast cancer.[16] However, contrary to the situation for ovarian and endometrial cancer, no protective effect was seen.[16] During the 1980s evidence was accumulated that early OC use increases the risk of premenopausal breast cancer.[16] Early use, whether defined as a low starting age of OC use,[52] duration of use prior to the first pregnancy,[53-55] or duration of use before 25 years of age[55] or overall duration of use[54] have in individual studies been associated with augmented breast cancer risk. The reasons for the previous inconsistency have been lively debated.[55-66] A possible explanation for this has been offered by McPherson et al.,[67] suggesting that due to different prescription habits, studies not yet showing a risk may have been carried out in geographical areas with too short a latency time for breast cancer development. Reanalyses of studies originally not displaying a risk[53,68] and a cohort showing an increasing risk[69] have made the hypothesis that early use increases the risk more probable. Findings that early users who later develop breast cancer also have larger primary breast tumors, more often have axillary metastases, more often have tumors lacking estrogen and progesterone receptors, and have a poorer survival[59,70-72] further support a relationship.

The studies of early OC use describing an increased premenopausal breast cancer risk so far relate to artificial hormone use during the 1960s and early 1970s. Another 15 to 20 years of follow-up have to elapse before we are able to assess the risk for premenopausal breast cancer after low dose OC use and peri- and postmenopausal risk after high dose OC use.

7. Exogenous Hormones Perimenopausally

Recent studies on perimenopausal hormone use have indicated that the risk of developing breast cancer postmenopausally is moderately increased after perimenopausal OC use and estrogen use.[73-77] An increased risk was evident for duration of hormone use[73,74,77] and longer time between use and diagnosis (latency time).[73]

8. Dietary Factors

In animal studies, a diet high in fat increases the risk for developing breast tumors.[78,79] While studies correlating fat and protein consumption in different countries and breast cancer incidence show a high association, case controls studies designed to measure fat intake on an individual basis have failed to provide conclusive evidence that fat intake increases the risk of human breast cancer.[6] One possibility for the difficulty in these latter studies may be that the fat intake does not differ sufficiently in industrialized countries for detecting a difference between cases and referents.

9. Constitutional Factors

Patients with postmenopausal breast cancer are, on average, heavier than healthy referents, while premenopausal patients tend to weigh less than healthy referents.[80-82] This may indicate that the increased fat tissue plays a role in converting adrenal steroids into estrogens in postmenopausal cases.[83,84] An increased risk for development of postmenopausal breast cancer in women cholecystectomized 30 years prior to the breast cancer diagnosis[85] may also be due to the above mechanism as the risk of gallstones is higher in obese women.[85]

10. Familial Factors

Breast cancer in certain families shows a monogenic inheritance.[86,87] The proportion of cases showing this extreme disposition could be as high as 8 to 10%. In such families, cumulatively up to 50% of the females develops breast cancer. In other families the disposition is related to a mixture of ovarian and breast tumors, or a mixture of endometrial, colon cancer, and breast cancer, and in still other families brain tumors, sarcomas, leukemia, and breast cancer occur together.[86] Familial cases often present at an earlier age, have a tendency to bilaterality and multifocal involvement of the breast, and cases show a somewhat better prognosis than sporadic ones.[86,87] Estimates of the risk for a woman to develop breast cancer have been done in relation to number of first degree relatives with breast cancer, the age at diagnosis of first degree relative, and whether the tumor in the relative was bilateral. A woman, with two first degree relatives with breast cancer before 60 years of age and with at least one of the relatives with bilateral cancer, could have a cumulative risk of 50% to develop breast cancer.[88]

In general, the familial influence for breast cancer is less (in many investigations only doubling or tripling the risk of breast cancer).[89] In separate investigations it has also been found that age at menarche, low parity, and age at first full-term pregnancy are not risk factors for familial cases.[90-92] In our own investigation, familial cases were found to have shorter than average menstrual cycles than controls,[91] again raising the possibility that the cumulative number of cycles is of importance for the risk.

11. Trends in Incidence

The incidence of breast cancer is generally now increasing in developing countries.[11,93] Screening activities increase the incidence for women over 50 years of age. In young women (unscreened age groups), an increased incidence has also been seen.[59,94,95] It has been postulated that the increase could be due to previous early OC use, because conventional risk factors cannot explain the change.[93,95]

12. Male Breast Cancer

In men with breast cancer, beside familial factors, exposure to ionizing irradiation and the XXY constitutional karyotype, factors affecting gonadal function,[96,97] and plasma prolactin levels[97] have been hypothesized to increase breast cancer risk.

C. AGE, TUMOR BIOLOGY, AND PROGNOSIS

1. Tumor Biology

Young women with breast cancer have a higher proliferation rate in their breast tumors,[98-103] and a tendency for more aneuploid tumors.[104] Estrogen receptor content is lower in premenopausal women than in postmenopausal women.[105] Early users of OCs have a lower estrogen receptor content in their primary tumor and in benign uterine mucosae compared with later users and never users.[70,72]

Before the first full-term pregnancy women who have used OCs have a higher proliferation rate of normal breast epithelium than nonusers, while after the first pregnancy no difference is seen.[18] An hypothesis has been forwarded that both animal and human data indicate that reproductive events taking place early in reproductive life may have an important influence on growth characteristics and reproductive hormone regulation in both normal and neoplastic tissue investigated later in life.[44] Thus, tumors occurring in younger women may be more undifferentiated due to their origin from a less differentiated epithelia and tumor characteristics at diagnosis at least partly reflect the normal physiology at time of initiation.

2. Prognosis

The prognosis of breast cancer is worse in very young and very old patients.[106,107] In young women this may point to a more "aggressive tumor biology" reflecting, according to the above hypothesis, a more undifferentiated normal tissue at the time of initiation. The worse prognosis in elderly patients could be due to delayed diagnosis and less intensive treatment. Young women with breast cancer who at an early age have used OCs have a worse prognosis[69,72] even after adjusting for age at diagnosis, stage, and adjuvant treatment given.[72] These women also show a lower hormone receptor concentration in their primary tumors.[70,72] Patients diagnosed during pregnancy have a worse prognosis compared with age- and stage-matched patients.[108,109] This could reflect that tumors originating in breast epithelium not fully differentiated through the pregnancy have a worse outcome. Again, more receptor negative tumors (especially low in progesterone receptors) are seen.[109] This probably reflects similar findings in mice that receptor development in not fully differentiated mammary epithelium does not yet show the estrogen dependent progesterone receptor.[110]

The prognosis of breast cancer detected postmenopausally in women with a history of estrogen substitution for menopausal symptoms, has not yet been investigated. However, from the above reasoning it could be postulated that these tumors occur in a more differentiated tissue and thus ought to have a better prognosis than tumors initiated at a younger age.

II. PROSTATIC CARCINOMA

A. AGE AND INCIDENCE

The incidence of prostatic carcinoma increases with age (Figure 1) and constitutes the most common tumor type in the male.[8] In contrast to cancer of the female breast, the incidence curve for prostatic tumors does not show any important changes in the trend in relation to the reproductive years of the male (Figure 1). Around 20% of all malignant tumors in men arise in the prostatic gland[7] and become very common in older men often diagnosed as latent carcinoma without prior symptoms as an incidental finding or at autopsy.[111,112]

B. AGE AND RISK FACTORS

Although little is known about etiologic factors, some general statements can be formulated. Carcinoma of the prostate is virtually unknown in castrates.[113] The tumor often shows a hormone dependency and castration often is a valuable therapeutic adjunct in patients where the disease becomes generalized.[111] The current hypothesis about its development assigns the male sexual hormone, testosterone, a central role.[114] Hormonal and dietary factors may promote the disease.

However, little is known about initiating agents. The reproductive years, especially the early reproductive years, may be of great importance for disease occurrence. American blacks display the highest incidence of prostatic carcinoma. In studies of adolescent boys in California, higher levels of testosterone at a given age were found in black boys compared with other ethnic groups who later display a lower prostatic carcinoma incidence.[114] In a recent study on body mass and prostatic cancer, it was found that the muscle mass more than the amount of fat tissue correlated with the risk of the disease,[115] a finding that again implicates the role of androgens in the occurrence of the disease.

C. AGE, TUMOR BIOLOGY, AND PROGNOSIS

Patient age at diagnosis is not significantly related to crude survival,[116] however, in patients above 70 years of age a larger tumor volume is associated with a significantly increased number of poorly differentiated tumors.[116] Again, an elderly black population shows a more striking predominance of these tumors than the older white population.[116]

III. TESTICULAR CANCER

A. AGE AND INCIDENCE

Cancer of the testis shows a markedly different incidence distribution over age compared with tumors not associated with reproductive organs, such as cancer of the lung and stomach. Its peak incidence is in early reproductive life, 20 to 40 years (Figure 1). The two main histological groups, malignant teratomas and seminomas, have a somewhat different age spectra; teratomas present on the average 10 years earlier than seminomas.[117,118] Cancer of the testis registered in older men has often been lymphomas wrongly diagnosed and misclassified as true testicular tumors.[119] There is a marked geographic variation of the incidence with areas in Scandinavia, especially Denmark, displaying the highest incidence in the world.[118] The incidence in Europe and North America has been reported to be increasing.[118]

B. AGE AND RISK FACTORS

Men born with a cryptorchid testis have a higher risk of developing testicular cancer.[118] The risk also extends to men with hydrocele and congenital hernias.[118,120,121] Recent investigations have focused on the possibility that the hormonal milieu during pregnancy may be of importance for a later risk of testis cancer.[118] Mothers of patients more often report a history of taking hormonal drugs such as DES, estrogen, and contraceptive pills during pregnancy.[117,118,120] Further, abnormal weight gain and nausea during pregnancy more often is reported by the mothers, suggested to be due to excessive estrogen levels.[118] An hypothesis has been forwarded that excessive estrogen exposure to the fetus increases the risk for both cryptorchism, hydrocele, congenital hernia, and testis cancer.[118] Of special interest in this regard is the registration of an increase in the incidence of cryptorchism in England accompanied by an increase in testis cancer incidence.[118]

C. AGE, TUMOR BIOLOGY, AND PROGNOSIS

The prognosis of testicular cancer has greatly improved.[122] Because patients with testicular cancers have a rather low mean age, the very intensive treatments are often possible to undertake in a successful manner. Although data are scarce, it is possible that older patients, due to difficulties in tolerating radiation and chemotherapy, may have a somewhat worse prognosis.

IV. OVARIAN CANCER

A. AGE AND INCIDENCE

Incidence of ovarian carcinoma of the epithelial type increases with age (see Figure 1),[8] while germ cell tumors peak in young adulthood.[123] Northern European women have a high incidence of epithelial ovarian cancer in contrast to a low incidence among Indian, Japanese, and African women.[123]

B. AGE AND RISK FACTORS

Nulliparous women as well as women with a low parity have a higher risk of developing cancer of the ovary.[123] This have given rise to an hypothesis that the number of ovulations is related to the risk.[123] One possible reason for the increased risk may be microtrauma at each ovulation increasing the proliferation of the ovarian stroma. OC use reduces the risk of ovarian cancer by up to 50%.[123] Familial factors may in some instances be quite strong. In some families a monogenic pattern can be seen.[123] Sometimes this hereditary pattern includes tumor development in other organs, especially the breast.[86,122]

Germ cell tumors may share risk factors with testicular germ cell tumors in males.[124] As such, the hormonal environment in the mother and exogenous hormone use during pregnancy may predipose the fetus for later development of a germ cell tumor.[124]

C. AGE, TUMOR BIOLOGY, AND PROGNOSIS

Prognosis is better among young patients both with respect to relapse and death.[125] The lower risk of relapse in young patients is due to an earlier stage at diagnosis, a more favorable histology, and less residuum.[125]

V. ENDOMETRIAL CANCER

A. AGE AND INCIDENCE

Endometrial cancer increases with age (see Figure 1) and is rare prior to menopause.[8] There is a suggested relationship between affluence of the country and endometrial cancer incidence.[126] There has been an increase in incidence of this cancer worldwide.[126]

B. AGE AND RISK FACTORS

Nulliparous and obese women experience a higher risk.[126] Also, diseases occurring in conjunction with obesity such as diabetes and hypertension are more frequent among cases.[126] Estrogens prescribed during menopause increase endometrial cancer risk in a dose-dependent fashion.[127-132] OC use prior to menopause reduces the risk of endometrial cancer substantially.[5] The present theory regarding development of endometrial cancer focuses on "the unopposed estrogen hypothesis".[5]

C. AGE, TUMOR BIOLOGY, AND PROGNOSIS

Older patients have deeper myometrial invasion, more poorly differentiated tumors, more advanced stages of the disease, lower operability rates, and a poorer survival (even after correction for intercurrent deaths).[125]

Endometrial cancer developing after estrogen supplementation perimenopausally may have a better prognosis,[133-136] although not all investigations have been consistent.[137,138]

VI. CANCER OF THE UTERINE CERVIX

A. AGE AND INCIDENCE

The incidence of cervical cancer (Figure 1) characteristically peaks between 40 to 60 years of age.[8] The worldwide incidence varies greatly, with high risk areas such as Colombia (where women may have a lifetime risk of over 6%) to low risk areas such as Jewish women in Israel (lifetime risk 1% or less).[139] In North America and northern European countries, possibly due to early screening and a change in lifestyle factors, the incidence of cancer of the cervix has been declining.[139] This has been true for squamous cell carcinoma, but not for adenocarcinoma, where an increased incidence instead is seen, especially among very young women.[140-142]

B. AGE AND RISK FACTORS

Studies on risk factors have converged on the importance of sexual habits. It has been found that an early age at first coitus, a history of multiple partners, and unmarried women experience a higher risk of squamous cell carcinoma.[139] Populations in which circumcisions of males are practiced have a lower incidence of cancer of the uterine cervix.[139] The above factors support a hypothesis between an infectious risk factor and cervical cancer. Infections with human papillomavirus have also been linked to occurrence of the disease.[143] A history of smoking is more common in cases,[143,144] as is also a history of prior OC use.[143,145,146]

Due to its rareness, it has been difficult to investigate the epidemiology in cases of adenocarcinoma. However, so far it seems as if the infectious risk factors do not apply to these cases,[147,148] and instead, a hypothesis that early OC use may increase the incidence of adenocarcinoma and thus explain the rise in incidence among young women, has been forwarded.[140]

C. AGE, TUMOR BIOLOGY, AND PROGNOSIS

Cases detected by screening generally show a less advanced stage and an improved prognosis.[139] Survival in this disease seems to be less a function of age than the disease itself and therapy response is as good in elderly as in younger patients.[149]

VII. THYROID CARCINOMA

A. AGE AND INCIDENCE

The incidence (Figure 1) increases with age with a rapid increase in late reproductive life.[8] Females have a higher risk of developing thyroid cancer, which is especially evident during the reproductive years.[150] A large geographical variation in incidence is seen, with high-risk areas such as Iceland and Hawaii.[150] The diagnosis of thyroid carcinoma may pose difficulties as it is sometimes difficult to differentiate the malignant tumor from a benign adenoma.[150] The prevalence of thyroid carcinoma at autopsy may vary between countries from 0.3% to 28% even after the slides have been reviewed. Cases diagnosed at autopsy show an almost equal sex ratio.[150]

B. AGE AND RISK FACTORS

A history of prior irradiation, especially in childhood, increases the risk of thyroid carcinoma.[151-157] In general, the association with radiation has been stronger for the papillary type than the follicular type of cancer.[150]

Reproductive factors have also been postulated to be of importance as women experience a higher risk.[158] Such factors increasing the risk include the number of pregnancies and if the first pregnancy ended in miscarriage . A hypothesis was forwarded by the same authors that elevated levels of female sex hormone led to elevated levels of thyroid stimulating hormone and that this promoted hyperplasia of the thyroid and that hyperplasia in turn was associated with an increased risk of cancer.[158]

The reason for the high incidence in some coastal areas is unknown.

Around 20% of medullary carcinomas belong to the genetic syndrome, multiple endocrine neoplasia.[150] The heritable form of medullary carcinoma is diagnosed around 30 years of age, which is about 50 years earlier than for the nonfamilial form.[150]

C. AGE, TUMOR BIOLOGY, AND PROGNOSIS

The survival in older cases with papillary and follicular carcinoma is lower than for younger patients;[159] however, this can probably be accounted for by larger tumors and a higher intercurrent death rate.[159,160]

ACKNOWLEDGMENT

I am indebted to Associate Professor T. R. Möller, Director of the Southern Swedish Regional Tumour Registry, Lund, Sweden, for helpful discussion and critical reading of the manuscript.

TABLE 1
Summary of Hypotheses Relating Exogeneous Administration of Artificial Steroid Hormones to Later Cancer Risk

Time period	Increased risk	Decreased risk
In utero		
Diethylstilbestrol (mother)	Cervical cancer (daughter)	
	Vaginal cancer (daughter)	
	Testicular cancer (son)	
	Ovarian germ cell tumors (daughter)	
Estrogen (mother)	Testicular cancer (son)	
	Ovarian germ cell tumors (daughter)	
Estrogen+progestin (mother)	Testicular cancer (son)	
	Ovarian germ cell tumors (daughter)	
Childhood		
Anabolic steroids	Liver cancer?	
Puberty/before first child		
Oral contraceptives	Breast cancer	Ovarian cancer?
	Cervical cancer?	Endometrial cancer?
Pregnancy		
DES	Breast cancer?	
Adulthood/after first child		
Oral contraceptives	Cervical cancer?	Ovarian cancer
		Endometrial cancer
"Fertile years"		
Oral contraceptives	Liver cancer?	
	Bile duct carcinoma?	
	Malignant melanoma?	
Estrogens	Breast cancer (males)?	
Anabolic steroids	Liver cancer?	
Peri-/postmenopausal age		
Oral contraceptives	Breast cancer?	
Estrogen	Endometrial cancer	
(+/– progestin)	Breast cancer	
DES	Endometrial cancer	

Note: The time period for the artificial hormone exposure is shown in relation to an increased or decreased risk for malignant tumors.

TABLE 2
Summary of Hypotheses Relating Endogeneous "Excessive" or "Reduced" Levels of Steroid Hormones to Later Cancer Risk

Time period (Responsible Hormone)	Risk factor	Increased risk	Decreased risk
In utero			
Estrogens (mother)?	Obesity, excessive nausea	Testicular cancer (son) Ovarian germ cell tumors (daughters)	
Puberty/before first child			
Estrogens (with progestins?)	Early menarche Number of regular menstrual cycles Short menstrual cycles Early abortions Late first pregnancy Obesity?	Breast cancer Breast cancer (postmenopausal)	
Estrogen stimulating S-TSH[a]?	Early abortions Multiple pregnancies	Thyroid cancer	
Testosterone	High levels in risk group	Prostatic cancer	
Adulthood/after first child			
Estrogens (with progestins?)	Nulliparity/low parity Obesity	Endometrial cancer	
	Nulliparity/low parity Obesity	Breast cancer (postmenopausal)	
Estrogen stimulating S-TSH?	Early abortions Multiple pregnancies	Thyroid cancer	
Testosterone	Castration		Prostatic carcinoma
"Fertile years"			
Estrogens (–progestins?)	Castration		Breast cancer
Peri-/postmenopausal age			
–Estrogens (–progestins?)	Early castration or early cessation of menses cancer		Breast cancer Endometrial
+Estrogens (with progestins?)	Late cessation of menses	Breast cancer Endometrial cancer	
Estrogens	Obesity	Breast cancer Endometrial cancer	

Note: The time period for the responsible hormone exposure and risk factor (-s) is shown in relation to the risk for various tumors.

[a]S-TSH = thyroid stimulating hormone.

REFERENCES

1. **Doll, R.,** The age distribution of cancer: implications for models of carcinogenesis, *J. R. Stat. Soc. Ser. A,* 134, 133, 1971.
2. **Pike, M. C.,** Age related factors in cancers of the breast, ovary and endometrium, *J. Chronic Dis.,* 40(Suppl. 2), 59S, 1987.
3. **Pike, M. C., Krailo, M. D., Henderson, B. E., Casagrande, J. J., and Hoel D. G.,** 'Hormonal' risk factors, 'breast tissue age' and the age incidence of breast cancer, *Nature,* 303, 767, 1983.
4. **Key, T. J. A. and Pike, M. C.,** The role of oestrogens and progestagens in the epidemiology and prevention of breast cancer, *Eur. J. Cancer Clin. Oncol.,* 24, 1, 29, 1988.
5. **Key, T. J. A. and Pike, M. C.,** The dose-effect relationship between 'unopposed' oestrogens and endometrial mitotic rate: its central role in explaining and predicting endometrial cancer risk, *Br. J. Cancer,* 57, 205, 1988.
6. **Miller, A. B. and Bulbrook, R. D.,** UICC multidisciplinary project on breast cancer: the epidemiology, aetiology and prevention of breast cancer, *Int. J. Cancer,* 37, 173, 1986.
7. The Cancer Registry, National Board of Health and Welfare, *Cancer Incidence of Sweden,* 1984, Stockholm.
8. **Møller Jensen, O., Carstensen, B., Glattre, E., Malker, B., Pukkala, E., and Tulinius, H.,** *Atlas of Cancer Incidence in the Nordic Countries,* Nordic Cancer Union, Copenhagen, 1988.
9. **Clemmesen, J.,** *Statistical Studies in Malignant Neoplasms,* Vol. 1, Munksgaard, Copenhagen, 1965, 260.
10. **Ewertz, M., Holmberg, L., Karjalainen, S., Trettli, S., and Adami, H.-O.,** Incidence of male breast cancer in Scandinavia 1943-1982, *Int. J. Cancer,* 43, 27, 1989.
11. **Petrakis, N. L., Ernster, V., and King, M.-C.,** Breast, in *Cancer Epidemiology and Prevention,* Schottenfeld, D. and Fraumeni, J. F., Eds., WB Saunders, Philadelphia, 1982, 855.
12. **Vorherr, H.,** Breast Cancer, Epidemiology, Endocrinology, Biochemistry and Pathobiology, Urban & Schwarzenberg, Baltimore, 1980, 3.
13. **Klein, P. A. and Smith, R. T.,** The role of oncogenic viruses in neoplasia, *Ann. Rev. Med.,* 28, 311, 1977.
14. **Albanes, D. and Winick, M.,** Are cell number and cell proliferation risk factors for cancer?, *J. Natl. Cancer Inst.,* 80, 772, 1988.
15. **Thomas, D.,** Do hormones cause breast cancer?, *Cancer,* 53, 595, 1984.
16. **Olsson, H.,** Oral contraceptives and breast cancer, a review, *Acta Oncol.,* 28, 849, 1989.
17. **Russo, J., Calaf, G., Roi, L., and Russo, I. H.,** Influence of age and gland topography in cell kinetics of normal human breast, *JNCI,* 78, 413, 1987.
18. **Battersby, S., Andersson, T. J., and King, R. J. B.,** Influence of oral contraceptives on normal breast epithelial proliferation, *J. Steroid Biochem.,* 28, 4S, 1987.
19. **Tokunaga, M., Norman, J. E., Asano, M., Tokuoko, S., Ezaki, H., Nishimori, I., and Tsuji, Y.,** Malignant breast tumours among atomic bomb survivors, Hiroshima and Nagasaki, 1950-1974, *J. Natl Cancer Inst.,* 62, 1347, 1979.
20. **Boice, J.,** Risk estimates for breast cancer, in *Proceedings of the 7th Annual Meeting,* Critical issues in setting radiation dose limits, National Council on Radiation Protection and Measurements, Bethesda, MD, 1981, 164.
21. **Fournier, D. V., Weber, W., Hoeffken, W., Bauer, M., Kulbi, F., and Barth, V.,** Growth rate of 147 mammary carcinoma, *Cancer,* 45, 2198, 1980.
22. **Koscielny, S., Tubiana, M., and Valleron, A.J.,** A simulation model of the natural history of human breast cancer, *Br. J. Cancer,* 52, 515, 1987.
23. **Baral, E., Larsson, L. E., and Mattsson, B.,** Breast cancer following irradiation of the breast, *Cancer,* 40, 2905, 1977.
24. **Hankey, B. F., Curtis, R. E., Naughton, M. D., Boice, J. D., and Flannery, J. T.,** Retrospective cohort analysis of second breast cancer risk for primary breast cancer patients with an assessment of the effect of radiation therapy, *J. Natl. Cancer Inst.,* 70, 797, 1983.
25. **Harvey, E. B., and Brinton, L. A.,** Second cancer following cancer of the breast in Connecticut, 1935-1982, in Multiple primary cancers in Connecticut and Denmark, *Natl. Cancer Inst. Monogr.,* 68, 99,.1985.
26. **MacMahon, B., Cole, P., Lin, T. M., Lowe, C. R., Mirra, A. P., Ravnihar, B., Valaoras, V. G., and Yuasa, S.,** Age at first birth and breast cancer risk, *Bull. WHO,* 43, 209, 1970.
27. **Adami, H. O., Rimsten, Å., Stenkvist, B., and Vegelius, J.,** Reproductive history and risk of breast cancer, *Cancer,* 41, 747, 1978.
28. **Ewertz, M. and Duffy, S. W.,** Risk of breast cancer in relation to reproductive factors, *Br. J. Cancer,* 58, 99, 1988.
29. **Kvåle, G. and Heuch, I.,** A prospective study of reproductive factors and breast cancer. II. Age at first and last birth, *Am. J. Epidemiol.,* 126, 5, 842, 1987.
30. **Tulinius, H., Day, N. E., Johannesson, G., Bjarnson, O., and Gonzales, M.,** Reproductive factors and risk of breast cancer, *Int. J. Cancer,* 21, 724, 1978.
31. **Olsson, H., Landin Olsson, M., and Gullberg, B.,** Retrospective assessment of menstrual cycle length in patients with breast cancer, benign breast disease and in women without breast disease, *J. Natl. Cancer Inst.,* 70, 17, 1983.

32. **Johansson, E. D. B.,** The sterile menstrual cycle: driving force behind pathology in reproductive organs, *Acta Obstet. Gynecol. Scand.,* (Suppl.) 123, 147, 1984.

33. **Henderson, B. E., Ross, R. K., Judd, H. L., Krailo, M. D., and Pike, M. C.,** Do regular cycles increase breast cancer risk?, *Cancer,* 56, 1206, 1985.

34. **Olsson, H., Ranstam, J., and Landin-Olsson, M.,** The number of menstrual cycles prior to the first full-term pregnancy - an important risk factor of breast cancer?, *Acta Oncol.,* 5, 387, 1987.

35. **Kvåle, G. and Heuch, I.,** Menstrual factors and breast cancer risk, *Cancer,* 62, 1625, 1988.

36. **La Vecchia, C., Decarli, A., Di Pietro, S., Franceschi, S., Negri, E., and Parazzini, F.,** Menstrual cycle patterns and the risk of breast disease, *Eur. J. Cancer Clin. Oncol.,* 21, 417, 1985.

37. **Battersby S., Anderson T. J., King R. J. B., and Going J.,** Influence of oral contraceptives on normal human breast epithelial proliferation, *J. Steroid Biochem.,* 28(Suppl.), 4S, 1987.

38. **La Vecchia, C., Decarli, A., Parazzini, F., Gentile, A., Negri, E., Cecchetti, G., and Franceschi, S.,** General epidemiology of breast cancer in Northern Italy, *Int. J. Epidemiol.,* 16(3), 347, 1987.

39. **Yuan, J. -M., Yu, M. C., Ross, R. K., Gao, Y.- T., and Henderson, B. E.,** Risk factors for breast cancer in chinese women in Shanghai, *Cancer Res.,* 48, 1949, 1988.

40. **De Waard, F. and Trichopoulos, D.,** A unifying concept of the aetiology of breast cancer, *Int. J. Cancer,* 41, 666, 1988.

41. **Simpson, H. W., Candlish, W., Pauson, A. W., McArdle, C. S., Griffiths, K., and Small, R. G.,** Genesis of breast cancer is in the premenopause, *Lancet,* 2, 74, 1988.

42. **Krailo, M., Thomas, D. C., and Pike, M. C.,** Fitting models of carcinogenesis to a case-control study of breast cancer, *J. Chron. Dis.,* 40(Suppl.), 181S, 1987.

43. **Moolgavkar, S. H., Day, N. E., and Stevens, R. G.,** Two-stage models for carcinogenesis: epidemiology of breast cancer in females, *J. Natl. Cancer Inst.,* 65, 559, 1980.

44. **Olsson, H.,** Reproductive events, occurring in adolescence at the time of development of reproductive organs and at the time of tumour initiation, have a bearing on growth characteristics and reproductive hormone regulation in normal and tumour tissue investigated decades later- a hypothesis, *Med. Hypotheses,* 28, 93, 1989.

45. **Bruzzi, P., Negri, E., La Vecchia, C., Decarli, A., Palli, D., Parazzini, F., and Del Turco, M. R.,** Short term increase in risk of breast cancer after full term pregnancy, *Br. Med. J.,* 297, 1096, 1988.

46. **MacMahon, B., Cole, P., and Brown, J.,** Etiology of human breast cancer: a review, *J. Natl. Cancer Inst.,* 50, 21, 1973.

47. **Byers, T., Graham, S., Rzepka, T., and Marshall, J.,** Lactation and breast cancer: evidence for a negative association in premenopausal women, *Am. J. Epidemiol.,* 12, 664, 1985.

48. **McTiernan, A. and Thomas, D. B.,** Evidence for a protective effect of lactation on risk of breast cancer in young women: results from a case-control study, *Am. J. Epidemiol.,* 124, 353, 1986.

49. **Pike, M. C., Henderson, B. E., Casagrande, J. T., Rosario, I., and Gray, G. E.,** Oral contraceptive use and early abortion as risk factors for breast cancer in young women, *Br. J. Cancer,* 43, 72, 1981.

50. **Hadjimichael, O. C., Boyle, C. A., and Meigs, J. W.,** Abortions before first live birth and risk of breast cancer, *Br. J. Cancer,* 53, 281, 1986.

51. **Ewertz, M. and Duffy, S. W.,** Risk of breast cancer in relation to reproductive factors in Denmark, *Br. J. Cancer,* 58, 99, 1988.

52. **Olsson, H., Möller, T., and Ranstam, J.,** Early oral contraceptive use and premenopausal breast cancer - final report from a study in southern Sweden, *JCNI,* 81, 1000, 1989.

53. **McPherson, K., Vessey, M. P., Neil, A., Doll, R., Jones, L., and Roberts, M.,** Early oral contraceptive use and breast cancer. Results of another case-control study, *Br. J. Cancer,* 5, 653, 1987.

54. **Meirik, O., Lund, E., Adami, H. O., Bergström, R., Christofferson, T., and Bergsjö, P.,** Oral contraceptive use and breast cancer in young women, A joint national case-control study in Sweden and Norway, *Lancet,* 2, 650, 1986.

55. **Pike, M. C., Henderson, B. E., Krailo, M. D., and Duke, A.,** Breast cancer in young women and use of oral contraceptives: possible effect of formulation and age at use, *Lancet,* 22, 926, 1983.

56. **Meirik, O., Lund, E., and Adami, H.-O.,** Oral contraceptives and breast cancer, *Lancet,* 2, 1272, 1986.

57. **Meirik, O., Lund, E., Adami, H.- O., Bergström, R., Christofferson, T., and Bergsjö, P.,** Oral contraceptives and breast cancer, *Lancet,* 1, 1042, 1987.

58. **McPherson, K. and Coope, P. A.,** Early oral contraceptive use and breast cancer risk, *Lancet,* 1, 685, 1986.

59. **Olsson, H., Ranstam, J., and Möller, T. R.,** Breast cancer and oral contraceptives, *Lancet,* 2, 1181, 1985.

60. **Ranstam, J., Möller, T. R., and Olsson, H.,** Oral contraceptives and breast cancer, *Lancet,* 2, 923, 1986.

61. **Ranstam, J., Olsson, H., and Möller, T.,** Oral contraceptive use and the risk of breast cancer, *N. Engl. J. Med.,* 316, 162, 1987.

62. **Ranstam, J. and Olsson, H.,** Oral contraceptives and breast cancer, *Lancet,* 1, 636, 1987.

63. **Stadel, B. V. and Schlesselman, J. J.,** Oral contraceptives and breast cancer, *Lancet,* 2, 922, 1986.

64. **Pike, M. C.,** Breast cancer and oral contraceptives, *Lancet,* 2, 1180, 1985.

65. **McPherson, K., and Drife, J. O.,** The pill and breast cancer: why the uncertainty?, Editorial, *Br. Med. J.,* Sept. 20, 709, 1986.

66. **Peto, J.,** Oral contraceptives and breast cancer: is the CASH study really negative?, *Lancet,* 1, 552, 1989.

67. **McPherson, K., Coope, P. A., and Vessey, M. P.,** Early oral contraceptive use and breast cancer: theoretical effects of latency, *J. Epidemiol. Community Health,* 40, 289, 1986.

68. **Stadel, B. V., Lai, S., Schlesselman, J. J., and Murray, P.,** Oral contraceptives and premenopausal breast cancer in nulliparous women, *Contraception,* 3, 287, 1988.

69. **Kay, C. R. and Hannaford, P. C.,** Breast cancer and the pill-a further report from the Royal College of General Practitioners' oral contraceptive study, *Br. J. Cancer,* 58, 675, 1988.

70. **Olsson, H., Borg, Å., Ewers, S.- B., Fernö, M., Möller, T., and Ranstam, J.,** A biological marker strongly associated with early oral contraceptive use, for the selection of a high risk group for premenopausal breast cancer, *Med. Oncol. Tumor Pharmacother.,* 3(2), 77, 1986.

71. **Olsson, H. and Ranstam, J.,** Breast cancer and the pill, *Br. J. Cancer,* 59, 834, 1989.

72. **Olsson, H., Möller, T. R., Ranstam, J., Borg, Å., and Fernö, M.,** Early oral contraceptive use as a prognostic factor in breast cancer, *Anticancer Res.,* 8, 29, 1988.

73. **Hoover, R., Glass, A., Finkle, W. D., Azevedo, D., and Milne, K.,** Conjugated estrogens and breast cancer risk in women, *J. Natl. Cancer Inst.,* 67, 815, 1981.

74. **Brinton, L. A., Hoover, R., and Fraumeni, J. F.,** Menopausal oestrogens and breast cancer risk: an expanded case-control study, *Br. J. Cancer,* 54, 825, 1986.

75. **Hennekens, C. H., Speizer, F. E., Lipnick, R. J., Rosner, B., Bain, C., Belanger, C., Stampfer, M. J., Willett, W., and Peto, R.,** A case-control study of oral contraceptive use and breast cancer, *JNCI,* 72, 39, 1984.

76. **Jick, H., Walker, A. M., Watkins, R. N., D'Ewart, D. C., Hunter, J .R., Danford, A., Madsen, S., Dinan, B. J., and Rothman, K.,** Oral contraceptives and breast cancer, *Am. J. Epidemiol.,* 112, 577, 1980.

77. **Hunt, K., Vessey, M., McPherson, K., and Coleman, M.,** Long term surveillance of mortality and cancer incidence in women receiving hormone replacement therapy, *Br. J. Obstet. Gynecol.,* 94, 620, 1987.

78. **Welsch, C. W. and Aylsworth, C. F.,** Enhancement of murine mammary tumorigenesis by feeding high levels of dietary fat: a hormonal mechanism?, *J. Natl. Cancer Inst.,* 70, 215, 1983.

79. **Wynder, E. and Rose, D. P.,** Diet and breast cancer, in *Cancer, Diet and Nutrition. A Comprehensive Sourcebook,* Greenwald, P., Eershow, A. G., Novelli, W. D., and Benton, C. M., Eds., Marquis Who's Who, Chicago, 1985, 178.

80. **Willett, W. C., Browne, M. L., Bain, C., Lipnick, R. J., Stampfer, M. J., Rosner, B., Colditz, G. A., Hennekens, C. H., and Speizer, F. E.,** Relative weight and risk of breast cancer among premenopausal women, *Am. J. Epidemiol.,* 122, 731, 1985.

81. **Lubin, F., Ruder, A. M., Wax, Y., and Modan, B.,** Overweight and changes in weight throughout adult life in breast cancer etiology. A case-control study, *Am. J. Epidemiol.,* 122, 579, 1985.

82. **Törnberg, S. A., Holm, L. -E., and Carstensen, J. M.,** Breast cancer risk in relation to serum cholesterol. serum B-lipoprotein, height, weight and blood pressure, *Acta Oncol.,* 27, 31, 1988.

83. **Siiteri, P. K., Schwartz, B. E., and MacDonald, P. C.,** Estrogen receptors and the estrone hypothesis in relation to endometrial and breast cancer, *Gynecol. Oncol.,* 2, 228, 1974.

84. **De Waard, F., Baanders-van Halewijn, E. A., and Huizinga, J.,** The bimodal age distribution of patients with mammary carcinoma, *Cancer,* 17, 141, 1964.

85. **Gudmundsson, S., Möller, T., and Olsson, H.,** Cancer incidence after cholecystectomy—a cohort study with thirty years of follow up, *Eur. J. Surg. Oncol.,* 15, 113, 1989.

86. **Lynch, H. T. and Lynch, J. F.,** Breast cancer genetics, in *Familial Cancer, 1st International Research Conference Basel, 1985,* Müller, H. J. and Weber, W., Eds., S. Karger, Basel, 1985, 20.

87. **Anderson, D. E.,** Breast cancer, in *Familial Cancer, 1st International Research Conference, Basel, 1985,* Müller, H. J. and Weber, W., Eds., S. Karger, Basel, 1985, 17.

88. **Schwartz, A. G., King, M.-C., Belle, S. H., Satarino, W. A., and Swanson, G. M.,** Risk of breast cancer to relatives of young breast cancer patients, *J. Natl. Cancer Inst.,* 75, 665, 1985.

89. **Kalache, A. and Vessey, M.,** Risk factors for breast cancer, in *Clinics in Oncology,* W.B. Saunders, Philadelphia, 1982, 661.

90. **Brinton, L. A., Hoover, R., and Fraumeni, J. F., Jr.,** Interaction of familial and hormonal risk factors for breast cancer, *JNCI,* 69, 817, 1982.

91. **Olsson, H., Landin Olsson, M., Kristoffersson, U., and Ranstam, J.,** Risk factors of breast cancer in relation to a family history of breast cancer in southern Sweden, in *Familial Cancer, 1st International Research Conference, Basel, 1985,* Müller, H.J. and Weber, W., Eds., S. Karger, Basel, 1985, 34.

92. **Negri, E., La Vecchia, C., Bruzzi, P., Dardanoni, G., Decarli, A., Palli, D., Parazzini, F., and Rosselli del Turco, M.,** Risk factors for breast cancer: pooled results from three Italian case-control studies, *Am. J. Epidemiol.,* 128, 1207, 1988.

93. **Ranstam, J., Janzon, L., and Olsson, H.,** Rising incidence of breast cancer among young women in Sweden, *Br. J. Cancer,* 61, 120, 1990.

94. **Anon.,** *National Cancer Institute 1986 Annual Cancer Statistics Review,* NIH Publ. 87-2789, National Institutes of Health, Bethesda, MD, 1986, III.A.2.

95. **White, E., Daling, J. R., Norstedt, T. L., and Chu, J.,** Rising incidence of breast cancer among young women in Washington State, *JNCI,* 79, 239, 1987.

96. **Mabuchi, K., Bross, D. S., and Kessler, L.,** Risk factors for male breast cancer, *J. Natl. Cancer Inst.*, 74, 375, 1985.

97. **Olsson, H. and Ranstam, J.,** Head trauma and exposure to prolactin-elevating drugs as risk factors for male breast cancer, *J. Natl. Cancer Inst.*, 80, 679, 1988.

98. **Meyer, J. S., McDivitt, R. W., Stone, K. R., Prey, M. U., and Bauer, W. C.,** Practical breast carcinoma cell kinetics: review and update, *Breast Cancer Res. Treat.*, 4, 79, 1984.

99. **Silvestrini, R., Daidone, M. G., and Gasparini, G.,** Cell kinetics as a prognostic marker in node negative breast cancer, *Cancer,* 56, p. 1982, 1985.

100. **Gentile, C., Sanfilippo, O., and Silvestrini, R.,** Cell proliferation and its relationship to clinical features and relapse in breast cancers, *Cancer,* 48, 974, 1981.

101. **Schiffer, L. M., Braunschweiger, P. G., Stragand, J. J., and Poulakos, L.,** The cell kinetics of human mammary cancers, *Cancer,* 43, 1707, 1979.

102. **Moran, R. E., Black, M. M., Alpert, L., and Straus, M. J.,** Correlation of cell-cycle kinetics, hormone receptors, histopathology, and nodal status in human breast cancer, *Cancer,* 54, 1586, 1984.

103. **Kute, T. E., Muss, H. B., Hopkins, M., Marshall, R., Case, D., and Kammire, L.,** Relationship of flow cytometry results to clinical and steroid receptor status in human breast cancer, *Breast Cancer Res. Treat.*, 6, 113, 1985.

104. **Von Rosen, A., Fallenius, A., Sundelin, B., and Auer, G.,** Nuclear DNA content in mammary carcinomas in women aged 35 or younger, *Am. J. Clin. Oncol. (CCT)*, 9(5), 382, 1986.

105. **Seibert, K. and Lippman, M. E.,** Hormone receptors in breast cancer, in *Breast Cancer,* Vol. 1, Baum, M., Ed., W. B. Saunders, London, 1983, 751.

106. **Adami, H.- O., Malker, B., Holmberg, L., Persson, I., and Stone, B.,** The relation between survival and age at diagnosis in breast cancer, *N. Engl. J. Med.*, 315, 559, 1986.

107. **Høst, H. and Lund, E.,** Age as a prognostic factor in breast cancer, *Cancer,* 57, 2217, 1986.

108. **Tretli, S., Kvalheim, G., Thoresen, S., and Höst, H.,** Survival of breast cancer patients diagnosed during pregnancy or lactation, *Br. J. Cancer,* 58, 382, 1988.

109. **Olsson, H., Borg, Å., Fernö, M., Möller, T. R., and Sigurdsson, H.,** Breast cancer, developing during pregnancy, its relationship to hormone receptors in the primary tumour and survival, paper presented at Australian Bicentennial Breast Cancer Conference, A Westmead Hospital Symposium, Nov. 18-21, 1988, 14.

110. **Haslam, S. Z.,** Acquistion of estrogen-dependent progesterone receptors by normal mouse mammary gland, ontogeny of mammary progesterone receptors, *J. Steroid Biochem.*, 31, 9, 1988.

111. **Mandel, J. S. and Schuman, L. M.,** Epidemiology of cancer of the prostate, in *Reviews in Cancer Epidemiology,* Lilienfeld, A., Ed., Elsevier/North-Holland, New York, 1980, 1.

112. **Greenwald, P.,** Prostate, in *Cancer Epidemiology and Prevention,* Schottenfeld, D. and Fraumeni, J. F., Jr., Eds., W.B. Saunders, Philadelphia, 1982, 938.

113. IARC Monographs of the Evaluation on Carcinogenic Rrisks to Humans, Overall evaluations of carcinogenicity, an update of IARC monographs volumes 1-42, Androgenic Anabolic Steroids, Suppl. 7, International Agency for Research on Cancer, Lyon, 1987, 96.

114. **Ross, R. K., Paganini-Hill, A., and Henderson, B. E.,** Epidemiology of prostatic cancer, in *Diagnosis and Management of Genitourinary Cancer,* Skinner, D. G. and Lieskovsky, G., Eds., W.B. Saunders , Philadelphia, 1988, 40.

115. **Seversson, R. K., Grove, J. S., Nomura, A. M. Y., and Stemmerman, G. N.,** Body mass and prostatic cancer: a prospecitve study, *Br. Med. J.*, 297, 713, 1988.

116. **Williams, G.,** Prognostic indices in prostatic cancer, in *Pointers to Cancer Prognosis,* Stoll, B. A., Ed., Martinus Nijhoff, Boston, 1987, 230.

117. **Schottenfeld, D., and Wasshauer, M. E.,** Testis, in *Cancer Epidemiology and Prevention,* Schottenfeld, D. and Fraumeni, J.F., Eds., W.B. Saunders , Philadelphia, 1982, 947.

118. **Henderson, B. E., Ross, R. K., and Pike, M. C.,** Epidemiology of testicular cancer, in *Diagnosis and Management of Genitourinary Cancer,* Skinner , D. G. and Lieskovsky, G., Eds., W.B. Saunders, Philadelphia, 1988, 46.

119. **Pike, M. C., Chilvers, C. E. D., and Bobrow, L. G.,** Classification of testicular cancer in incidence and mortality statistics, *Br. J. Cancer,* 56, 83, 1987.

120. **Depue, R. H., Pike, M. C., and Henderson, B. E.,** Estrogen exposure during gestation and risk of testicular cancer, *J. Natl. Cancer Inst.*, 71, 1151, 1983.

121. **Swerdlow, A. J., Huttly, S. R. A., and Smith, P. G.,** Testicular cancer and antecedent diseases, *Br. J. Cancer,* 55, 97, 1987.

122. **Skinner, D. G. and Lieskovsky, G.,** Management of early stage nonseminomatous germ cell tumours of the testis, in *Diagnosis and Management of Genitourinary Cancer,* Skinner, D. G. and Lieskovsky, G., Eds., W.B. Saunders, Philadelphia, 1988, 516.

123. **Weiss, N. S.,** Ovary, in *Cancer Epidemiology and Prevention,* Schottenfeld, D. and Fraumeni, J. F., Eds., W. B. Saunders, Philadelphia, 1982, 871.

124. **Walker, A. H., Ross, R. K., Haile, R. W. C., and Henderson, B. E.,** Hormonal factors and risk of ovarian germ cell cancer in young women, *Br. J. Cancer,* 57, 418, 1988.

125. **Dembo, A. J., Thomas, G. M., and Friedlander, M. L.,** Prognostic indices in gynecologic cancer, in *Pointers to Cancer Prognosis,* Stoll, B. A., Ed., Martinus Nijhoff, Boston, 1987, 230.

126. **De Waard, F.,** Uterine corpus, in *Cancer Epidemiology and Prevention,* Schottenfeld, D. and Fraumeni, J.F., Eds., W.B. Saunders, Philadelphia, 1982, 901.

127. **Mack, T. M., Pike, M.C., Henderson, B. E., Pfeffer, R .I., Gerkins, V. R., and Arthur, M.,** Estrogens and endometrial cancer in a retirement community, *N. Engl. J. Med.,* 294, 1262, 1976.

128. **McDonald, T. W., Annegers, J. F., O'Fallon, W. M., Dockerty, M. B., Malkasian, G. D., and Kurland, L. T.,** Exogenous estrogen and endometrial carcinoma, *Am. J. Obstet. Gynecol.,* 127, 572, 1977.

129. **Weiss, N. S., Szekely, D. R., English, D. R., and Schweid, A. I.,** Endometrial cancer in relation to patterns of menopausal estrogen use, *JAMA,* 242, 261, 1979.

130. **Antunes, S., Williams, V., and Vessey, M. P.,** Cardiovascular disease and hormone replacement treatment: a pilot study, *Br. Med. J.,* 282, 1277, 1981.

131. **Hulka, B. S., Grimson, R. C., Greenberg, B. G., Kaufman, D. G., Fowler, W. C., Hogue, C.J ., Berger, G. S., and Pulliam, C. C.,** "Alternative" controls in a case-control study of endometrial cancer and exogenous estrogen, *Am. J. Epidemiol.,* 112, 376, 1980.

132. **Persson, I., Adami, H.- O., Bergkvist, L., Lindgren, A., Pettersson, B., Hoover, R., and Schairer, C.,** Risk of endometrial cancer after treatment with oestrogens alone or in a conjunction with progesterone: results of a prospective study, *Br. Med. J.,* 298, 147, 1989.

133. **Schwartzraum, J. A., Hulka, B. S., Fowler, W. C., Kaufman, D. G., and Hoberman, D.,** The influence of exogenous estrogen use on survival after diagnosis of endometrial cancer, *Am. J. Epidemiol.,* 126, 851, 1987.

134. **Collins, J., Donner, A., Allen, A. H., Donner, A., Allen, L .H., and Adams, O.,** Oestrogen use and survival in endometrial cancer, *Lancet,* 2, 961, 1980.

135. **Chu, J., Prentice,.R. L., and Bauermeister, D. E.,** Endometrial carcinoma: histopathology, survival and exogenous estrogens, *Gynecol. Obstet. Invest.,* 12, 161, 1981.

136. **Underwood, P. B., Miller, N. L., Kreutner, A., Joyner, C. A., and Lutz, M. H.,** Endometrial carcinoma: the effect of estrogens, *Gynecol. Oncol.,* 8, 60, 1979.

137. **Robbey, G. J. and Bradley, R.,** Changing trends and prognostic features in endometrial cancer associated with exogenous estrogen therapy, *Obstet. Gynecol.,* 54, 269, 1979.

138. **Smith, D. C., Prentice, P. L., and Bauermeister, D. E.,** Endometrial carcinoma: histopathology, survival and exogenous estrogens, *Gynecol. Obstet.Invest.,* 12, 161, 1981.

139. **Cramer, D. W.,** Uterine cervix, in *Cancer Epidemiology and Prevention,* Schottenfeld, D. and Fraumeni, J.F., Eds., W.B. Saunders, Philadelphia, 1982, 837.

140. **Peters, R. K., Chao, A., Mack, T., Thomas, D., Bernstein, L., and Henderson, B.,** Increased frequency of adenocarcinoma of the uterine cervix in young women in Los Angeles County, *JNCI,* 76, 423, 1986.

141. **Eide, T. J.,** Cancer of the uterine cervix in Norway by histologic type, 1970-1984, *JNCI,* 79, 199, 1987.

142. **Schwartz, S. M. and Weiss, N. S.,** Increased incidence of adenocarcinoma of the cervix in young women in the United States, *Am. J. Epidemiol.,* 6, 1045, 1986.

143. **Brinton, L. A. and Fraumeni, J. F., Jr.,** Epidemiology of uterine cervical cancer, *J. Chronic Dis.,* 1986; 39, 1051, 1986.

144. **Greenberg, E. R., Vessey, M., McPherson, K., and Yeates, D.,** Cigarette smoking and cancer of the uterine cervix, *Br. J. Cancer,* 51, 139, 1985.

145. **Beral, V., Hannaford, P., and Kay, C.,** Oral contraceptive use and malignancies of the genital tract. Results from the RCGP oral contraceptive study, *Lancet,* 2, 1331, 1988.

146. **Ebeling, K., Nischan, P., and Schindler, Ch.,** Use of oral contraceptives and risk of invasive cervical cancer in previously screened women, *Int. J. Cancer,* 39, 427, 1987.

147. **Brinton, L., Tashima, K. T., Lehman, H. F., Levine, R. S., Mallin, K., Savitz, D. A., Stolley, P. D., and Fraumeni, J. F., Jr.,** Epidemiology of cervical cancer by cell type, *Cancer Res.,* 47, 1706, 1987.

148. **Kvåle, G., Heuch, I., and Nilssen, S.,** Reproductive factors and risk of cervical cancer by cell type, *Br. J. Cancer,* 58, 820, 1988.

149. **Holmes, F. F.,** *Cancer and Aging,* Springer-Verlag, Heidelberg, 1983, 38.

150. **Ron, E., and Modan, B.,** Thyroid, in *Cancer Epidemiology and Prevention,* Schottenfeld, D. and Fraumeni, J. F.,,Jr., Eds., W. B. Saunders, Philadelphia, 1982, 833.

151. **Hempelmann, L. H., Hall, W. J., Phillips, M., Cooper, R. A., and Ames, W. R.,** Neoplasms in persons treated with x-ray in infancy: fourth survey in 20 years, *JNCI,* 55, 519, 1975.

152. **Favus, M. J., Schneider, A. B., Strachura, M. E., Arnold, J. E., Ryo, U. Y., Pinsky, S. M., Colman, M., Arnold, M. J., and Frohman, L. A.,** Thyroid cancer occurring as a late consequence of head and neck irradiation. Evulation of 1056 patients, *N. Engl. J. Med.,* 294, 1019, 1976.

153. **Ron, E., and Modan, B.,** Thyroid and other neoplasma following childhood scalp irradiation, in *Radiation Carcinogenesis. Epidemiology and Biological Significance,* Boice, J. B. and Fraumeni, J. F., Jr., Eds., Raven Press, New York, 1984, 139.

154. **Modan, B.,** Evaluation of risks in medical radiation exposure — the thyroid story, in *Radiation Research. Proceedings of the Sixth International Congress of Radiation Research,* Okada, S., Imamura, S., Tenshima, T., and Yamasuchi, H., Eds., Japanese Association for Radiation Research, Tokyo, 1979, 968.

155. **Prentice, R. L., Kato, H., Yoshimoto, K., and Mason, M.,** Radiation exposure and thyroid cancer incidence among Hiroshima and Nagasaki residents, *Natl. Cancer Inst. Monogr.,* 62, 207, 1982.

156. **Fürst, C. J., Lundell, M., Holm, L. -E., and Silfverswärd, C.,** Cancer incidence after radiotherapy for skin hemangioma: a retrospective cohort study in Sweden, *JNCI,* 88, 1387, 1988.

157. **Olsson, H., Brandt, L., Möller, T., and Ranstam, J.,** Prior irradiation as a risk factor for various tumour types, in *Radiation and Cancer Risks,* Brustad, T., Langmark, F., and Reitan, J., Eds., Hemisphere, New York, 1990, 131.

158. **Preston-Martin, S., Bernstein, L., Pike, M. C., Maldonado, A. A., and Henderson, B. E.,** Thyroid cancer among young women related to prior thyroid disease and pregnancy history, *Br. J. Cancer,* 55, 191, 1987.

159. **Tennvall, J., Björklund, A., Möller, T., Ranstam, J., and Åkerman, M.,** Prognostic factors of papillary, follicular, and medullary carcinomas of the thyroid. Retrospective multivariate analysis of 221 patients with a follow-up of 11 years, *Acta Radiol. Oncol.,* 24, 17, 1985.

160. **Tennvall, J., Björklund, A., Möller, T., Ranstam, J., and Åkerman, M.,** Is the EORTC-prognostic index of thyroid cancer valid in differentiated thyroid carcinoma? Retrospective multivariate analysis of differentiated thyroid carcinoma with long follow-up, *Cancer,* 57, 1405, 1986.

Chapter 7

DEHYDROEPIANDROSTERONE: A NATURALLY OCCURRING STEROID WITH CANCER PREVENTIVE ACTIVITY

Arthur G. Schwartz, Marvin L. Lewbart, and Laura L. Pashko

TABLE OF CONTENTS

I. INTRODUCTION

Although dehydroepiandrosterone (DHEA) was first isolated from human urine over 50 years ago, the biological significance of this steroid and its sulfate ester (DHEAS) is still a mystery. DHEA and DHEAS are secreted by the human adrenal cortex in amounts at least as great as cortisol.[1] Fetal adrenal DHEAS is the principal precursor for placental estrogen biosynthesis in the human.[2] Aside from this biological activity, the role of these steroids in the male and nonpregnant female is not understood.[3]

In the human, the plasma levels of DHEA and DHEAS are at their highest level around age 20 to 25 and thereafter undergo a progressive age-related decline, reaching 10% to 20% of their maximal levels in the eighth decade.[4,5]

II. DHEA AND BREAST CANCER SUSCEPTIBILITY

In 1962 Bulbrook et al. reported that women with primary operable breast cancer excrete subnormal amounts of 11-deoxy-17-ketosteroids (derived primarily from DHEA and DHEAS) prior to mastectomy and suggested that this steroid abnormality might precede the onset of the disease.[6] In order to test this hypothesis, Bulbrook et al. undertook a 9-year prospective study on approximately 5000 women with no apparent breast cancer, and they found that women who excrete subnormal urinary quantities of androsterone and etiocholanolone are at enhanced risk for developing the disease.[7]

With the development of suitable analytical techniques, several laboratories have undertaken determinations of DHEAS plasma levels in women with breast cancer and in matched controls. Several retrospective studies have shown subnormal plasma levels of DHEA and DHEAS in advanced breast cancer patients.[8-10] The findings of Zumoff et al.[11] are of particular interest since these investigators addressed the problem of the marked fluctuations in DHEA levels over a 24-h cycle. DHEA and cortisol are secreted episodically and synchronously, and their levels may vary by as much as 100% on individual spot determinations; DHEAS levels, however, show much less variability.[12] Zumoff et al. measured 24-h mean plasma concentrations of DHEA and DHEAS by sampling blood every 20 min, pooling aliquots of the 72 samples, and determining the concentration of steroid in the pooled samples. When these determinations were made on plasma from women with primary operable breast cancer and from 37 normal women, ages 21 to 75, they found that in contrast to the marked and progressive decline of DHEA and DHEAS concentrations with age in the normal women, the concentrations of both steroids were age-invariant in the cancer patients. The premenopausal patients had subnormal plasma DHEA and DHEAS levels, whereas the postmenopausal patients had supranormal levels.

III. PROTECTION OF CULTURED CELLS AGAINST CHEMICAL CARCINOGENS

One of the first observations suggesting that DHEA might have cancer preventive activity was the finding, made in 1975, that the steroid protected cultured hamster fibroblasts and rat liver epithelial-like cells against the cytotoxic and transforming effects of 7,12-dimethylbenz(a)anthracene (DMBA) and aflatoxin B_1.[13] Treatment of cultured cells with DHEA also inhibited the rate of metabolism of [^{3}H] DMBA to water-soluble products.[13] Carcinogens such as DMBA and aflatoxin B_1 are metabolically activated, through the NADPH-dependent mixed-function oxidases, to reactive epidoxes, which undergo further transformation to substances which are water soluble.[14,15] The inhibition of conversion of [^{3}H] DMBA to water-soluble derivatives by DHEA suggested that the steroid was interfering with carcinogen metabolism, and very possibly DHEA protected cells against carcinogen-induced toxicity and transformation by inhibiting the formation of reactive intermediates.

A. GLUCOSE-6-PHOSPHATE DEHYDROGENASE INHIBITION

DHEA was first shown in 1960 to be a potent inhibitor of glucose-6-phosphate dehydrogenases (G6PDH) from various mammalian sources, but did not inhibit the enzyme from yeast or spinach.[16] This inhibition was subsequently shown to be of the rare uncompetitive type with respect to both NADP and glucose-6-phosphate.[17] Not only do DHEA and specific steroids in the androstane series inhibit glucose-6-phosphate dehydrogenase but so do pregnenolone and related pregnane steroids. In the androstane series, a keto group at C-17 is required for inhibition; steroids possessing either no functional group at C-17 or a hydroxy or carboxy group at this position are inactive as inhibitors. The introduction of a double bond between C-5 and C-6 reduces inhibitory activity; DHEA (3β-hydroxy-5-androsten-17-one) is a less effective inhibitor than epiandrosterone (3β-hydroxy-5α-androstan-17-one). The presence of a 16α bromide (Br) group in the androstan series markedly enhances inhibitory action. 16α-Br-epiandrosterone (Epi-Br) has an inhibitory constant (K_i) of 0.571 μM for epiandrosterone and 18.4 μM for DHEA.[17] Similarly, greater potency is seen with bovine adrenal G6PDH; a K_i of 0.3 μM and 17.6 μM is obtained with Epi-Br and DHEA, respectively.[18]

G6PDH is the rate-limiting enzyme in the pentose-phosphate pathway, which is a major source of ribose-5-phosphate as well as extramitochondrial NADPH, a coenzyme required for reductive biosyntheses. We suggested in 1975 that DHEA protected cultured cells against the toxic and transforming effects of DMBA and protected cultured cells against the toxic and transforming effects of DMBA and aflatoxin B$_1$ by inhibiting G6PDH and reducing the availability of NADPH required for the metabolic activation of these carcinogens. In support of this hypothesis was the finding that epiandrosterone, a more potent G6PDH inhibitor than DHEA, was also more effective than DHEA in reducing the rate of conversion of [³H]DMBA to water-soluble metabolites.[13]

B. GLUCOSE-6-PHOSPHATE DEHYDROGENASE DEFICIENCY

Feo and collaborators, using cultured cells from G6PDH-deficient individuals, have provided strong experimental evidence that a reduction in G6PDH activity renders cells less sensitive to the transforming and toxic actions of various chemical carcinogens.

G6PDH deficiency is a sex-linked hereditary defect occurring with high frequency in certain populations. Among the most prevalent deficiency mutants are the Mediterranean variant, found primarily among Sephardic Jews, Greeks, and Sardinians, and G6PDH A⁻, common in Black populations. The Mediterranean deficiency is more severe than the A⁻ deficiency and occurs in many cells and tissues other than erythrocytes, including fibroblasts, lymphocytes, neutrophils, liver, adrenals, kidneys, and lens of the eye.[19]

Feo et al.[21,22] reported that cultured fibroblasts and lymphocytes from individuals with the Mediterranean variant of G6PDH deficiency are less sensitive to the cytotoxic and transforming effects of benzo(a)pyrene (BP) and are less efficient in metabolizing [³H]BP to water-soluble products than are fibroblasts from normal individuals. Treatment of normal fibroblasts or lymphocytes with DHEA mimicked the effect of the G6PDH deficiency. However, G6PDH deficient fibroblasts were as sensitive as control fibroblasts to cytotoxicity produced by methylnitrosourea (MNU), a carcinogen not requiring metabolic activation, nor did DHEA protect control cells against MNU-induced cytotoxicity. The authors also reported a marked reduction in pentose-phosphate shunt activity and a lowering of the NADPH/NADP pool ratio in the G6PDH-deficient cell.

IV. ANTI-OBESITY ACTION

In 1977 Yen et al. demonstrated that DHEA treatment of VY mice carrying the A^{vy} mutation, which produces a metabolic obesity, inhibited weight gain.[22] DHEA was also effective, although somewhat less so, in reducing weight gain of the nonobese VY mouse. Measurements of food consumption indicated that treated and untreated mice consumed equivalent amounts of food and that consequently DHEA produced its antiweight effect through a metabolic alteration in the efficiency of food utilization rather than as a result of appetite suppression.

Several other laboratories have confirmed and extended the initial finding of Yen et al. DHEA, when administered orally as a suspension in sesame oil at a dose of 450 mg/kg thrice weekly or given in the diet (0.2% to 0.6%), inhibited the weight gain of many different strains of mice and rats.[23-25]

Yen et al. originally hypothesized that DHEA treatment reduced weight gain through G6PDH inhibition, which might reduce fatty acid synthesis by limiting the availability of NADPH. However, subsequent work in other laboratories makes it unlikely that G6PDH inhibition is the primary mechanism of anti-obesity action.[25,26] A more likely mechanism is that DHEA treatment enhances thermogenesis through the stimulation of futile cycles or other energy-dissipating pathways.[27,28]

V. CANCER PREVENTIVE EFFECT

DHEA produced two biological effects that suggested that it might demonstrate cancer preventive activity *in vivo*: the steroid protected cultured cells against chemical carcinogen-induced cytotoxicity and transformation, and DHEA treatment of mice produced a striking antiweight effect, primarily through a reduction in caloric efficiency rather than through appetite suppression. Reducing weight gain of laboratory mice and rats through food restriction produces what may be the most marked cancer preventive action of any known regimen.[29] Spontaneous, chemically induced, and radiation-induced tumors in many different organs are all reduced in frequency in food-restricted rodents. Not only does underfeeding inhibit tumor development, it retards the rate of appearance of many age-related pathological changes and is believed to slow the rate of aging.[30,31] The fundamental mechanism by which underfeeding protects against such a broad spectrum of pathological changes is obscure, and its elucidation is of the greatest importance.

We did indeed find that long-term DHEA treatment inhibited the development of spontaneous breast cancer in C3H-A^{vy}/A (obese) and C3H-A/A (nonobese mice[23,32] (Table 1), DMBA- and urethane-induced lung adenomas in A/J mice[33] (Table 2), and 1,2-dimethylhydrazine-induced colon tumors in BALB/c mice.[34] Garcea et al.[35] reported that DHEA administration to Wistar rats inhibited the development of liver preneoplastic foci induced by diethylnitrosamine initiation followed by partial hepatectomy and treatment with *N*-acetylaminofluorene and phenobarbital. Similarly Moore et al.[36] found that DHEA administration to F344 rats previously treated with dihydroxy-di-*n*-propylnitrosamine inhibited the development of thyroid tumors and preneoplastic liver foci, and Weber et al.[37] reported that DHEA treatment reduced the frequency of *N*-nitrosomorpholine-induced hemangiosarcomas in Sprague-Dawley rats.

In all of the above studies in which DHEA was administered orally and inhibited tumor development, there was a concomitant antiweight effect. Although this reduction in weight gain was not simply a result of food restriction, it is possible that reducing weight, even through a metabolic alteration in the efficiency of food utilization, might inhibit tumor development through a mechanism similar to that of restricting food intake. In order to determine if DHEA has any directly acting anticarcinogenic activity, we employed the two-stage procedure for induction of skin papillomas (DMBA initiation and TPA promotion)[38] and the complete model (weekly applications of DMBA to skin) for induction of skin papillomas and carcinomas.[39] In these experiments DHEA was applied topically to mouse skin 1 h before DMBA or TPA treatment. Under these conditions of topical treatment, DHEA has no effect on body weight and it is likely that any inhibition of tumor development by DHEA results from a direct action of the steroid on cells in the skin. We found that topical DHEA application (100 to 400 µg) to the skin of CD-1 mice inhibited DMBA-initiated and TPA-promoted papilloma formation at both the

TABLE 1
Effects of Long-Term DHEA Treatment on Breast Cancer Incidence in C3H-A/A and C3H-A^{vy}/A Mice

	Length of treatment (months)														
	4	5	6	7	8	9	10	11	12	13	14	15	16	17	18
C3H-A/A															
No. controls living	78	78	75	72	67	60	54	49	42	35	35	33	30	29	20
No. controls with cancer (cumulative)	0	0	1	3	4	6	6	7	8	13	13	13	13	14	21
No. DHEA living	77	76	75	75	75	73	63	54	52	48	44	42	38	32	29
No. DHEA with cancer (cumulative)	0	1	1	1	1	1	1	3	4	5	6	6	7	7	9
C3H A^{vy}/A															
No. controls living	27	26	26	24	21	17	15	12	11	9	7	7			
No.controls with cancer (cumulative)	0	0	0	2	5	9	11	14	15	17	19	19			
No. DHEA living	23	23	22	22	21	19	19	16	16	15	12	9			
No. DHEA with cancer (cumulative)	0	0	0	0	0	0	0	0	0	1	4	5			

Note: DHEA-treated mice received 450 mg/kg of DHEA (prepared as a suspension in sesameoil) by peroral intubation 3 times weekly. Spontaneous breast tumors were detected by weekly palpation.

(From Schwartz, A. G., Hard, G. C., Pashko, L. L., Abou-Gharbia, M., and Swern, D., *Nutr. Cancer,* 3, 46, 1981. With permission.)

initiation and promotion stages and inhibited DMBA-induced papilloma and carcinoma development in the complete carcinogenesis model.[40,41]

Topical application of 100 or 400 µg of DHEA to the skin of mice (doses that inhibited papilloma formation when applied 1 h before DMBA) also inhibited the amount of topically applied [^{3}H]DMBA bound to skin DNA over a 12-h period.[40] Very probably the antitumor initiating activity of DHEA in mouse skin results from inhibition of G6PDH activity and depression of carcinogen activation, as was likely the mechanism by which DHEA protected cells against DMBA- and aflatoxin B$_1$-induced toxicity and transformation.

A. INHIBITION OF TUMOR PROMOTION

Topical DHEA treatment also inhibits papilloma formation when applied 1 h before each TPA application, indicating that the steroid also blocks tumor promotion. DHEA and specific structural analogs block three steps that appear to play an important role in the tumor promoting action of TPA. These include:

1. Inhibition of TPA-induced stimulation of [^{3}H]thymidine incorporation into mouse epidermis
2. Inhibition of TPA-induced stimulation of superoxide anion (O_2^-) production by human neutrophils
3. Suppression of TPA-induced enhancement of mouse skin prostaglandin E$_2$ levels

Experimental evidence indicates that the first two effects, and possibly the third as well, result from an inhibition of G6PDH.

TABLE 2
Effect of DHEA on DMBA-and Urethane-Induced Lung Tumorigenesis

	No. of mice having indicated no. of tumors			
Tumors per mouse	DMBA alone	DMBA + DHEA	Urethane alone	Urethane + DHEA
0		3		
1		5		
2		5		
3	2	5		
4	1	1		1
5	1	1		
6	2	2		
8	3		1	2
9	3			1
10	2		1	
11	2	1		1
12			1	3
13				1
14	2			1
15	2		4	1
16	1		2	2
17	1		2	2
18			1	
19	2		3	
20			1	1
21			1	
22	1		1	1
23			1	2
24	1		2	
25			2	
26	1		1	
28				1
35	1			
No. of mice per group	28	23	24	20

Note: Groups of A/J mice were treated with either DMBA (0.5 mg in 0.2 ml sesame oil administered perorally) or urethane (1 mg/kg intraperitoneally of a sterile saline solution of urethane). Nine days after carcinogen treatment, mice received a diet containing 0.6% DHEA or a control diet. Fourteen weeks later, the mice were sacrificed and the number of lung adenomas was determined. DHEA produced a marked reduction in the incidence of lung tumors in DMBA-treated mice ($p < 0.001$, $X^2 = 25.2$) and a smaller effect in the urethane-treated animals ($p < 0.05$, $X^2 = 5.7$).

(From Schwartz, A. G. and Tannen, R. H., *Carcinogenesis*, 2, 1335, 1981. With permission.)

1. Inhibition of TPA Stimulated [³H]Thymidine Incorporation in Mouse Epidermis

TPA application to mouse skin stimulates epidermal DNA synthesis and hyperplasia.[42,43] The hyperplastic property of tumor promoters is apparently essential to their tumor promoting action, and it has been suggested that tumor promotion may simply result from clonal expansion of an altered, initiated cell which has a greater sensitivity than normal epidermal cells to the growth stimulatory effect of the promoter.[44]

A single i.p. injection of DHEA (10 mg/kg) into ICR mice immediately before TPA application abolishes the TPA stimulation in epidermal [³H]thymidine incorporation.[18] The synthetic steroid, Epi-Br, a compound that is about 30 times more potent than DHEA as an inhibitor of G6PDH,[17] is also much more active as an inhibitor of the TPA stimulation of [³H]thymidine incorporation — an injected dose of 0.4 mg/kg of Epi-Br is more effective than

10 mg/kg of DHEA.[18] The much greater activity of Epi-Br as both an inhibitor of G6PDH and as a suppressor of TPA stimulated [³H]thymidine incorporation led us to conclude that G6PDH inhibition very likely caused the suppression in [³H]thymidine incorporation.

DHEA is also effective in abolishing TPA stimulated [³H]thymidine incorporation in mouse epidermis when topically applied (100 to 400µg) or when administered p.o. (400 mg/kg). The requirement for a much greater oral (400 mg/kg) than i.p. (10 mg/kg) dose of DHEA may be a result of steroid degradation in the liver following the oral route of administration.

2. Inhibition of 3T3 Fibroblast Differentiation

Specific 3T3 fibroblast clones can, under carefully defined conditions, be stimulated to undergo highly efficient differentiation into adipocytes.[45] Adipocyte differentiation is a multistep process, the mechanism of which is unclear. Increases in thymidine incorporation, in cell number, and in translatable mRNAs precede the elevation of marker enzymes of lipid synthesis, and of increased incorporation of acetate into lipid.[45] Using the above assay of conversion of 3T3 preadipocytes to adipocytes, Gordon et al.[46] found that DHEA and Epi-Br blocked the conversion to adipocytes of the 3T3-L1 and 3T3-F442A mouse embryo fibroblast clones. They also observed that Epi-Br was much more potent than DHEA in blocking conversion and suggested that G6PDH inhibition by these steroids very likely accounted for this effect.

Two major functions usually ascribed to the oxidative branch of the pentose phosphate cycle are the generation of NADPH for reductive biosynthesis and other specific metabolic reactions as well as the formation of ribose-5-phosphate, which is utilized in nucleotide biosynthesis via the intermediate 5-phosporibosyl-1-pyrophosphate. Purine ribonucleotide and thymidylic acid biosynthesis are dependent upon tetrahydrofolic acid, which requires NADPH for its reductive synthesis from folic acid. Also, the enzymatic formation of deoxyribonucleotide diphosphates from their corresponding ribonucleotide diphosphates by ribonucleotide reductase is NADPH dependent.

If DHEA and related steroids repress DNA synthesis in cells by reducing ribonucleotide and deoxyribonucleotide synthesis as a result of G6PDH inhibition, then provision of these nucleotides would be expected to reverse the DHEA-induced inhibition. This was indeed shown to be the case with cultured HeLa TCRC-2 cells. DHEA at a concentration of 10^{-5} M inhibited the growth rate of these cells in culture, and this growth inhibition was almost completely overcome by adding to the culture medium a mixture of the deoxynucleosides of adenine, guanine, thymine, and cytosine.[47] Gordon et al.[48] have also found that the addition of the four ribonucleosides (uridine, cytidine, adenosine, and guanosine) to cultured 3T3-L1 cells almost completely prevented the blocking action of Epi-Br on the differentiation of these cells to adipocytes.

Garcea et al. have made the interesting observation that nucleosides reverse the DHEA blocking action on preneoplastic foci development in rat liver. Preneoplastic foci are readily induced in rat liver by a single injection of DMN followed by treatment with 2-acetylaminofluorene, partial hepatectomy, and then phenobarbital.[49] If DHEA is administered during the period of phenobarbital treatment, there is a reduction both in the size of these foci (53%) as well as in the [³H]thymidine labeling indices of focus cells (48%). A regimen of three daily injections of the four ribo- or deoxyribonucleosides completely reversed the DHEA inhibition in both focus size and in the [³H]thymidine labeling index of focus cells.[49]

3. Inhibition of TPA-Induced Stimulated Superoxide Anion Formation

Unlike tumor initiators,which are mutagenic to bacterial and mammalian cells, TPA is apparently not intrinsically mutagenic.[50] However, TPA induces sister chromatid exchanges in cultured hamster fibroblasts[51] and chromosomal aberrations in cultured mouse keratinocytes,[52] in primary human leukocyte cultures,[53] and in human fibroblast cultures.[54]

There is evidence that TPA treatment stimulates the formation of various forms of reactive oxygen, such as superoxide anion (O_2^-) and hydroxyl radical as well as various hydroxy and hydroperoxy fatty acids, which are responsible for the clastogenic action of the tumor promoter.[55] Two sources of reactive oxygen which are stimulated by TPA are an O_2^--generating oxidase found in phagocytic cells[56] and the arachidonic acid cascade, which produces hydroperoxy and hydroxy fatty acids through the action of either cyclooxygenase or lipoxygenase.[57]

An alternative to the hypothesis that tumor promoter-induced reactive oxygen produces mutagenic or clastogenic effects in initiated epidermal cells, which transforms them into papilloma cells, is that reactive oxygen might simply act as a mitogen to initiated cells, stimulating their growth into benign tumors. Craven et al.[58] have obtained experimental evidence that in rat colonic mucosa the stimulation of reactive oxygen formation by deoxycholate is critical to the enhancement in [^{3}H]thymidine incorporation produced by the bile salt. Intracolonic instillation of deoxycholate, a substance which promotes experimental colon tumorigenesis, stimulates [^{3}H]thymidine incorporation into colonic mucosa. This response to deoxycholate is abolished by the superoxide mimetic copper (II) (3,5-diisopropylsalicylic acid)$_2$ (CuDIPS), a result which indicates that reactive oxygen, and particularly O_2^-, plays an essential role in the stimulation of [^{3}H]thymidine incorporation. Similarly, Bull et al.[59] reported that intrarectal instillation of various hydroxy and hydroperoxy derivatives of arachidonic and linoleic acid stimulate [^{3}H]thymidine incorporation into rat colonic mucosa.

Suppression of TPA-promoted skin papilloma formation in mice by treatment with CuDIPS strongly suggests an essential role for reactive oxygen in TPA-promoted tumorigenesis.[60] Various lipoxygenase inhibitors are also effective in inhibiting TPA-promoted papillomas in mice.[61] On the contrary, indomethacin, a cyclooxygenase inhibitor, enhances tumor formation at topical doses of less than 100 µg with inhibition occurring at higher doses.[62]

TPA treatment of human neutrophils *in vitro* produces a rapid increase in the formation of O_2^-,[56] which is generated by an NADPH-dependent oxidase.[63] DHEA inhibits this stimulation of O_2^- formation, and the synthetic steroid, Epi-Br, is a more potent inhibitor, a result again suggesting that G6PDH inhibition and a reduction in NADPH pool size is the probable mechanism of inhibition.[64] Further support for this mechanism of inhibition of O_2^- production is the finding that neutrophils from individuals with the Mediterranean variant of G6PDH deficiency produce less O_2^- (58% decrease) when stimulated with TPA than do neutrophils from normal individuals.[65]

There are three processes which contribute to tumor development: (1) metabolic activation of a carcinogen through the action of mixed-function oxidases, (2) tumor promoter stimulation of cell proliferation, and (3) tumor promoter stimulation of O_2^- formation are all inhibited by DHEA, probably as a result of G6PDH inhibition and a lowering of the NADPH and ribose-5-phosphate cellular pools. We have recently obtained evidence indicating that these first two processes are inhibited in mouse epidermis following a regimen of 40% food restriction for 2 weeks, suggesting a similarity in the mechanism by which underfeeding and DHEA inhibit tumorigenesis. Specifically, reducing the food intake of A/J mice (60% of *ad libitum* fed) for 2 weeks inhibits the rate of binding of [^{3}H]DMBA to mouse skin DNA by 50%.[66] A similar reduction in [^{3}H]DMBA binding to skin DNA is produced by topical application of DHEA 1 h before DMBA treatment. The TPA stimulation in the rate of [^{3}H]thymidine incorporation in mouse epidermis is also abolished in food-restricted animals, an effect that is also seen with topical DHEA treatment. We found that mouse epidermal G6PDH activity was depressed by 60% following 2 weeks of food restriction,[66] and when one considers the evidence that the inhibition of [^{3}H]DMBA binding to DNA and the suppression of TPA stimulation in [^{3}H]thymidine incorporation by DHEA very likely results from G6PDH inhibition, it is reasonable to assume that the depression in epidermal G6PDH activity following underfeeding may exert a similar effect.

VI. DHEA ANALOGS

Certain side effects have been observed following treatment of mice and rats with DHEA. DHEA can be metabolized into testosterone and esterone, and treatment of rats with biologically active doses of DHEA produces both uterine enlargement in females[67] and seminal vesicle enlargement in males.[26] In addition, DHEA treatment causes hepatomegaly and increases liver catalase activity,[26] effects that are also produced by a group of hypolipedemic drugs that are peroxisome proliferators.[68]

We have developed two synthetic analogs of DHEA, 16α-fluoro-5-androsten-17-one (8354) and 16α-fluoro-5α-androstan-17-one(8356) (Figure 1), which do not demonstrate the estrogenic, androgenic, and liver-enlarging effects of DHEA and are also more potent G6PDH inhibitors than the parent steroid.[26] When orally administered to mice, 8354 and 8356 are at least four times as potent as DHEA in inhibiting the binding of [^{3}H]DMBA to skin DNA and in suppressing the TPA stimulation in epidermal [^{3}H]thymidine incorporation.[26] Compounds 8354 and 8356 are also more active than DHEA in blocking DMBA-initiated and TPA-promoted skin papilloma development in mice at both the initiation and promotion stage.[69] Compound 8354 has about three times the anti-obesity activity of DHEA, whereas 8356 is about equally potent.

VII. INHIBITION OF TPA STIMULATION OF SKIN PROSTAGLANDIN LEVELS

The arachidonic acid cascade produces various eicosanoids through both the lipoxygenase pathway, which generates various hydroxy fatty acids, leukotrienes, and the cyclooxygenase pathway, which is the source of specific prostaglandins, prostacyclins, and thromboxanes. There is evidence that both of these pathways in arachidonic acid metabolism are important in the tumor-promoting action of TPA. Inhibitors of lipoxygenase block TPA-induced tumor promotion,[61] and the work of Fischer and Adams[57] suggests that a major source of TPA-stimulated reactive oxygen produced in isolated mouse epidermal cells is due to the metabolism of arachidonic acid via the lipoxygenase pathway. Fürstenberger and Marks [70] have found that TPA-induced increases in prostaglandin E$_2$ (PGE$_2$) content in mouse epidermis may be an obligatory event in the TPA enhancement of the DNA synthesis rate, which plays a critical role in tumor promotion. Indomethacin treatment blocks both the TPA stimulation in epidermal PGE$_2$ content as well as the stimulation in [^{3}H]thymidine incorporation. This inhibition by indomethacin can be reversed by topical application of PGE$_2$ simultaneously with TPA.

We have found that treatment of CD-1 mice with DHEA, and even more so with compounds 8354 and 8356, inhibits TPA stimulation of skin PGE$_2$ levels.[71] Four steroids were tested for their capacity to affect TPA stimulation of skin PGE$_2$ content: 8356, 8354, DHEA, and etiocholanolone. Both 8356 and 8354 are more potent inhibitors of G6PDH than DHEA, whereas etiocholanolone, one of the primary degradative metabolites of DHEA in the human, is a very weak inhibitor.[17] We found that treatment of CD-1 mice for 14 d with diet containing either 0.2% 8354 or 0.2% 8356 prior to TPA application completely abolished the elevation in skin PGE$_2$ content produced 24 h after TPA treatment.[71] DHEA treatment was significantly less effective, whereas etiocholanolone produced little, if any, suppression in the enhancement of PGE$_2$ content.

The overall correlation among the four tested steroids between G6PDH inhibitory activity and potency in blocking stimulation of skin PGE$_2$ content again suggests a role for G6PDH inhibition in the mechanism of this effect. Arachidonic acid, the fatty acid precursor of PGE$_2$, is biosynthesized from linoleic acid by an NADH-NADPH dependent desaturase and elongase.[72,73] One possibility is that steroid treatment reduces the pool of arachidonic acid available for prostaglandin synthesis. However, further work is necessary to clarify the mechanism of this inhibition.

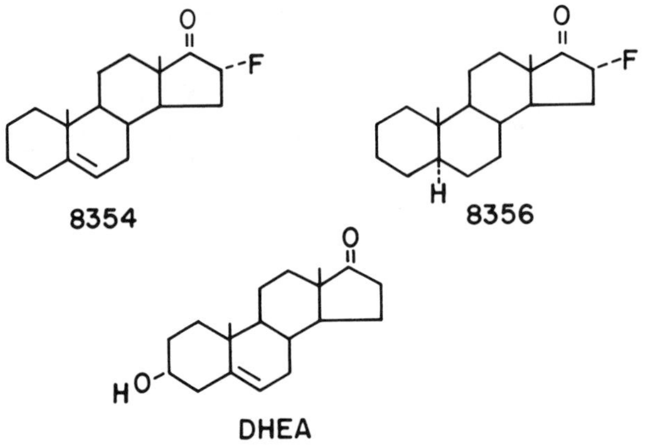

FIGURE 1.   Structure of steroids.

VIII. ANTI-ATHEROGENIC EFFECT

A recently reported epidemiologic study by Barrett-Connor et al.[74] suggests that high plasma concentrations of DHEA may protect men against the development of atherosclerotic heart disease. These investigators reported the results of a prospective study that examined the relationship of plasma DHEAS levels to subsequent 12 year mortality in a population-based cohort of 242 men aged 50 to 79 years. After adjusting for age, systolic blood pressure, serum cholesterol level, obesity, fasting plasma glucose level, cigarette smoking status, and personal history of heart disease, they found that DHEAS level was independently and inversely related to death from any cause and death from cardiovascular disease in particular in men over age 50.

Gordon et al. found that DHEA treatment of rabbits protected them against the development of experimentally induced atherosclerosis, a finding that may be related to the above epidemiologic observation.[75] The authors used a model in which severe aortic atherosclerosis occurs. A 2% cholesterol diet was given to ten New Zealand white male rabbits for 11 weeks: five received 0.5% DHEA in the diet, five did not. After 1 week on the diet, a balloon catheter-induced aortic intimal injury was performed on all animals. On day 77 the rabbits were sacrificed, the aortas were removed, and atherosclerosis was assessed by Sudan strain. Plaque thickness in five regions were quantified, and the authors noted a 39% decrease in plaque thickness in the DHEA-treated group. The effect was not due to differences in food intake, body weight, total serum cholesterol, or triglycerides.

Not only was plaque formation in the aorta inhibited by DHEA treatment, but fatty infiltration of the heart and liver was also markedly reduced, suggesting a possible effect of DHEA on the uptake of lipoproteins. Low density lipoprotein (LDL) that is modified by reactive oxygen generated by endothelial cells, smooth muscle cells, or phagocytes is taken up in an unregulated manner via a scavenger receptor on macrophages, and this may lead to the formation of foam cells, an important component of the atherosclerotic lesion.[76] In monocytes an important source of reactive oxygen which modifies LDL may be O_2^- produced by an NADPH-dependent oxidase.[77] As suggested by Gordon et al., DHEA inhibits O_2^- formation in TPA-stimulated neutrophils,[64] and this effect of DHEA may contribute to its anti-atherogenic effect.

In summary, DHEA has demonstrated cancer preventive and anti-atherogenic activity in laboratory animals, which make it a potentially very useful drug for human use. The elimination of certain undesirable side effects associated with DHEA treatment and the retention of biologic activity, as demonstrated with the synthetic compounds, 16α-fluoro-5-androsten-17-one and 16α-fluoro-5α-androstan-17-one, suggests that relatively safe compounds with DHEA-like activity can be developed, and such compounds may have important therapeutic applications in the human.

REFERENCES

1. **Baulieu, E. E.,** Studies of conjugated 17-ketosteroids in a case of adrenal tumor, *J. Clin. Endocrinol. Metab.,* 22, 501, 1962.
2. **Siiteri, P. K. and MacDonald, P. C.,** Placental estrogen biosynthesis during human pregnancy, *J. Clin. Endocrinol. Metab.,* 26, 751, 1966.
3. **Vande Wiele, R. and Lieberman, S.,** The metabolism of dehydroisoandrosterone, in *Biological Activity of Steroids in Relation to Cancer,* Pincus, G. and Vollmer, E., Eds., Academic Press, New York, 1960, 93.
4. **Zumoff, B., Rosenfeld, R. S., Strain, G. W., Levin, J., and Fukushima, D. K.,** Sex differences in the twenty-four-hour mean plasma concentrations of dehydroisoandrosterone (DHA), dehydroisoandrosterone sulfate (DHAS), and the DHA to DHAS ratio in normal adults, *J. Clin. Endocrinol. Metab.,* 51, 330, 1980.
5. **Orentreich, N., Brind, J. L., Rizer, R. L., and Vogelman, J. H.,** Age changes and sex differences in serum dehydroepiandrosterone sulfate concentrations throughout adulthood, *J. Clin., Endocrinol. Metab.,* 59, 551, 1984.
6. **Bulbrook, R. D., Hayward, J. L., Spicer, C. C., and Thomas, B. S.,** Abnormal excretion of urinary steroids by women with early breast cancer, *Lancet,* 2, 1238, 1962.
7. **Bulbrook, R. D., Hayward, J. L., and Spicer, C. C.,** Relation between urinary androgen and corticoid excretion and subsequent breast cancer, *Lancet,* 2, 395, 1971.
8. **Brownsey, B., Cameron, E. H. D., Griffiths, K., Gleave, E. N., Forest, A. P. M., and Campbell, H.,** Plasma dehydroepiandrosterone sulfate levels in patients with benign and malignant breast disease, *Eur. J. Cancer,* 8, 131, 1972.
9. **Rose, D. P., Stauber, P., Thiel, A., Crawley, J. J., and Milbrath, J. R.,** Plasma dehydroepiandrosterone sulfate, androstenedione and cortisol, and urinary free cortisol excretion in breast cancer, *Eur. J. Cancer,* 13, 43, 1977.
10. **Wang, D. Y., Bulbrook R. D., Herian, M., and Hayward, J. L.,** Studies on the sulphate esters of dehydroepiandrosterone and androsterone in the blood of women with breast cancer, *Eur. J. Cancer,* 10, 477, 1974.
11. **Zumoff, B., Levin, J., Rosenfeld, R. S., Markham, M., Strain, G. W., and Fukushima, D. K.,** Abnormal 24-hr mean plasma concentrations of dehydroisoandrosterone and dehydroisoandrosterone sulfate in women with primary operable breast cancer, *Cancer Res.,* 41, 3360, 1981.
12. **Rosenfeld, R. S., Rosenberg, B. J., Fukushima, D. K., and Hellman, L.,** 24-hour secretory pattern of dehydroisoandrosterone and dehydroisoandrosterone sulfate, *J. Clin. Endocrinol. Metab.,* 40, 850, 1975.
13. **Schwartz, A. G. and Perantoni, A.,** Protective effect of dehydroepiandrosterone against aflatoxin B_1- and 7,12-dimethylbenz(a)anthracene-induced cytotoxicity and transformation in cultured cells, *Cancer Res.,* 35, 2482, 1975.
14. **Kinoshita, N. and Gelboin, H. V.,** Aryl hydrocarbon hydroxylase and polycyclic hydrocarbon tumorigenesis: effect of the enzyme inhibitor 7,8-benzoflavone on tumorigenesis and macromolecule binding, *Proc. Natl. Acad. Sci. U.S.A.,* 69, 824, 1972.
15. **Swenson, D. H., Miller, J. A., and Miller, E. C.,** 2,3-Dihydro-2,3-dihydroxy aflatoxin B_1: an acid hydrolysis product of an RNA-aflatoxin B_1 adduct formed by hamster and rat liver microsomes *in vitro, Biochem. Biophys. Res. Commun.,* 53, 1260, 1973.
16. **Marks, P. A. and Banks, J.,** Inhibition of mammalian glucose-6-phosphate dehydrogenase by steroids, *Proc. Natl. Acad. Sci. U.S.A.,* 46, 447, 1960.
17. **Raineri, R. and Levy, H. R.,** On the specificity of steroid interaction with mammalian glucose-6-phosphate dehydrogenase, *Biochemistry,* 9, 2233, 1970.
18. **Pashko, L. L., Schwartz, A. G., Abou-Gharbia, M., and Swern, D.,** Inhibition of DNA synthesis in mouse epidermis and breast epithelium by dehydroepiandrosterone and related steroids, *Carcinogensis,* 2, 717, 1981.
19. **Beutler, E.,** Glucose-6-phosphate dehydrogenase deficiency, in *The Metabolic Basis of Inherited Disease,* Stambury, J. B., Wingaarden, J. B., Fredrikson, D. S., Goldstein, J. L., and Brown, M. S., Eds., McGraw-Hill, New York, 1983, 1625.
20. **Feo, F., Pirisi, L., Pascale, R., Daino, L., Frassetto, S., Garcea, R., and Gaspa, L.,** Modulatory effect of glucose-6-phosphate dehydrogenase deficiency on the benzo(a)pyrene toxicity and transforming activity for *in vitro* cultured human skin fibroblasts, *Cancer Res.,* 38, 3419, 1984.
21. **Feo, R., Ruggiu, M. E., Lenzerini, L., Garcea, R., Daino, L., Frassetto, S., Addis, V., Gaspa, L., and Pascale, R.,** Benzo(a)pyrene metabolism by lymphocytes from normal individuals carrying the Mediterranean variant of glucose-6-phosphate dehydrogenase, *Int. J. Cancer,* 39, 560, 1987.
22. **Yen, T. T., Allan, J. V., Pearson, D. V., Acton, J. M., and Greenberg, M.,** Prevention of obesity in $A^{vy/a}$ mice by dehydroepiandrosterone, *Lipids,* 12, 409, 1977.
23. **Schwartz, A. G., Hard, G. C. Pashko, L .L:, Abou-Gharbia, M., and Swern, D.,** Dehydroepiandrosterone: an anti-obesity and anti-carcinogenic agent, *Nutr. Cancer,* 3, 46, 1981.
24. **Cleary, M. P., Fox, N., Lazin, B., and Billheimer, J.,** A comparison of the effects of dehydroepiandrosterone treatment to ad libitum and pair-feeding in the obese Zucker rat, *Nutr.Cancer Res.,* 5, 1247, 1985.

25. **Coleman, D. L., Schwizer, R. W., and Leiter, E. H.,** Effects of genetic background on the therapeutic effects of dehydroepiandrosterone (DHEA) in diabetes-obesity mutants and in aged mice, *Diabetes,* 33, 26, 1984.

26. **Schwartz, A. G., Lewbart, M. L., and Pashko, L. L.,** Novel dehydroepiandrosterone analogues with enhanced biological activity and reduced side effects in mice and rats, *Cancer Res.,* 48, 4817, 1988.

27. **Clearly, M. P., Hood, S. S., Chando, C., Hansen, C. T., and Billheimer, J. T.,** Response of sucrose-fed BHE rats to dehydroepiandrosterone, *Nutr. Res.,* 4, 485, 1984.

28. **Lardy, H., Su, C.-Y., Kneer, N., and Wielgus, S.,** Dehydroepiandrosterone induces enzymes that permit thermogenesis and decrease metabolic efficiency, in *Hormones, Thermogenesis, and Obesity,* Lardy, H. and Stratman, F., Eds., Elsevier, New York, 1988, 415.

29. **Tannenbaum, A. and Silverstone, H.,** Nutrition in relation to cancer, *Adv. Cancer Res.,* 1, 451, 1953.

30. **McCay, C. M., Crowell, M. F., and Maynard, L. M.,** The effect of retarded growth upon the length of life-span and upon the ultimate body size, *J. Nutr.,* 10, 63, 1935.

31. **Yu, B. P., Masoro, E. J., Murata, I., Bertrand, H., and Lynd, F. T.,** Life span study of SPF Fischer 344 male rats fed *ad libitum* or restricted diets: longevity, growth, lean body mass and disease, *J. Gerontol.,* 37, 130, 1982.

32. **Schwartz, A. G.,** Inhibition of spontaneous breast cancer formation in female C³H (A$^{vy/A}$) mice by long-term treatment with dehydroepiandrosterone, 39, 1129, 1979.

33. **Schwartz, A. G. and Tannen R. H.,** Inhibition of 7,12-dimethylbenz(a)anthracene- and urethane-induced lung tumor formation in A/J mice by long term treatment with dehydroepiandrosterone, *Carcinogenesis,* 2, 1335, 1981.

34. **Nyce, J. W., Magee, P. N., Hard, G. C., and Schwartz, A. G.,** Inhibition of 1,2-dimethylhydrazine-induced colon tumorigenesis in BALB/c mice by dehydroepiandrosterone, *Carcinogenesis,* 5, 57, 1984.

35. **Garcea, R., Daino, L., Pascale, R., Frassetto, S., Cozzolino, P., Ruggiu, M. E, and Feo, F.,** Inhibition by dehydroepiandrosterone of liver putative preneoplastic foci formation in rats subjected to the initiation-selection process of experimental carcinogenesis, *Toxicol. Pathol.,* 15, 164, 1987.

36. **Moore, M. A., Thamavit, W., Tsuda, H., Sato, K., Ichihara, A., and Ito, N.,** Modifying influence of dehydroepiandrosterone on the development of di-hydroxy-di-n-propylnitrosamine-initiated lesions in the thyroid, lung, and liver of F344 rats, *Carcinogenesis,* 7, 311, 1986.

37. **Weber, E., Moore, M. A., and Bannasch, P.,** Phenotypic modulation of hepatocarcinogenesis and reduction in N-nitrosomorpholine-induced hemangiosarcomas and adrenal lesion development in Sprague-Dawley rats by dehydroepiandrosterone, *Carcinogenesis,* 9, 1191, 1988.

38. **Boutwell, R. K.,** The function and mechanism of promoters of carcinogenesis, *CRC Crit. Rev. Toxicol.,* 2, 419, 1964.

39. **Terracini, B., Shubik P., and Della Porta, G.,** A study of skin carcinogenesis in the mouse with single applications of 9,10-dimethyl-1,2-benzanthracene at different dosages, *Cancer Res.,* 20, 1538, 1960.

40. **Pashko, L. L., Rovito, R. J., Williams, J.R., Sobel, E. L., and Schwartz, A. G.,** Dehydroepiandrosterone (DHEA) and 3 β-methylandrost-5-en-17-one: inhibitors of 7,12-dimethylbenz(a)anthracene (DMBA)-initiated and 12-O-tetra-decanoylphorbol-13-acetate (TPA)-promoted skin papilloma formation in mice, *Carcinogenesis,* 5, 463, 1984.

41. **Pashko, L. L., Hard, G. C., Rovito, R. J., Williams, J. R., Sobel, E. L., and Schwartz, A. G.,** Inhibition of 7,12-dimethylbenz(a)anthracene-induced skin papillomas and carcinomas by dehydroepiandrosterone and 3 β-methylandrost-5-en-17-one in mice, *Cancer Res.,* 45, 164, 1985.

42. **Argyris, T. S.,** Epidermal growth following a single application of 12-O-tetradecanoyl-phorbol-13-acetate in mice, *Am. J. Pathol,* 98, 639, 1980.

43. **Baird, W. M., Sedgwick J. A., and Boutwell, R. K.,** Effects of phorbol and four diesters of phorbol on the incorporation of tritiated precursors into DNA, RNA, and protein in mouse epidermis, *Cancer Res.,* 31, 1434, 1971.

44. **Hennings, H. and Yuspa, S. H.,** Two-stage tumor promotion in mouse skin: an alternative interpretation, *J. Natl. Cancer Inst.,* 74, 735, 1985.

45. **Green, H. and Kehinde, O.,** An established preadipose cell line and its differentiation in culture. II. Factors affecting the adipose conversion, *Cell,* 5, 19, 1975.

46. **Gordon, G. B., Newitt, J. A., Shantz, L. M., Weng, D. E., and Talalay, P.,** Inhibition of the conversion of 3T3 fibroblast clones to adipocytes by dehydroepiandrosterone and related anticarcinogenic steroids, *Cancer Res.,* 46, 3389, 1986.

47. **Dworkin, C. R., Gorman, S. D., Pashko, L. L., Cristofalo, V. J., and Schwartz, A. G.,** Inhibition of growth of HeLa and Wi-38 cells by dehydroepiandrosterone and its reversal by ribo- and deoxyribonucleosides, *Life Sci.,* 38, 1451, 1986.

48. **Gordon, G. B., Shantz, L. M., and Talalay, P.,** Modulation of growth, differentiation and carcinogenesis by dehydroepiandrosterone, *Adv. Enzyme Regul.,* 26, 355, 1987.

49. **Garcea, R., Daino, L., Frassetto, S., Cozzolino, P., Ruggiu, M. E., Vannini, M. G., Pascale, R., Lenzerini, L., Simile, M. M., Puddu, M., and Feo, F.,** Reversal by ribo- and deoxyribonucleosides of dehydroepiandrosterone-induced inhibition of enzyme altered foci in the liver of rats subjected to the initation-selection process of experimental carcinogenesis, *Carcinogenesis,* 9, 931, 1988.

50. **Lankas, G. R., Baxter, C. S., and Christian, R. T.,** Effect of tumor promoting agents on mutation frequencies in cultured V79 Chinese hamster cells, *Mutat. Res.,* 45, 153, 1977.

51. **Kinsella, A. R. and Radman, M.,** Tumor promoter induces sister chromatid exchange: relevance to mechanisms of carcinogenesis, *Proc. Natl. Acad. Sci. U.S.A.,* 75, 6149, 1978.

52. **Dzarlieva-Petrusevska, R. T. and Fuesnig, N. E.,** Tumor promoter 12-O-tetra-decanoylphorbol-13-acetate (TPA)-induced chromosome aberrations in mouse keratinocyte cell lines: a possible genetic mechanism of tumor promotion, *Carcinogenesis,* 6,1447, 1985.

53. **Emerit, I. and Cerutti, P.,** Tumor promoter phorbol-12-myristate-13-acetate induces chromosomal damage via indirect action, *Nature,* 293, 144, 1981.

54. **Kinsella, A. R., Gaines, H. S., and Butter, J.,** Investigation of a possible role for superoxide anion production in tumor promotion, *Carcinogenesis,* 4, 717, 1983.

55. **Cerutti, P. A.,** Prooxidant states and tumor promotion, *Science,* 227, 375, 1985.

56. **Goldstein, B. D., Witz, G., Amoruso, M., Stone, D. S., and Troll, W.,** Stimulation of human polymorphonuclear leukocyte superoxide anion radical by tumor promoters, *Cancer Lett.,* 11, 257, 1981.

57. **Fischer, S. M. and Adams, L. M.,** Suppression of tumor promoter-induced chemiluminescence in mouse epidermal cells by several inhibitors of arachidonic acid metabolism, *Cancer Res.,* 45, 3130, 1985.

58. **Craven, P. A., Pfanstiel, J., and DeRubertis, F.R.,** Role of reactive oxygen in bile salt stimulation of colonic epithelial proliferation, *J. Clin. Invest.,* 77, 850, 1986.

59. **Bull, A. W., Negro, N. D., Golembieski, W.A ., Crissman, J. D., and Marnett, L. J.,** *In vivo* stimulation of DNA synthesis and induction of ornithine decarboxylase activity in rat colon by hydroperoxides, autooxidation products of unsaturated fatty acids, *Cancer Res.,* 44, 4924, 1984.

60. **Kensler, T. W., Bush, D. M., and Kozumbo, W. J.,** Inhibition of tumor promotion by a biomimetic superoxide dismutase, *Science,* 221, 75, 1983.

61. **Aizu, E., Nakadate, T., Yamamoto, S., and Kato, R.,** Inhibition of 12-O-tetradecanoylphorbol-13-acetate-mediated epidermal ornithine decarboxylase induction and skin tumor promotion by new lipoxygenase inhibitors lacking protein kinase C inhibitory effects, *Carcinogenesis,* 7, 1809, 1986.

62. **Fischer, S. M., Gleason, G. L., Mills, G. D., and Slaga, T. J.,** Indomethacin enhancement of TPA tumor promotion in mice, *Cancer Lett.,* 10, 343, 1980.

63. **Babior, B. M.,** The enzymatic basis for O_2^- production by human neutrophils, *Can. J. Physiol. Pharmacol.,* 60, 1353, 1982.

64. **Whitcomb, J. M. and Schwartz, A. G.,** Dehydroepiandrosterone and 16α-Br-epiandrosterone inhibit 12-O-tetradecanoylphorbol-13-acetate stimulation of superoxide radical production by human polymorphonuclear leukocytes, *Carcinogenesis,* 6, 33, 1985.

65. **Pascale, R., Garcea, R., Ruggiu, M. E., Daino, L., Frasseto, S., Vannini, M. G., Cozzolino, P., Lenzerini, L., Feo, L., and Schwartz, A. G.,** Decreased stimulation by 12-O-tetradecanoylphorbol-13-acetate of superoxide radical production by polymorphonuclear leukocytes carrying the Mediterranean variant of glucose-6-phosphate dehydrogenase, *Carcinogenesis,* 8, 1567, 1987.

66. **Schwartz, A. G. and Pashko, L. L.,** Food restriction inhibits [^{3}H]7,12-dimethylbenz(a)-anthracene binding to mouse skin and tetradecanoylphorbol-13-acetate stimulation of epidermal [^{3}H]thymidine incorporation, *Anticancer Res.,* 6, 1279, 1986.

67. **Knudsen, T. T. and Mahesh, V. B.,** Initiation of precocious sexual maturation in the immature rat treated with dehydroepiandrosterone, *Endocrinology,* 97, 458, 1975.

68. **Reddy, J. K., Warren J. R., Reddy, M. K., and Lalwani, N. D.,** Hepatic and renal effects of peroxisome proliferators: biological implications, *Ann. N.Y. Acad. Sci.,* 386, 81, 1982.

69. **Schwartz, A. G., Fairman, D. K., Polansky, M., Lewbart, M. L., and Pashko, L. L.,** Inhibition of 7,12-dimethylbenz(a)anthracene-initiated and tetra-decanoylphorbol-13-acetate-promoted skin papilloma formation in mice by dehydroepiandrosterone and two synthetic analogs, *Carcinogenesis,* 10, 1809, 1989.

70. **Fürstenberger, G. and Marks, F.,** Indomethracin inhibition of cell proliferation induced by the phorbolester TPA is reversed by prostaglandin E_2 in mouse epidermis, *Biochem. Biophys. Res. Commun.,* 84, 1103, 1978.

71. **Hastings, L. A., Pashko, L. L., Lewbart, M. L., and Schwartz, A. G.,** Dehydroepiandrosterone and two structural analogs inhibit 12-O-tetradecanoyl-phorbol-13-acetate stimulation of prostaglandin E_2 content in mouse skin, *Carcinogenesis,* 9, 1099, 1988.

72. **Brenner, R.R.,** The desaturation step in animal biosynthesis of polysaturated fatty acids, *Lipids,* 6, 567, 1971.

73. **Nagao, M., Ishibashi, T., Okayasu, T., and Imai, Y.,** Possible involvement of NADPH-cytochrome P450 reductase and cytochrome b_5 on β-ketostearoyl-CoA reduction in microsomal fatty acid chain elongation supported by NADPH, *FEBS Lett.,* 155, 11, 1983.

74. **Barrett-Connor, E., Khaw, K.-T, and Yen, S. C.,** A prospective study of dehydroepiandrosterone sulfate, mortality, and cardiovascular disease, *N. Engl. J. Med.,* 315, 1519, 1986.

75. **Gordon, G. B., Bush, D. E., and Weisman, H. F.,** Reduction of atherosclerosis by administration of dehydroepiandrosterone, *J. Clin. Invest.,*82, 712, 1988.

76. **Fogelman, A. M., Schecter, I., Seager, J., Hokum, M., Child, J. S., and Edwards, P. A.,** Malondialdehyde alteration of low density lipoproteins leads to cholesteryl ester accumulation in human monocyte-macrophages, *Proc. Natl. Acad. Sci. U.S.A.,* 77, 2214, 1980.

77. **Hiramatsu, K., Rosen, H., Heinecke, J. W., Wolfbauer, G., and Chait, A.,** Superoxide initiates oxidation of low density lipoprotein by human monocytes, *Arteriosclerosis,* 7, 55, 1987.

Part I:
Factors Affecting the
Age Incidence of Cancer

IB: Genetic Diseases

Chapter 8

COLORECTAL CANCER IN FAMILIAL POLYPOSIS COLI

Tomas M. Heimann

TABLE OF CONTENTS

Familial polyposis coli is a condition that results from an inherited predisposition to develop colorectal polyps and cancer. Although there are some variations in the presenting symptoms, the development of myriads of colonic adenomatous polyps is the hallmark of this disease. When untreated, nearly all patients develop colorectal cancer at a mean age of approximately 40 years, or about 25 years earlier than the general population.[1] Although polyposis coli is not a common disease, study of these patients is important since it may provide significant information regarding the pathogenesis of colorectal cancer in the general population.

I. DIAGNOSIS

Familial polyposis coli is inherited in an autosomal dominant fashion resulting in the development of multiple colonic polyps and eventually colorectal cancer. Usually the colonic polyps become apparent during the second decade of life and the colorectal cancer potential increases in proportion to the age of the patient. The disease process produces relatively few symptoms and the conditions under which new patients are discovered can be grouped into several clinically significant categories. New cases which may result from primary genetic mutations or unknown previous family history are usually found at a later age and are more likely to have an associated colorectal cancer (Figure 1). Occasionally, polyposis coli is diagnosed incidentally when a detailed history is obtained in patients seeking medical treatment for seemingly unrelated problems such as an inguinal hernia, or when polyps are palpated during a rectal exam. Patients with Gardner's syndrome may present with multiple sebaceous cysts, osteomas, or desmoid tumors and this may alert the physician to the correct diagnosis (Figures 2 and 3). Once multiple polyposis is found, examination of the family members at risk will allow detection of other asymptomatic patients. This last group often consists of children and siblings, they tend to be younger, and have a lower risk of having a colonic cancer at the time of diagnosis (Figure 4).

II. CANCER RISK

The colorectal cancer risk in familial polyposis coli is directly proportional to the age of the patient. The mean age for patients with polyposis undergoing colectomy at The Mount Sinai Hospital in New York between 1947 and 1970 was 38 years and nearly 40% had colorectal cancer. Since 1970, the mean age at operation has decreased to 29 and the cancer incidence has dropped to 22%.[2] Review of the medical records of 100 patients with polyposis coli shows that none of the patients operated before age 20 had an invasive cancer. The incidence of colorectal cancer in the third decade, however, is already 25% and this rate increases to nearly 40% in older patients.

Multiple colorectal cancers also occur more frequently in patients with polyposis. Synchronous cancers were present in 15% of the patients with cancer, and the mean age of the patients in this group was 51 years.[3] In patients with colonic cancer undergoing subtotal colectomy with ileorectal anastomosis, the incidence of metachronous second cancers was 33%. The propensity to develop a second cancer in the rectum is even more pronounced when patients who died from the first neoplasm are excluded thereby increasing the incidence to 46%.[4] The mean interval between the initial colonic resection and the development of the second rectal cancer was only 5 years. The mean age at the time of diagnosis of the second cancer was 57 years. Rectal cancer also occurred in 10% of patients who did not have a colonic tumor at the time of colectomy. The mean age of the patients in this group was 60 years but the mean interval from colectomy to development of rectal cancer of 18 years was much longer than in the patients with a previous colonic cancer (Figure 5).[5]

The Dukes classification of 37 colorectal cancers seen in 31 patients with familial polyposis

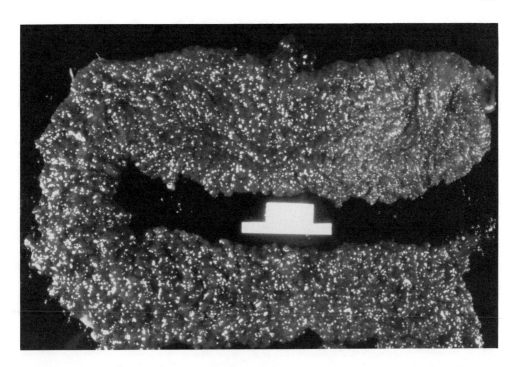

FIGURE 1. Colectomy specimen from 37-year-old female with familial polyposis coli. The entire colon and rectum are carpeted with polyps of various sizes. The largest polyp in the sigmoid colon contains early carcinomatous changes.

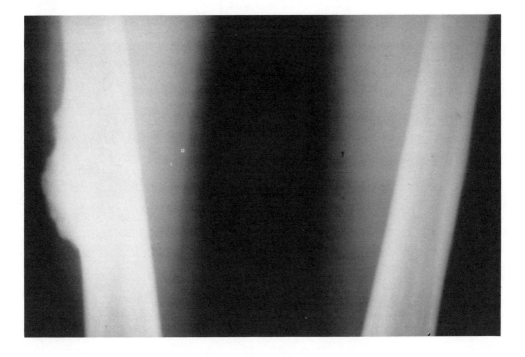

FIGURE 2. Osteoma of the femur in a 47-year-old patient with Gardner's syndrome. The patient also had multiple previous excisions of sebaceous cysts before the diagnosis of Gardner's syndrome was made when a cecal carcinoma was discovered.

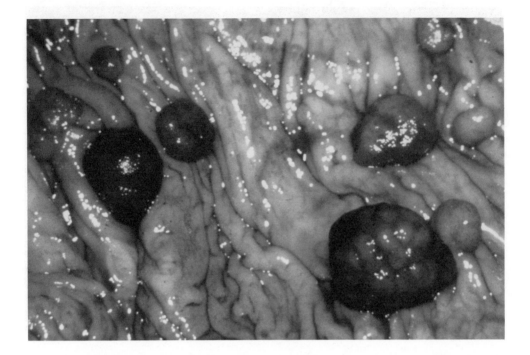

FIGURE 3.   Multiple colonic polyps in a patient with Gardner's syndrome. The colonic mucosa between the polyps appears normal.

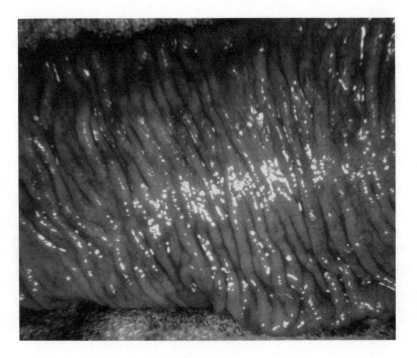

FIGURE 4.   Colon and rectum from a 13-year-old patient with familial polyposis coli treated with an ileoanal pullthrough. Multiple foci of adenomatous hyperplasia and small adenomatous polyps are present throughout the specimen.

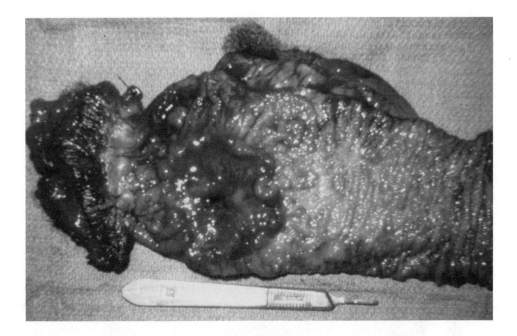

FIGURE 5. Large rectal carcinoma in a 64-year-old patient with familial polyposis who underwent a subtotal colectomy 21 years earlier. This is a poorly differentiated deeply infiltrating lesion with multiple positive nodes. The patient is alive and free of recurrent disease 8 years after abdominoperineal resection.

shows a similar distribution to that seen in the general population: 11% were Dukes' A lesions, 30% were Dukes' B, 27% were Dukes' C, and 32% had distant metastasis. Nearly 50% of all Dukes' C and D lesions occurred in patients who developed rectal cancer after subtotal colectomy. None of the patients in this group had early lesions. It is not easily understood why metachronous rectal cancers have such a poor prognosis. Although the finding of advanced lesions may be partly explained on the basis of poor follow-up, advanced lesions have also been discovered in patients returning for frequent endoscopic surveillance (Figure 6). Patients without pedunculated rectal polyps and those with regression of polyps after subtotal colectomy are still at risk to develop a carcinoma since careful inspection of the rectal mucosa often demonstrates diffuse adenomatous changes (Figure 7).

III. CHOICE OF OPERATION

It is apparent that patients who undergo subtotal colectomy at an early age have initially a fairly low incidence of developing rectal cancer. The cancer rate seems to increase significantly as the patients become older and careful surveillance every 3 to 6 months becomes necessary in all patients over 40 years of age. Complete prevention of development of rectal cancer is only possible if all rectal mucosa is removed. Total proctocolectomy and ileostomy is usually not an attractive alternative for a young asymptomatic patient with polyposis coli. It may, however, be an acceptable choice in the treatment of patients over age 40 where the risk of rectal cancer may be increasing and frequent endoscopic surveillance is not possible.

Recently, mucosal proctectomy with ileoanal anastomosis has become another alternative in the surgical treatment of patients with polyposis coli.[6,7] The best results with this operation are obtained in young patients undergoing a simultaneous total colectomy. Patients with a previous subtotal colectomy who are approaching 40 years of age are also candidates for this operation. However, several factors may make the conversion from ileorectal to ileoanal anastomosis less

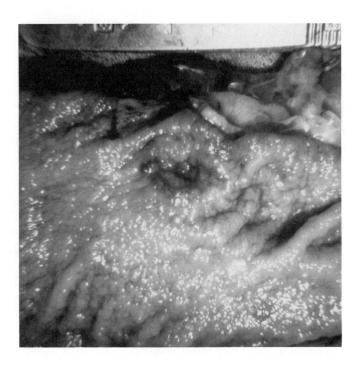

FIGURE 6. Small rectal cancer present in a 50-year-old patient with familial polyposis coli. The patient had a subtotal colectomy 5 years ago and subsequently developed regression of the remaining rectal polyps. Previous endoscopy 6 months earlier revealed three adenomatous polyps which were removed. This tumor invaded the serosa and one lymph node was positive. Patient is alive and well 9 years after abdominoperineal resection.

satisfactory. In a significant number of patients the mucosal stripping is difficult to perform due to scarring from previous fulguration.[8] Also, in patients with Gardner's syndrome, mesenteric fibrosis and shortening of the ileal mesentery make identification of the arterial blood supply impossible. This can create serious problems in achieving sufficient length to perform an ileoanal anastomosis without tension. Occasionally the development of large mesenteric desmoids may not allow the conversion to an ileoanal anastomosis (Figure 8). Mucosal proctectomy and ileoanal anastomosis produces best results when performed in a young patient with polyposis coli as the initial operative procedure. When used in older patients following a subtotal colectomy, the complication rate is higher and the functional results are often less satisfactory. It is also important to note that failure to completely remove the rectal mucosa down to the level of the dentate line will often give rise to new polyps and therefore some risk of cancer formation remains.

IV. TIMING OF OPERATION

The cancer risk in familial polyposis coli is closely associated with the age of the patient on a statistical basis. These parameters may be used as guidelines for timing of cancer surveillance and for operation. It is clear, however, that on an individual basis cancer risk and timing for operation is difficult to determine. In general, colectomy with either ileorectal or ileoanal anastomosis should be performed soon after the diagnosis of polyposis coli is made. Older patients and those with a colonic cancer should have a total proctocolectomy and ileostomy or ileoanal anastomosis since retaining the rectum carries a fairly high risk of developing rectal cancer. Timing and selection of older patients with a previous subtotal colectomy for further

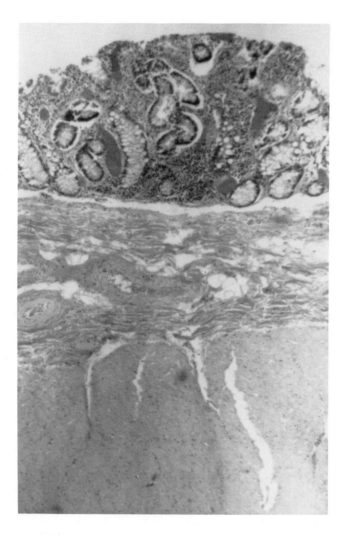

FIGURE 7. Adenomatous hyperplasia seen throughout the colon and rectum in patients with polyposis coli. These areas are still present in patients who undergo subtotal colectomy and appear to have regression of rectal polyps.

operation to avoid development of rectal cancer remains a controversial subject which will defy solution until a reliable parameter to assess cancer risk becomes available.

V. CANCER SURVEILLANCE

Patients with polyposis coli are often reluctant to accept surgical treatment because they are essentially asymptomatic. Although the cancer risk is present in all afflicted family members, it may not be sufficient to convince the patient to undergo a colectomy until a family member develops colorectal cancer. Knowledge of colorectal cancer distribution in patients who have had a colon resection is essential to determine the best diagnostic modality. Over 50% of the cancers are located in the rectum and sigmoid, while the remainder are evenly distributed throughout the colon. The polyps are usually distributed throughout the colon and rectum, and therefore sigmoidoscopy with biopsy of one of the polyps is usually sufficient to establish the diagnosis of polyposis coli. In children, the initial adenomatous changes may be difficult to detect and some degree of magnification may be necessary to see the mucosal irregularities

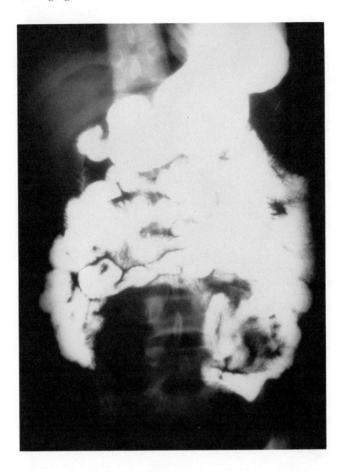

FIGURE 8.   Large mesenteric desmoid in a 27-year-old patient with Gardner's syndrome. The tumor extends from pelvis to diaphragm and compresses the ureters bilaterally. It developed within 18 months of a colectomy.

clearly. If the findings are unclear, repeat endoscopy in 1 year may show larger pedunculated polyps (Figure 9).

Assessment of cancer risk may be made empirically from the number of polyps present, size and villous component. All of these increase with age, but timing of cancer development seems to remain a chance occurrence. Once the patient has developed one colorectal cancer, it is unwise to leave any colorectal mucosa regardless of the age of the patient since risk of second cancer formation within a relatively short period of time is significant.

VI. CONCLUSION

Elimination of the risk of colorectal cancer is the primary goal in the surgical treatment of patients with familial polyposis coli. With the advent of flexible colonoscopy and understanding of the inheritance patterns of this condition, the incidence of colorectal cancer has decreased significantly. It is still unclear which operation produces the best results in this group of patients, and there are advocates for both subtotal colectomy with ileorectal anastomosis and mucosal proctectomy with ileoanal anastomosis. Long-term follow-up of patients with polyposis coli has demonstrated that there is also a propensity to develop other tumors of the intestinal tract such as duodenal and small intestinal cancers. These also seem to arise from adenomatous polyps.[9,10] Elimination of colorectal cancer in this population allows for a longer life expectancy and

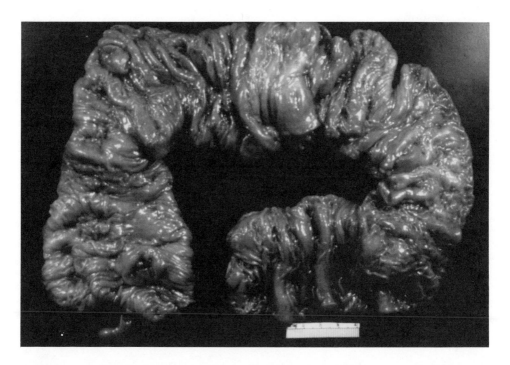

FIGURE 9. Small sessile adenomatous polyps in a 17-year-old patient with familial polyposis coli. Preoperative colonoscopy with multiple biopsies was necessary to confirm the diagnosis.

therefore an increased incidence of other associated tumors. While upper gastrointestinal endoscopy and polypectomy may be beneficial, surveillance of the small bowel remains difficult to perform and the incidence of adenomatous polyps in the jejunum and ileum is probably underestimated.

REFERENCES

1. **Bussey, H. J. R.,** *Familial Polyposis Coli,* Johns Hopkins University Press, Baltimore, 1975.
2. **Heimann, T. M., Greenstein, A. J., Bolnick, K., et al.,** Colorectal cancer in familial polyposis coli and ulcerative colitis, *Dis. Colon Rectum,* 28, 658, 1985.
3. **Greenstein, A.J., Slater, G., Heimann, T. M., et al.,** Comparison of multiple synchronous colorectal cancer in ulcerative colitis, familial polyposis coli, and de novo cancer, *Ann. Surg.,* 203, 123, 1986.
4. **Heimann, T. M., Bolnick, K., and Aufses, A. H., Jr.,** Results of surgical treatment for familial polyposis coli, *Am. J. Surg.* 152, 276, 1986.
5. **Moertel, C. G., Hill, J. R., and Adson, M. A.,** Surgical management of multiple polyposis: the problem of cancer in the retained bowel segment, *Arch. Surg.,* 100, 521, 1970.
6. **Heimann, T. M., Beck, A. R., and Greenstein, A.J.,** Familial polyposis coli: management by total colectomy with preservation of continence, *Arch. Surg.,* 113, 1104, 1978.
7. **Heimann, T. M., Gelernt, I., Salky, B., et al.,** Familial polyposis coli: results of mucosal proctectomy with ileoanal anastomosis, *Dis. Colon Rectum.,* 30, 424, 1987.
8. **Heimann, T. M., Slater, G., Kurtz, R. J., et al.,** Ultrasonic fragmentation: a new technique for mucosal proctectomy, *Arch. Surg.,* 120, 1200, 1985.
9. **Jarvinen, H., Nyberg, M., and Peltokallio, P.,** Upper gastrointestinal tract polyps in familial adenomatosis coli, *Gut,* 24, 333, 1983.
10. **Burt, R. W., Berenson, M. M., Lee, R. G., et al.,** Upper gastrointestinal polyps in Gardner's syndrome, *Gastroenterology,* 86, 295, 1984.

Chapter 9

PROGEROID SYNDROMES AND CANCER

Makoto Goto

TABLE OF CONTENTS

I. INTRODUCTION

Cancer diathesis in aged populations is well recognized,[1] although the exact role of aging per se on the development of cancer remains an open question. Extensive investigation has suggested that carcinogenesis may be affected by the duration of exposure to the carcinogenic agent(s), homeostasis of the internal environment, and intrinsic factors such as genetic influence. The effect of intrinsic factors on carcinogenesis may be further clarified by the study of genetic diseases characterized by accelerated aging, the so-called progeroid syndromes or premature aging syndromes. From among the premature aging syndromes listed in Table 1, Martin[2] has described genetic syndromes with multiple aspects (or segments) of the senescent phenotype as "segmental progeroid syndromes" and differentiated them from "unimodal progeroid syndromes" with a single aspect of the senescent phenotype, such as Alzheimer's disease (premature senile dementia), xeroderma pigmentosum (premature aging of skin), familial hypercholesterolemia (premature atherosclerosis), and type III amyloidosis (premature cardiac amyloidosis).

Other examples of segmental progeroid syndromes include Down syndrome, Hutchinson-Gilford syndrome (progeria), and ataxia telangiectasia. This chapter reviews cancer diathesis in some of the segmental progeroid syndromes.

II. WERNER'S SYNDROME

A. CLINICAL FEATURES

Werner's syndrome is recognized by several signs and symptoms,[3] some of which are similar to natural aging:

1. Characteristic habitus (slender extremities with a stocky trunk), short stature, and light body weight are common findings (Figure 1). All patients appear to be normal at birth and in childhood. Their growth stops shortly before adolescence, but the body parts are proportional in size.
2. Scleroderma-like skin changes include atrophic skin and muscle, circumscribed hyperkeratosis, telangiectasia, skin ulcers, and localized calcification.
3. Precocious aging is characterized by a bird-like appearance, alopecia, graying of the hair, skin hyperpigmentation, hoarseness, arteriosclerosis, cataracts, and osteoporosis.
4. Endocrinologic abnormalities are mainly diabetes mellitus and hypogonadism.
5. Consanguineous marriage between first cousins is noted in a majority of the patients' parents (Figure 2). Familial occurrence of this syndrome in both sexes is frequently reported.[4]
6. Malignant tumors in Werner's syndrome are described in Section II.D.

B. CLINICAL COURSE

The mean age at which patients are first diagnosed as having Werner's syndrome is 36.7 years (range of 15 to 70 years). However, the mean age at which patients or their families recognize certain characteristic manifestations of Werner's syndrome is 20 years (range of 2 to 40 years). The earliest sign is graying of the hair or alopecia, at a mean age of 20.3 years, followed in order by voice changes (22.5), skin changes (24 years), cataracts (29.6), diabetes mellitus (31.7 years), and skin ulcers (34.7 years).

The average life span of patients with Werner's syndrome is 43.5 years (range of 29 to 70 years), and the majority die of malignancies of various kinds; however, data relating to the age and cause of death are limited.

TABLE 1
Selected Premature Aging Syndrome

1. Werner's syndrome (adult progeria)
2. Hutchinson-Gilford syndrome (progeria)
3. Cockayne syndrome
4. Down syndrome
5. Turner syndrome
6. Louis-Bar syndrome (Ataxia telangiectasia)
7. Rothmund-Thomson syndrome
8. Diabetes mellitus

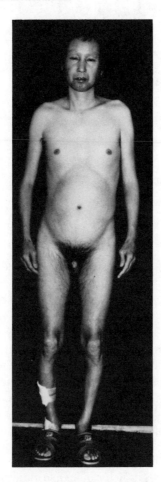

FIGURE 1.   Forty-two-year-old male. Note the characteristic habitus and stature characterized by Cushingoid appearance (body height: 158 cm, body weight: 45 kg).

C. CLINICO-PATHOLOGICAL DIFFERENCES BETWEEN NATURAL AGING AND WERNER'S SYNDROME

As Werner's syndrome is the most common syndrome of premature aging, it shares many of the features characteristic of natural aging. However, several signs and symptoms associated

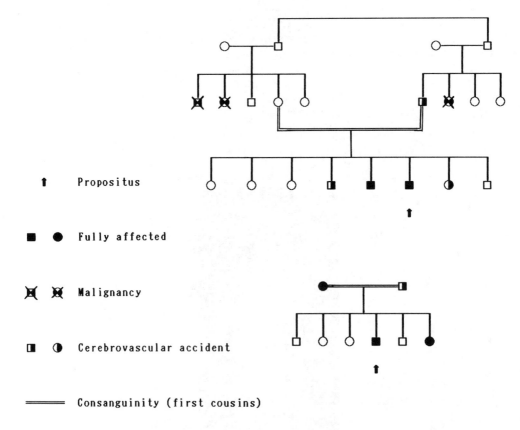

FIGURE 2.   Representative pedigree charts of Werner's syndrome and keys to symbols.

with natural aging occur earlier and sometimes with greater severity in Werner's syndrome (Table 2), while other features occur to a much lesser degree or not at all (Table 3). Immune dysfunctions similar to those of natural aging have also been reported. These include a high incidence of autoantibodies, depressed natural killer cell activity, and decreased percentages of T-cell subsets.[5-7] Although natural aging and Werner's syndrome bear a striking resemblance, at least superficially, closer inspection reveals many differences between the two entities in terms of the nature and degree of their various features. For example, dwarfism is primary in Werner's syndrome, but acquired in natural aging. Ocular cataracts in Werner's syndrome are cortical and subcapsular ("dystrophic type"), while those in natural aging are cortical or nuclear ("senile type"). Generalized osteoporosis is frequently found in the periphery in patients with Werner's syndrome, but is particularly severe in the spine in natural aging. Skin ulceration resulting in gangrene, subcutaneous calcification, hyperuricemia,[8] and hyaluronuria[9] are not usually associated with natural aging. In contrast, Werner's syndrome patients do not suffer from senile dementia or prostatic hypertrophy, which are frequently found in natural aging.

D. CANCER IN WERNER'S SYNDROME

The association between Werner's syndrome and neoplasia was first recognized by Agatston and Gartner in 1939.[11] They reported a case of Werner's syndrome with fibrosarcoma. Subsequently, Oppenheimer and Kugel[12] drew attention to the frequent association of Werner's syndrome with malignancy. Petrohelos[13] summarized the cases reported up to 1963, and stressed the increased occurrence of sarcomas in Werner's syndrome. Since then, an increasing number of reports have suggested that individuals with Werner's syndrome are at high risk for the development of cancer.

TABLE 2
Clinico-Pathological Characteristics of
Natural Aging and Werner's Syndrome

	Natural aging	Werner's syndrome
Dwarfism	+	#
Gray hair, hair loss	+	#
Skin hyperpigmentation	+	#
Voice change	+	#
Atherosclerosis	+	#
Cataract	+	#
Osteoporosis	+	#
Skin atrophy	+	#
Diabetes mellitus	+	#
Malignancy	+	#
Hypogonadism	+	#
Autoantibodies	+	#
Hyperlipidemia	+	#
Diminished replicative life span of fibroblast	+	#

TABLE 3
Clinico-Pathological Characteristics of
Natural Aging and Werner's Syndrome

	Natural aging	Werner's syndrome
Senile dementia	+	—
Prostatic hypertrophy	+	—
Skin ulcer	—	#
Subcutaneous calcification	—	#
Hyperuricemia	—	+
Hyaluronuria	—	#
Lymphopenia	+	+
Amyloid deposition	+	+
Lipofuscin deposition	+	+

The majority of patients with Werner's syndrome reported in the world literature have been of Japanese origin. About 300 cases of this disease have been documented in Japan since 1917,[4,15] and several immunological dysfunctions comparable to natural aging have also been described.[5-7] Cancer diathesis, especially of lymphoreticular origin in primary immunodeficiency syndromes, has been well documented[16] (Table 4). In contrast to primary immunodeficiency syndrome, Werner's syndrome is characterized by a high incidence of neoplasmas of mesenchymal origin,[14] a finding confirmed by the Japanese study.[4] However, the high frequency of different types of malignancies in this syndrome, including carcinomas as well as tumors of mesenchymal origin, should be stressed.[10]

Characteristic findings of the malignancies in Werner's syndrome are listed in Table 5, which is based on the Japanese study. The most prevalent cancers in the general Japanese population are stomach cancer, liver and biliary duct carcinoma, and lung and bronchial cancer in males, and stomach cancer, uterine cancer, and liver and biliary duct carcinoma in females.[1] However, these types of malignancies are rarely found in Japanese patients with Werner's syndrome. In addition, while cancers of the prostate and pancreas are frequent in the normal aged population, no Werner's syndrome patient has been reported to suffer from such cancers. Neither childhood cancers nor malignancies with embryonal characteristics have been described in Werner's

TABLE 4
Malignancies Associated with Immune Dysfunction[16]

	Epithelial	Leukemia lymphoreticular	Mesenchymal	Nervous system	Total
Werner's syndrome	20[a] (46.5%)[b]	3 (7%)	18 (41.9%)	2 (5%)	43
Primary immunodeficiency syndrome[c]	21 (18%)	88 (74.5%)	4 (3.5%)	5 (4%)	118

[a]   No. of cases.
[b]   Percentage of the type of malignancy in total patients with malignancy.
[c]   Includes Wiskott-Aldrich, congenital X-linked immunodeficiency, severe combined immunodeficiency, ataxia telangiectasia, common variable immunodeficiency, and IgA deficiency syndromes.

TABLE 5
Characteristics of Malignancies in Werner's Syndrome

1.   Malignancies frequent among normal Japanese are rare; no cases of carcinoma of the uterus, only one of stomach cancer, and two of lung cancer.
2.   Malignancies frequent among normal aged individuals are rare; no cases of carcinoma of the prostate or pancreas.
3.   No cases of childhood cancer or teratocarcinoma.
4.   Malignancies usually develop after the patients are fully affected.

syndrome. Malignancies usually develop after the patients have manifested most of the signs and symptoms described in previous chapters. The youngest patients associated with malignancies were 26 years old. These findings suggest that Werner's syndrome is not merely an accelerated form of natural aging, but rather a caricature of aging.

III. OTHER PROGEROID SYNDROMES AND CANCER

Down syndrome (21-trisomy) is characterized by short stature, short neck, typical facies, narrow palate, muscular hypotonia, and congenital heart diseases which lead to death in infancy in some cases. This syndrome is also well recognized as having a high risk of leukemia, particularly acute lymphoblastic leukemia, the incidence being 10 to 20 times higher than in the normal population.[17]

Cockayne syndrome, which is inherited in an autosomal manner, is characterized by dwarfism, pigmentary degeneration of the retina, optic atrophy, deafness, cataracts, extreme inanition, secondary hypogonadism, diabetes mellitus, atherosclerosis, sparse scalp hair, and severly retarded mental development. The average life span of patients with Cockayne syndrome is about 12 years. A central pathogenic mechanism in this syndrome may be the inability to repair long-patch errors in DNA sequence (the type of error induced by ultraviolet radiation and a number of chemicals), though no evidence of a high incidence of malignancy has been described.[18,19]

Rothmund-Thomson syndrome (poikiloderma congenita) is an autosomal recessive disorder associated with ectodermal dysplasia, juvenile-onset cataracts, hypogonadism, short stature, sparse scalp hair, and reduced life span. This syndrome is sometimes associated with squamous cell carcinoma, osteosarcoma, and fibrosarcoma.[20] The biochemical basis of Rothmund-Thomson syndrome is unknown. A defect in DNA-repair mechanisms that would explain the photosensitivity and the apparently increased risk for malignancy has been postulated.[21]

Ataxia-telangiectasia (Louis-Bar syndrome) is an autosomal recessive multisystem disorder comprising progressive oculocutaneous telangiectasia, cerebellar ataxia, bronchopulmonary disease, and lymphoreticular neoplasia. The close association with leukemia and malignant lymphoma is likely attributable to the immunodeficiency observed in ataxia telangiectasia. Possible chromosomal rearrangement encompassing an immunoglobulin gene on chromosome 14 could be responsible for the high incidence of malignancy in this disease.[22]

Hutchinson-Gilford syndrome (progeria) is characterized by a combination of infantilism and premature senility that is associated with alopecia, atrophy of subcutaneous fat and muscle, dwarfism, and propensity to fatal atherosclerotic complications during the first 2 or 3 decades of life. The cause and mechanism are unknown. There is no obvious increase in neoplasia in Hutchinson-Gilford syndrome.[23]

Xeroderma pigmentosum, which is categorized as a unimodal progeroid syndrome, is characterized by premature aging of the skin and a high incidence of skin cancer. This cancer-prone disease is inherited as an autosomal recessive trait. Because xeroderma pigmentosum cells are more readily mutated and transformed by ultraviolet radiation than normal cells, skin cancers in patients with xeroderma pigmentosum are definitely caused by the ultraviolet light in sunlight.[24]

IV. CONCLUSION

Some progeroid syndromes such as Werner's syndrome, Down syndrome, Rothmund-Thomson syndrome, ataxia-telangiectasia, and Xeroderma pigmentosum have a cancer diathesis. Of these, a high incidence of malignancies of mesenchymal origin is well recognized in patients with Werner's syndrome, while patients with Down syndrome have a high risk of leukemia. Analysis of the central pathogenic mechanisms in these progeroid syndromes may shed a new light on the relationship between aging and cancer.

REFERENCES

1. **Segi, M. and Kurihara, M.,** *Cancer Mortality for Selected Sites in 24 Countries,* Japanese Cancer Society, Tokyo, 1972.
2. **Martin, G. M.,** Genetic syndromes in man with potential relevance to the pathobiology of aging, *Birth Defects Orig. Series, Genetics of Aging,* 14, 5, 1977.
3. **Goto, M., Horiuchi, Y., Tanimoto, K., Ishii, T., and Nakashima, H.,** Werner's syndrome: analysis of 15 cases with a review of the Japanese literature, *J. Am. Geriat. Soc.,* 26, 341, 1978.
4. **Goto, M., Tanimoto, K., Horiuchi, Y., and Sasazuki, T.,** Family analysis of Werner's syndrome: a survey of 42 Japanese families with a review of the literature, *Clin. Genet.,* 19, 8, 1981.
5. **Goto, M., Horiuchi, Y., Okumura, K., and Tada, T.,** Immunological abnormalities of aging. An analysis of T lymphocyte subpopulations of Werner's syndrome, *J. Clin. Invest.,* 64, 685, 1979.
6. **Goto, M., Tanimoto, K., Aotsuka, S., Okawa, M., and Yokohari, R.,** Age-related changes in auto- and natural antibody in the Werner's syndrome, *Am. J. Med.,* 72, 607, 1982.
7. **Goto, M., Tanimoto, K., Horiuchi, Y., and Kuwata, T.,** Reduced natural killer cell activity of lymphocytes from patients with Werner's syndrome and recovery of its activity by purified human leukocyte interferon, *Scand. J. Immunol.,* 15, 389, 1982.
8. **Takeuchi, F., Kamatani, N., and Goto, M.,** Gout-like arthritis in patients with Werner's syndrome, *Jpn. J. Rheumatol.,* 1, 215, 1987.
9. **Goto, M. and Murata, K.,** Urinary excretion of macromolecular acidic glycosaminoglycans in Werner's syndrome, *Clin. Chim. Acta,* 85, 101, 1978.
10. **Sato, K., Goto, M., Nishioka, K., Arima, K., Hori, N., Yamashita, N., Fujimoto, Y., Nanko, H., and Ohara, K.,** Werner's syndrome associated with malignancies: five case reports with a survey of case histories in Japan, *Gerontology,* 34, 212, 1988.
11. **Agatston, S. A. and Gartner, S.,** Precocious cataracts and scleroderma, *Arch. Ophthal.,* 21, 492, 1939.

12. **Oppenheimer, B. S. and Kugel, V. H.,** Werner's syndrome: reports of the first necropsy and a family in a new case, *Am. J. Med. Soc.,* 202, 629, 1941.
13. **Petrohelos, M.,** Werner's syndrome: a survey of three cases, with review of the literature, *Am. J. Ophthal.,* 56, 941, 1963.
14. **Epstein, C. J., Martin, G. M., Schultz, A. L., and Motulsky, A. G.,** Werner's syndrome: a review of its symptomatology, natural history, pathologic features, genetics and relationship to the natural aging process, *Medicine,* 45, 197, 1966.
15. **Ishida, R.,** Cataracts associated with scleroderma, *Jpn. J. Opthalmol.,* 21, 1025, 1917.
16. **Kersey, J. H.,** in *Immunodeficiency in Men and Animals,* Bergsma, D. and Good, R. A., Eds., Saunderbird, MA, 1975, 289.
17. **Robinson, L. L., Nesbit, M. E., Sather, H. N., Level, C., Shahidi, N., Kennedy, A., and Hammond, D.,** Down syndrome and acute leukemia in children. A 10-year retrospective survey from childrens cancer study group, *J. Pediatr.,* 105, 235, 1984.
18. **Cockayne, E. A.,** Case reports: dwarfism with retinal atrophy and deafness, *Arch. Dis. Child.,* 21, 52, 1946.
19. **Otsuka, F. and Robbins, J. H.,** The Cockayne syndrome — an inherited multisystem disorder with cutaneous photosensitivity and defective repair of DNA, *Am. J. Dermatopathol.,* 7, 387, 1985.
20. **Thomson, M. S.,** Poikiloderma congenital: two cases for diagnosis, *Proc. R. Soc. Med.,* 29, 453, 1936.
21. **Smith, P. J. and Patterson, M. C.,** Enhanced radiosensitivity and defective DNA repair in cultured fibroblasts derived from Rothmond-Thomson syndrome, *Mutat. Res.,* 94, 213, 1982.
22. **Boder, E.,** Ataxia telangietasia, in *Neurocutaneous Diseases,* Gomez, M. R., Ed., Butterworths, Reading, MA, 1987, 95.
23. **DeBusk, F. L.,** The Hutchinson-Gilford syndrome, *J. Pediatr.,* 80, 697, 1972.
24. **Maher, V. M., Roman, L. A., and Siliuskins, K. C.,** Frequency of UV-induced neoplastic transformation of diploid human fibroblasts is higher in XP cells than in normal cells, *Proc. Natl. Acad. Sci. U.S.A.,* 79, 2613, 1982.

Part I:
Factors Affecting the
Age Incidence of Cancer

IC: Time After Exposure to the Carcinogen

Chapter 10

LATE RADIATION EFFECTS IN ATOMIC BOMB SURVIVORS: A REVIEW

Shoji Tokuoka and Kouki Inai

TABLE OF CONTENTS

On the 6th of August 1945, a uranium-235 bomb was detonated over Hiroshima City, releasing ionizing radiation consisting mostly of gamma rays and some neutrons. Three days later, a plutonium bomb was exploded over Nagasaki City, releasing similar radioactivity. It was estimated that about 60% of Hiroshima's population and about 30% of Nagasaki's population were exposed within 1000 m from ground zero and that about 64,000 citizens of the former and about 39,000 citizens of the latter died within 2 months after the bombing. The survival rate was estimated to be about 25% for persons exposed within 1000 m, about 50% for those exposed at 1300 m, and about 95% for those exposed at 2000 m from ground zero in both cities.[1]

Concerning the number of deaths among populations exposed to the bombings, including military employees, another report has estimated that the most probable number of deaths by the end of 1945 is approximately 90,000 to 120,000 persons among an exposed population of 330,000 in Hiroshima and 70,000 ± 10,000 among an exposed population of 270,000 persons in Nagasaki.[2]

In March 1947, the Atomic Bomb Casualty Commission (ABCC), a research institution for studying late radiation effects in atomic bomb survivors, was established in Hiroshima and Nagasaki by the U.S. National Academy of Sciences-National Research Council. In 1948, the National Institute of Health of the Japanese Ministry of Health and Welfare joined in the endeavor by starting joint Japan-U.S. research activities. Finally, in 1975, ABCC was reorganized and renamed the Radiation Effects Research Foundation (RERF), which is equally financed by Japan and the U.S.

Since 1947, many reports have been published on acute and late effects noted among atomic bomb survivors in the two cities. What follows is a general review of studies dealing with radiation carcinogenesis, as the most important delayed radiation effect, and with the acceleration of aging, if any, among atomic bomb survivors in both cities.

I. ATOMIC BOMB SURVIVORS AND CANCER

A. LEUKEMIA, LYMPHOMA, AND MYELOMA
1. Leukemia

It is now well known that many types of exposure to ionizing radiation may induce leukemia and other malignant neoplasms.[3-6] In atomic bomb survivors, leukemia incidence began to increase about 2 years after exposure to ionizing radiation in both cities,[7,8] and subsequently with a statistically significant linear increase that correlated inversely with exposure distance, particularly for persons exposed proximally from hypocenter.[9] Consequently, morbidity[10-12] and mortality[13] of leukemia reached a peak around 1951 in the survivors.

According to one of the earliest studies made by Folley et al.[14] on leukemia in the survivors, 29 cases of leukemia (19 from Hiroshima and 10 from Nagasaki) and 23 deaths due to leukemia (13 from Hiroshima and 10 from Nagasaki) were detected among 195,000 survivors during 1948 to 1950. While among 332,000 nonexposed persons during the same period, 20 leukemia deaths (11 from Hiroshima and 9 from Nagasaki) were identified. The increase in both leukemia incidence and mortality was statistically significant in the survivors, as compared with the nonexposed population ($p < 0.001$). Among the survivors, significantly higher leukemia incidence ($p < 0.001$) and mortality ($p < 0.001$) were noted among those exposed within 2000 m from ground zero than among those exposed at distance of 2000 m or greater.

Based on an analysis of 67 leukemia cases in Hiroshima, which were observed several years later, the annual incidence rate of leukemia per 10^5 persons by exposure distance from ground zero was estimated as 151.1 within 1000 m, 46.8 at 1000 to 1499 m, 5.0 at 1500 to 1999 m, 1.1 at 2000 to 2999 m, and 3.4 at 3000 m or over.[15]

Leukemia was encountered in all survivors age groups, from 6 to over 60 years of age, in both sexes,[16] with acute leukemia and chronic granulocytic leukemia being most prevalent.[7,17] In Hiroshima, chronic granulocytic leukemia was especially predominant in younger age groups exposed within 1500 m.[8,11] Chronic lymphocytic leukemia originally uncommon in Japan was very rare in both cities.[10,16,18]

Studies of leukemia in the Life Span Study (LSS) sample at ABCC (RERF) was begun in the late 1950s.[19] The LSS cohort is a fixed population, consisting of 73,000 residents and 27,000 nonresidents at the time of the bombing (ATB) in either Hiroshima or of Nagasaki, based on the 1950 Japanese National Census.[20] About 10,000 individuals were added later to the original population sample.[21,22] Death certificate information obtained through the Japanese family registration system provides the basic information for determining mortality rates in the LSS cohort.

Gamma and neutron doses have been estimated for all but 3% of the exposed persons in the cohort by means of a dosimetry called T65D. Exposure was expressed in rad as tissue kerma in air.[13,23-25] In March 1986, a new method for estimating individual doses was introduced, called Dosimetry System 1986 (DS86). The DS86 free-in-air gamma dose increases somewhat in Hiroshima, but decreases in Nagasaki in comparison with the previous T65D. The neutron dose decreases in both cities to about 10% of its former value in Hiroshima and 30% in Nagasaki.[26,27] The data reviewed herein were based on T65D except for cancer mortality during the years 1950 to 1985, which was based on DS86.[26,27]

Case ascertainment for leukemia in both cities is believed to be complete.[19,28] A group of highly qualified hematologists has recently been in close agreement for the types of leukemia in the registry in accord with the French-American-British classification.[29]

An analysis by Ishimaru et al.[30] on 149 cases of leukemia ascertained in the LSS cohort during 1950 to 1966 revealed that the risk of radiogenic leukemia increased with increasing exposure dose in Hiroshima, while it increased only in the group with exposure dose 100 rad or more in Nagasaki. The risk of chronic granulocytic leukemia increased significantly in the less than 50 rad exposure group in Hiroshima, whereas an increased risk was observed only in the over 200 rad exposure group in Nagasaki. It has been suggested that the difference in risk of leukemia from atomic bomb exposure in the two cities may be due to differences in composition of the bombs.[11,30] This explanation for differences between the cities seems not to be the case in view of recent reassessments of the radiation released from the bombs in each city which indicates that it was quite similar.[26,27]

Ichimaru et al.[31] have calculated the standardized annual incidence rate for all types of leukemia by dose and city during the years 1950 to 1978 for the 189 cases of leukemia (149 from Hiroshima and 40 from Nagasaki) in the LSS cohort (Figure 1). The age-ATB-adjusted mean annual incidence rate per 10^5 persons by exposure dose for that study period was 60.8 in the 100 rad or more group, 7.5 in the 1 to 99 rad group, and 4.3 in the nonexposed group in Hiroshima, whereas the rates for the same exposure groups in Nagasaki were 28.2, 4.4, and 4.3, respectively (Figure 2).

The age-ATB-specific annual incidence rate for acute leukemia was $43.7/10^5$ persons in the 100 rad or more group, 3.9 in the 1 to 99 rad group, and 3.5 in the nonexposed group in Hiroshima, while the rates in Nagasaki for the same exposure groups were 25.8, 2.7, and 3.8, respectively. On the other hand, the corresponding rates per 10^5 persons for chronic granulocytic leukemia in the same exposure groups in Hiroshima were 17.2, 3.6, and 0.8, respectively, and 2.4, 1.8, and 0, respectively, in Nagasaki. The mean bone marrow kerma for the A-bomb survivors in the 100 rad or more groups was 123.5 rad in Hiroshima and 135.6 rad in Nagasaki.

Some unusual features concerning the occurrence of leukemia in relationship to age ATB and amount of radiation exposure have been observed in the LSS cohort. The results suggest that the latent period for acute leukemia may have been inversely related to exposure group. A stronger relationship exists for age ATB and latent period for acute leukemia. Those who were very young ATB had short latent periods. Virtually all of the radiation effect for children who were less than 15 years of age ATB occurred before 1960. On the other hand, risk of leukemia appeared later and declined later for persons who were older ATB. For example, the increase

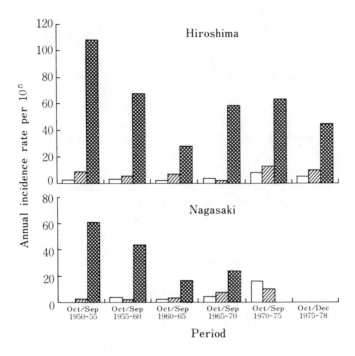

FIGURE 1. Standardized annual incidence rate for all types of leukemia in the RERF sample by dose, time period, and city, 1950—1978. ☐ = control; = ▨1-99 rad; ▦ = 100+ rad.[50]

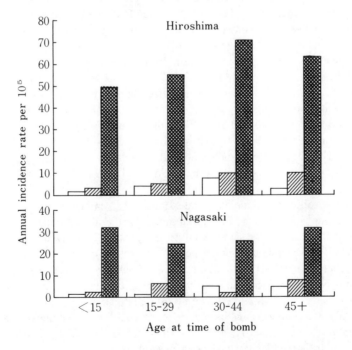

FIGURE 2. Age ATB specific annual incidence rate for all types of leukemia in the RERF sample by dose and city, 1950—1978. ☐= control; ▨= 1-99; ▦= 100+ rad.[50]

in risk for acute leukemia in persons over 45 ATB did not appear until 10 years after exposure with a peak incidence occurring 32 years after exposure,[31] followed by a slow decline.[32]

The annual incidence rate of acute leukemia for children less than age 15 ATB was 100.82/10^5 persons in the period 1950 to 1955, and rapidly declined to 53.88 in the period 1950 to 1960, and 0 in the period 1960 to 1971. In contrast, a gradual change in incidence, as 26.16, 66.52, and 41.28, respectively, was observed in the age group 30 to 44 years old ATB. For chronic granulocytic leukemia in the age group less than 15 years old ATB, the annual incidence rate which was 72.16/10^5 persons in 1950 to 1955, was 0 in the following two study periods. In contrast, the incidence rates were 25.89, 9.83, and 6.24, respectively, in the age group more than 30 years old ATB.[33] Note that the temporal patterns of acute leukemia and chronic granulocytic leukemia appear to be different, i.e., chronic granulocytic leukemia risk seems to have decreased even for the oldest survivors.

The large excess risk of leukemia in the groups of younger ages ATB rapidly decreased before 1960, and there was no longer any statistically significant difference of excess risk by age ATB in the high dose group by 1978.[31] In Hiroshima, the excess risk of leukemia continued into 1978, although it had decreased with time. In Nagasaki, it disappeared by 1970, 25 years after exposure. It has been predicted on this basis that radiation- induced leukemia in the high dose group would disappear almost completely within 40 years after atomic bomb exposure[31] (Figure 3).

In the LSS cohort, the change in leukemia deaths with elapsed time coincided well with the leukemia incidence described above. The 147 leukemia deaths in 1950 to 1970 were about 2.7 times higher than the expected value of 55.1, based on the leukemia mortality rate for all of Japan. The observed values were high particularly in the high dose groups, with the values being 8.6 times greater (observed 13, expected 1.50) in the 100 to 199 rad group and 29.4 times greater (observed 42, expected 1.43) in the 200 rad or more group, both rates being significantly higher ($p < 0.001$) in comparison to 3.5 times (observed 7, expected 1.99) in the 50 to 99 rad group.[22]

By city, a significant increase in leukemia deaths was observed in three dose groups, i.e., the 50 to 99 rad (observed 7, expected 1.37), 100 to 199 rad (observed 10, expected 0.88), and 200 rad or more (observed 27, expected 0.76) groups in Hiroshima, but only in the 200 rad or more group (observed 15, expected 0.67) in Nagasaki. When age ATB is considered, the mortality rate in the age group 0 to 9 years old ATB was 22.7 times greater in the 100 rad group and 66.5 times greater in the 200 rad or more group, respectively. The next highest mortality after the age group 0 to 9 years old ATB with 200 rad or more was noted in the age group more than 50 years old ATB exposure doses of 200 rad or more.

The radiation-induced leukemia mortality during the period 1950 to 1974 was 2.33/10^6 person/year/rad (PYR) in Hiroshima and 1.46 in Nagasaki, each showing a significant excess. The highest excess was seen during 1950 to 1954 (Hiroshima 4.11, Nagasaki 4.27), after which the mortality decreased gradually.[34] As seen with leukemia incidence, a significant excess mortality still persisted during the period 1975 to 1978 in Hiroshima. In contrast, no significant excess mortality was seen after the period 1963 to 1966 in Nagasaki.[13]

A recent mortality study by Preston et al.[35] on the LSS-E85 cohort, which consisted of an initial 120,000 members in 1985 with 11,500 more persons added later, ascertained 220 leukemia deaths among the exposed population during 1950 to 1982. The relative risk at 100 rads was 3.95 and was significantly high ($p < 0.001$). The excess risk per 10^6 (PYR) was 1.51, accounting for about 56% of the leukemia deaths. Under the newly revised dose system DS86, there was still a statistically significant leukemia excess during the period 1981 to 1985 in Hiroshima.[27]

In the studies of autopsied cases of leukemia, no morphological evidence was regarded as being specific to radiation induction.[36-40] Similarly, no evidence suggested radiogenic changes in autopsied cases of aplastic anemia among atomic bomb survivors.[41] In survivors exposed to high doses, chromosome abnormalities were found *in vitro* in peripheral hematopoietic stem

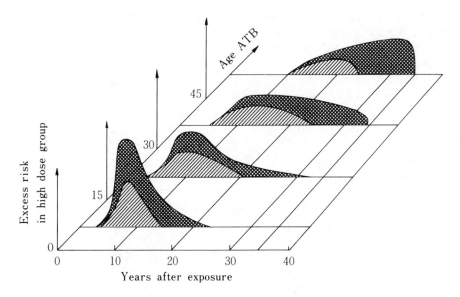

FIGURE 3.   Schematic diagram of the leukemogenic effect of A-bomb radiation by age ATB, elapsed years after exposure (latent period) and city. ▓▓ = Hiroshima: ▨ = Nagasaki.[50]

cells[42] and in peripheral lymphocytes,[43] even more than 30 years after exposure. Among the exposed members of the LSS cohort, the frequency of radiation-induced chromosome aberrations as well as an enzyme deficiency in *in vitro* peripheral lymphocytes increased in parallel with the magnitude of exposure dose.[44,45]

Persons who entered either Hiroshima or Nagasaki soon after the atomic bomb detonation could have been exposed to radiation mainly from fallout.[23] Since 1950, some leukemia cases were found among those who entered the city within 3 days after the detonation,[7,12,46-48] however, as far as the LSS cohort study is concerned, no findings have suggested any increased leukemia risk among those who entered either of the two cities within 1 month after the detonation.[19,49] No excess risk of leukemia has been observed in children exposed *in utero* either.[50]

2. Malignant Lymphoma

For malignant lymphoma, cases examined by Nishiyama et al.[51] in the LSS cohort during 1945 to 1965 (26 from Hiroshima and 12 from Nagasaki) revealed a high relative risk of 8.0 in the 100 rad or more group in Hiroshima. In consecutive mortality studies, however, no significant increase of deaths due to radiation-related malignant lymphoma was observed in the following study periods: 1950 to 1974,[34] 1950 to 1978,[13] 1950 to 1982,[35] and 1950 to 1985.[27]

3. Multiple Myeloma

An earlier histological review of surgically removed and autopsy materials accumulated during 1949 to 1962 in Hiroshima suggested an elevated prevalence of multiple myeloma in proximally exposed survivors.[52] However, another study of bone tumors during 1950 to 1965 failed to find any evidence suggesting an excess incidence of radiogenic multiple myeloma in either Hiroshima or Nagasaki.[53]

In an earlier mortality study of the LSS cohort, no evidence of elevated mortality due to multiple myeloma was observed during 1950 to 1974.[34] Shortly thereafter, however, the incidence of myeloma associated with increased exposure doses became statistically significant for the study period 1950 to 78. The number of estimated excess myeloma cases was 5.8 (29.0%) among approximately 80,000 survivors in the LSS cohort.[13]

According to Ichimaru et al.,[54] in the same cohort 22 (76%) of 29 multiple myelomas during

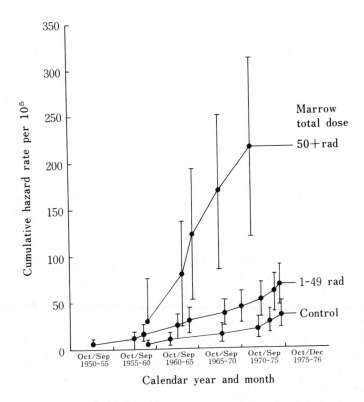

FIGURE 4. Cumulative hazard rate for multiple myeloma among A-bomb survivors and controls aged 20—59 years ATB in the RERF sample, Hiroshima and Nagasaki, 1950—1976.[50]

1950 to 1976 occurred in radiation-exposed persons. The annual incidence of myeloma per 10^3 population was 0.30 in the 1 to 99 rad group and 0.97 in the 100 rad or more group, as compared with an incidence of 0.21 in the less than 1 rad group. The incidence in the 100 rad or more group was significantly higher (about 4.6 times higher) than that in the less than 1 rad group.

An evident dose effect was noted in the age group 20 to 59 years old ATB. Increased risk in the group exposed to 50 rad or more became apparent 20 years after exposure[54] (Figure 4).

Recently, Shimizu et al.[27] indicated that the frequency of deaths due to multiple myeloma in the LSS-E85 cohort during 1950 to 1985 showed a significant correlation with newly revised DS86 exposure dose ($p = 0.002$), with 2.86 as the relative risk and $0.21/10^6$ PYR as the mean excess risk at the 100 rad dose level.

B. MALIGNANT TUMORS IN OTHER ORGANS

The LSS cohort studies are supported by the Tumor Registry (maintained by City Medical Associations) and the Tumor Tissue Registry (maintained by Prefectural Medical Associations), and the medical institutions, hospitals and universities of the two cities, in addition to the previously mentioned data collected from death certificates and the Japanese family registration system. Excess morbidity and mortality due to radiogenic leukemia in survivors continued to decline after peaking during the period 1950 to 1954, and the excess risk of leukemia persisted only in Hiroshima in 1981 to 1985. On the other hand, malignant tumors other than leukemia which have longer latent periods than leukemia[55] began to increase around 1960.[13]

When comparing the changes in the absolute risk of leukemia vs. the absolute risk of all other malignant tumors for the study periods of 1950 to 1955 and 1981 to 1985, for example, the absolute risk decreased from 3.6 to $1.6/10^6$ PYR for leukemia, but it increased from 3.1 to 17.4

for all malignant tumors other than leukemia.[56] Of the deaths in the LSS cohort due to all malignant tumors other than leukemia during 1950 to 1985, 7.86% (451/5734 cases) were regarded as deaths due to radiogenic cancers.[27]

To date, the organ-specific tumors causing statistically significant increases in mortality due to malignant tumors other than leukemia as well as multiple myeloma are cancers of the esophagus, stomach, colon, lung, breast, ovary, and urinary bladder.[26,27,35] A significantly increased morbidity rate for thyroid cancer has also been observed.[49]

Although it has not been determined statistically whether the gamma ray dose-response is linear or nonlinear, the relative biological effectiveness (RBE) of neutrons in cancers of the stomach, lung, and breast, together with leukemia, is 2 to 7 in a gamma linear model under T65D.[57] However, under recent DS86, neutron dose is very small even in Hiroshima, and attempts to measure separate effects of neutron by dose-response analysis with separately using gamma and neutron doses or to estimate their RBEs do not give any meaningful results.[26,27]

1. Cancer of the Esophagus

One hundred and thirty-three deaths due to esophageal cancer (105 from Hiroshima and 28 from Nagasaki) were ascertained in the LSS cohort during the study period 1950 to 1974, and a dose response was noted only in Hiroshima.[34] Although the number of excess deaths due to radiogenic esophageal cancer during 1950 to 1978 was estimated to be 8.4 (5.4%),[13] the number of actual deaths due to cancer of the esophagus was 176 in the LSS-E85 sample during 1950 to 1985, indicating a significant dose effect. In the 100 rad group, the relative risk was 1.43 and the absolute risk was 0.34/10⁶ PYR.[27]

2. Cancer of the Stomach

According to Obo,[58] the standardized mortality due to gastric cancer in atomic bomb survivors in Hiroshima for 1951 to 1959 was 75.56/10⁵ persons, as opposed to the figures of 54.54 in the nonexposed population, and 67.14 for all of Japan. Among cases registered with the Hiroshima Tumor Registry in 1957 to 1958, the number of gastric cancer cases recorded among those exposed within 1500 m from ground zero in Hiroshima was 1.93 times greater than the expected value.[59]

However, in Hiroshima several years after the detonation, no difference in gastric cancer incidence was observed between exposed and nonexposed groups in a study by Murphy and Yasuda[60] of 535 surgical and autopsy gastric cancer cases (187 from the exposed and 348 from the nonexposed). Nor was any remarkable difference observed in the results of Uraki[61] on 639 surgical gastric cancers at Hiroshima University Hospital 20 years after the bombing.

However, Ito et al.[62] recently studied gastric cancer morbidity in 7200 individuals who have been assigned estimated exposure doses among the 15,354 who received X-ray examinations at the Hiroshima Atomic Bomb Survivors Health Clinic during the period 1971 to 1982. They observed that gastric cancer morbidity increased with increasing dose and the risk in the 100 rad group relative to the 0 rad group was significantly high at 4.28 (for males 4.29 and for females 4.02). In the age group 20 to 34 years old, ATB with exposure doses of 10 rad or more, the incidence of gastric cancer morbidity was higher than among those more than 35 years old ATB having the same dose.

The cancer mortality in the LSS cohort during 1950 to 70 did not show any increase in the 100 to 199 rad group, but it showed a significant increase (observed 36, expected 21.1) in the 200 rad or more group.[22] During the extended study period of 1950 to 1973, the increase in mortality with increasing dose was highest in the 400 to 499 rad group in Hiroshima. In Nagasaki, the increase in mortality was observed only in the 500 rad or more group.[63] Gastric cancer risk due to radiation increased during the study periods 1950 to 1974[34] and 1950 to 1978[13] in the same cohort, and the number of excess gastric cancer deaths due to radiation in the same cohort in the latter study period was estimated as 41.6 cases (2.4%).

Age-adjusted prevalence of gastric cancer, based on 326 autopsied cases of gastric cancer in the LSS cohort during 1961 to 1968 (262 from Hiroshima and 64 from Nagasaki), was higher in Hiroshima females (Hiroshima, 9.9%; Nagasaki, 5.9%). In males, it was highest in the fifth decade.[64]

In a recent study by Matsuura et al.[65] of 2155 gastric cancer occurring cases during 1950 to 1977 (1720 from Hiroshima and 435 from Nagasaki), the dose response of incident gastric cancer was linear. The relative risk, 1.6, was significantly high in only the 200 rad or more group (Figure 5). Among those less than 30 years old ATB, excess risk of gastric cancer was high. The estimated risk of radiogenic gastric cancer was $1.24/10^6$ PYR (males, 1.46; females, 1.12). In the high dose group, no evidence suggested a shortened latent period for the development of stomach cancer. A poorly differentiated type of adenocarcinoma was observed more frequently rather than the well-differentiated one found in the high dose group.

A recent mortality study by Shimizu et al.[27] revealed that the relative risk of gastric cancer mortality at the dose level 100 rad in the LSS-E85 cohort during 1950 to 1985 was 1.23 (p <0.001) and the excess risk was $2.07/10^6$ PYR, which is the highest seen among specific cancers other than leukemia. In this cohort, deaths due to radiogenic gastric cancer accounted for only 6.3% of all gastric cancer deaths, reflecting the fact that stomach cancer is the most common cancer among Japanese, i.e., 35% of all deaths due to malignant neoplasms other than leukemia during this period.

3. Cancer of the Colon

In the LSS cohort, an excess risk of radiogenic colon cancer was first noted in the mortality study of 1950 to 1978 and was estimated as 15.8 cases (10.1%).[13]

According to a recent study by Nakatsuka et al.,[66,67] on the LSS cohort during 1950 to 1980, the distribution of 286 colon cancer cases (239 from Hiroshima and 47 from Nagasaki) by magnitude of exposure dose revealed a significant dose response (p <0.001), as shown in Figure 6. A relative risk of 2.0 in the 100 rad group, which consisted of 33 cases, was statistically significant as compared to that of the 0 rad group that totaled 99 cases (p <0.01). A relative risk of 4.5 referring 100+ rad to 0 rad was seen in the age group less than 20 years old ATB. When considered by site of cancer development, dose response evidence was strongest for the sigmoid because there were more cancers at this site than those in other segments of the colon, namely, the cecum and the ascending, transverse, and descending colon. No biased distribution was observed in the histological types of cancer by the magnitude of exposure dose.

In the mortality study of the LSS-E85 population during 1950 to 1985,[27] the number of deaths due to colon cancer correlated significantly with increasing dose (p <0.001), with the relative risk being 1.56 and the excess risk $0.56/10^6$ PYR in the 100 rad group. Differing from colon cancer, no significant dose response was observed for cancer of the rectum.[35,67]

4. Cancer of the Lung

In a study based on death certificates in Hiroshima around 1956, deaths due to lung cancer and digestive tract cancer increased inversely to exposure distance among atomic bomb survivors.[58] Furthermore, the number of observed cases of lung cancer among persons exposed within 1500 m from ground zero in Hiroshima filed with the Hiroshima Tumor Registry during 1957 to 1958, were four times more than expected.[59]

A mortality study of the LSS cohort showed that the development of radiation-related lung cancer began to appear around 1955 in the age group that was more than 35 years old ATB, having an estimated exposure dose of 50 rad or more.[68] The risk of lung cancer in the 90 rad or more group during 1961 to 1965 was shown to be 1.9 times higher than the expected value.[69]

In a pathology study by Mansur et al.[70] of 63 autopsied lung cancer cases in the LSS cohort during 1961 to 1964, a slight but significant increase of lung cancer in the 128 rad or more group was noted. Moreover, according to Cihak et al.,[71] who studied 204 autopsied lung cancer cases

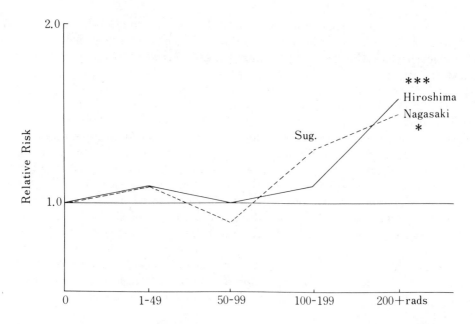

FIGURE 5. Stomach cancer incidence, by city and dose 1950—1977, relative risk. ———— = Hiroshima (1720 cases). - - - - - - - = Nagasaki (435 cases) (test for linear trend, Sug. $p < 0.1$, * $p < 0.05$, *** $p < 0.001$).[65]

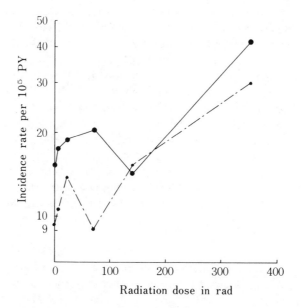

FIGURE 6. Colon cancer incidence rate by radiation dose and sex (adjusted for age ATB and city). ———— = male **(145 cases) -·-·- = female** (141 cases) (test for linear trend, ** $p < 0.01$; sex, age adjusted).[66]

during 1961 to 1970 (156 from Hiroshima and 48 from Nagasaki), the sex- and age-ATB-adjusted prevalence ratio (1.9) was significantly higher in the 200 rad or more group, consisting of 13 members, than in the less than 1 rad group, consisting of 61 members. There was no difference in the prevalence by city or sex.

Histological distribution of the predominant three types of lung cancer shows a high frequency of occurrence for adenocarcinoma (78/204 cases), squamous cell carcinoma (65/204 cases), and small cell carcinoma (39/204 cases). The relative risk of small cell carcinoma, however, was high in the 200 rad or more group. In the 400 or more rad group, all three cases were small cell type. Although the relative risk of lung cancer in A-bomb survivors who were heavy smokers who had consumed more than 20 cigarettes per day was more than seven times higher than that in nonsmokers, there was no evidence controversial to the development of radiogenic lung cancer among the atomic bomb survivors.[72]

Observing the trend of subsequent mortality due to lung cancer in the LSS cohort, the number of excess deaths, which was $0.35/10^6$ PYR in 1950 to 1974,[34] increased to $0.61/10^6$ PYR in a study period extended by 4 years to 1978. About 32 deaths (7.0%) were attributed to radiogenic lung cancer,[13] and correspondingly 50% of deaths in the high dose group (≥ 100 rad) could be regarded as of radiogenic cause.[32] Mortality due to lung cancer during 1950 to 1985 gave a relative risk of 1.46 and an excess risk of $1.52/10^6$ PYR[27] in the 100 rad group.

According to an analysis done by Yamamoto et al.[73] on 1057 autopsied cases of lung cancer in the LSS cohort during 1950 to 1980, the increase in lung cancer incidence was significant ($p < 0.0001$) with increasing exposure dose, and the relative risk was 2.4 in cases from Hiroshima and 1.5 from Nagasaki. The standardized incidence for the 100 rad or more group was 87.8 ± 10.5/year/10^5 population in Hiroshima and 71.9 ± 12.9 in Nagasaki. The relative risk was highest in the age group 10 to 29 years old ATB (Figure 7). The estimated excess of radiogenic lung cancers that had occurred during the study period was 76.2, equivalent to an absolute excess risk of 1.5 cases per 10^6 population per year.

Carcinomas of the squamous cell type and of the small cell type predominated in males and adenocarcinoma predominated in females. The estimated relative risk in the 100 rad group was 1.58 ± 0.25 for adenocarcinoma, 1.48 ± 0.26 for squamous cell carcinoma, and 2.14 ± 0.54 for small cell carcinoma. However, no significant difference in dose response between these three histological types was noted. In view of radiation carcinogenesis and the lung, an ongoing histological and epidemiological comparative study of lung cancer between A-bomb survivors and uranium miners in Colorado[74] may provide a difference in findings, reflecting either gamma or alpha radiations.[75]

No findings have suggested a radiation effect in the development of cancer in the upper respiratory tract.[76]

5. Cancer of the Breast

While the number of malignant tumors in persons exposed within 1500 m from ground zero was significantly greater than that in the nonexposed according to the Hiroshima Tumor Registry records for 1957 to 1958, observed breast cancers in females among those exposed within the same distance were two times more than the expected value.[59]

Among the 12,000 females of the Adult Health Study cohort (which consisted of a part of the LSS sample[1]) who received medical examination periodically at RERF, Wanebo et al.[77] reported an approximately fourfold increased risk in the 90 rad or more group (observed 9, expected 1.53) as compared to the 0 to 89 rad group (observed 9, expected 10.36) in 31 cases of breast cancer during 1946 to 1966.

In the mortality study, on the other hand, 104 deaths in females and 1 in males were considered due to breast cancer in the LSS cohort during 1950 to 1970. Although no deaths due to breast cancer occurred among females less than 10 years old ATB, there were 12 in the age group 10 to 19, 24 in the age group 20 to 34, 44 in the age group 35 to 49, and 24 in the age group more than 50 years old ATB. Two of the 12 in the age group 10 to 19 years old ATB were exposed to 200 rad or more and developed breast cancer during 1965 to 1970. Since the expected number of deaths due to breast cancer was 0.18 in the age group 10 to 19 years old in all of Japan, the mortality among the survivors was as much as 11 times higher in this age group than among the nonexposed.[22]

McGregor et al.,[78] who studied 231 cases of breast cancer in the LSS cohort during 1950 to

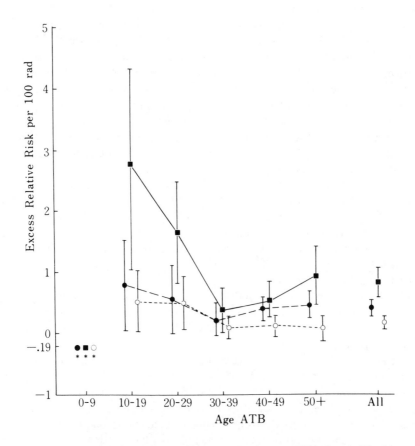

FIGURE 7.   Radiation dose-response of lung cancer by city, age ATB, and sex for Hiroshima (LSS-extended cohort, attained age 20+, 1950—1980).[73] ▬ ▬ ▬ = Hiroshima male; ▬ ▬ ▬ = Hiroshima female; —————— = Nagasaki both sexes. Plotted points show estimated relative risk at 100 rad ± 1 ~S.D., adjusted for attained age and interval of follow-up by the parametric background model. Asterisks indicate that relative risk or lower end of standard error bar is set at minimum feasible value.

1969, found no cases in the age group less than 10 years old, but found a linear increase of incident breast cancers with increasing exposure dose in the age group more than 10 years old. The excess risk of breast cancer at this period in the age group more than 10 years old ATB was $1.9/10^6$ PYR.

As early as 1969 (or 25 years after atomic bomb exposure), cases of breast cancer in females in the 100 rad or more group were found to approach or exceed the expected lifetime incidence based on cancer registry data from elsewhere in Japan. Of particular note was the far higher incidence of breast cancer 25 years after exposure to the bomb in the age group 10 to 19 years old ATB having moderate to high exposure doses than in the age group more than 35 years old ATB with the same exposure doses, suggesting that the mammary gland in the female was more radiosensitive in the second decade than in the third decade of life or later. No biased histological distribution of cancer types was observed by the magnitude of exposure dose.[79]

In a subsequent study of 360 cases of female breast cancer in the LSS cohort during 1950 to 1974 (291 from Hiroshima and 69 from Nagasaki) by Tokunaga et al.,[80] the highest relative risk (5.5) was seen in the age group 10 to 19 years old ATB, who had been assigned doses of 100 rad or more. The highest absolute risk was observed in the age group 30 to 39 years old ATB exposed to a dose of 200 rad or more. Histological diagnosis, as well as the classification of each cancer, was reconfirmed by Japanese and American pathologists.[81]

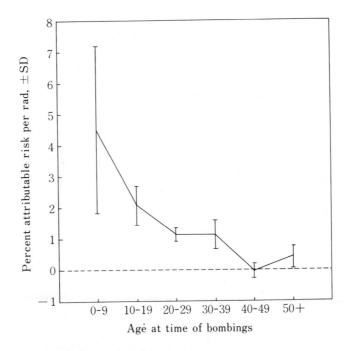

FIGURE 8. Linear regression estimates of excess relative risk per rad to breast tissue, by age ATB.[81]

An excess risk of radiation-related cancer of the breast was ascertained for the first time in females who were less than 10 years old ATB in a recent study of 564 cases of breast cancer in the LSS cohort during 1950 to 1980, conducted by Tokunaga et al.[82] Although a linear dose response was observed in the age groups that were 0 to 9, 10 to 19, 20 to 29, and 30 to 39 years old ATB, no such response was seen in the age groups 40 to 49 and 50 or more years old ATB[83] (Figure 8).

The p value of < 0.001 was correct when applied to a general decreasing trend in the relative risk of 50 rad or more group to the 0 to 9 rad group with increasing age ATB over the age range 0 to 39 years old. Of cases found in the age group 0 to 9 years old ATB, 70 to 90% having doses of 50 rad, and in the age group 10 to 30 years old ATB, having doses of 100 rad or more were attributed to radiation induction.[32] However, no evidence of radiogenic breast cancer was encountered at ages less than 30, an age range at which breast cancer development is rare in general.

Here, it should be emphasized that in regard to radiation carcinogenesis and the breast, the importance of age at radiation exposure is related more to the amount of hormonal stimulation following exposure and less to the developmental status of the breast tissue at the time of exposure.[82,83]

In a recent mortality study on breast cancer during 1950 to 1982, deaths due to breast cancer showed a significant relationship to exposure dose ($p < 0.001$). In the 100 rad group, the mean relative risk was 1.69 and the mean excess risk was $0.65/10^6$ PYR.[35]

A comparative study of breast cancer incidence in three populations of women exposed to ionizing radiation (atomic bomb survivors in Hiroshima and Nagasaki, patients who were exposed to multiple chest fluoroscopies in Massachusetts,[84] and patients who were treated by X-rays for acute postpartum mastitis in Rochester[85]) supported the finding that the radiation-induced cancer increased approximately linearly with increasing dose and depended heavily on age at exposure.[86]

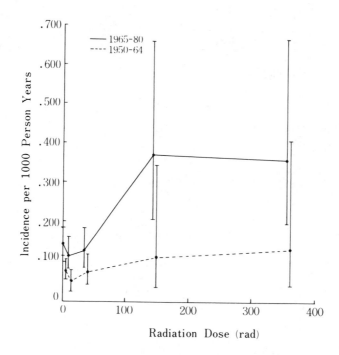

FIGURE 9. Incidence of ovarian cancer by radiation dose and study period, all cases. - - - - -, 1950—1964; ———— , 1965—1980. Bars, 90% confidence interval of incidence.[91]

6. Tumors of the Ovary

An early report[87] dealt with two female patients, each of whom was exposed at a distance about 1200 to 1300 m from ground zero in Hiroshima at 18 years of age, followed by such acute radiation symptoms as epilation, subcutaneous hemorrhage, and so on. One developed granulosa cell tumor of the ovary and the other serous cystadenocarcinoma of the ovary, 8 and 12 years after exposure, respectively.

Earlier projections of an elevated incidence of ovarian cancer among atomic bomb survivors in Hiroshima were based on findings in an analytical study of cancers filed during 1957 to 1958 in the Hiroshima Tumor Registry[59] and in a mortality study among exposed females in Hiroshima.[47,58,88] However, at that time no increased trend of ovarian cancer incidence was noted in a mortality study done in Nagasaki.[89]

For the first time in the study period 1950 to 1982,[49,90] a significant relationship was confirmed between ovarian cancer mortality and exposure dose in the LSS-E85 cohort. Deaths due to cancers of the ovary and other uterine adnexa in the exposed among 70,000 females of the cohort indicated a dose effect ($p = 0.05$) and a moderate mean excess risk: 0.27 deaths per 10^6 PYR. The estimated relative risk was 1.52 in the 100 rad group.

In a recent study of the period 1950 to 1980 by Tokuoka et al.[91] on 194 cases of ovarian cancer in the LSS-E85 cohort (139 from Hiroshima and 55 from Nagasaki), the age-adjusted incidence of ovarian cancer revealed a significant increase with increasing dose ($p < 0.01$), but by city the incidence was significant only for Hiroshima cases. As shown in Figure 9, the dose response was not evident in the first half of the study period (1950 to 1964); it was only significant ($p < 0.01$) in the latter half (1965 to 1980). The relative risk in the 100 rad or more group was the highest in the age group less than 20 years old ATB (Figure 10). No apparently biased histological distribution of cancer types reflecting radiation effect was found.

As to the incidence of benign ovarian tumors, 106 autopsy cases, with which benign ovarian

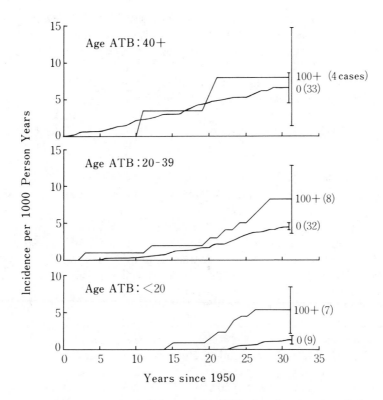

FIGURE 10.   Cumulative incidence rate (per 1000) of ovarian cancer by radiation dose and age ATB. Bars, 90% confidence interval of incidence.[91]

tumors were associated in the LSS-E85 cohort during the same study period (85 from Hiroshima and 21 from Nagasaki), revealed an increased incidence of benign tumors with increasing dose (p <0.05). However, the tendency was not significant in the microscopically confirmed cases (89/106 cases, 84%).[91] Further follow-up study including younger age groups ATB are needed to clarify this relationship.

7. Cancers of the Urinary Organs

The relative risk of mortality due to urinary cancers in the exposed of the LSS cohort during 1950 to 1974 was 2.16 and the excess death was 0.13/10⁶ PYR. Mortality was significantly elevated in the latter part of the study period, particularly during 1967 to 1970.[34] When the study period was extended to 1950 to 1978, the estimated excess deaths due to radiogenic urinary cancer increased to 7.9 cases (7.6%).[13] In the study period 1950 to 1982,[35] almost all of 113 urinary cancer deaths were found to be due to transitional cell carcinoma of the urinary bladder.[92]

In the LSS-E85 cohort during the study period 1950 to 1985,[27] for which the DS86 dosimetry system was adopted, relative risk of mortality due to urinary bladder cancer at a dose level of 100 rad was 2.13 and the excess risk per 10⁶ PYR was 0.41. In the same cohort during the same study period, deaths due to kidney cancer was not elevated significantly among participants who had been exposed to radiation.[27]

8. Cancer of the Prostate

A histological study (1961 to 1969) of 1357 LSS male autopsy cases, age 50 years or older at time of death, revealed 118 cases with prostate cancer, consisting of 90 cases of intraglandular cancer and 28 cases of cancer with extraglandular invasion. Although the prevalence of prostate cancer increased significantly with increasing age, the 19 cases of intraglandular cancer among 71 males assigned exposure doses of 100 rad or more indicated no difference in prevalence when compared to the number of cancer cases (39) among 142 males of either the nonexposed or 0 rad group.[93]

According to a mortality study by Preston et al.[35] for the period 1950 to 1982 on the LSS-E85 cohort, neither the mean excess relative risk nor the tendency for prostate cancer mortality to increase with time at a dose level of 100 rad were statistically significant. When the study period was extended to 1985 and the DS86 dose system was applied, no excess deaths due to prostate cancer were observed.[27]

9. Cancer of the Thyroid

Studies made on the RERF Adult Health Study population demonstrated a significantly high prevalence of thyroid cancer in members who were exposed to such high radiation doses that acute radiation symptoms developed.[94] Thyroid cancer also occurred more frequently in females[95] and relative risk increased significantly in females in the 50 rad or more group.[96] In addition, an examination of 536 thyroid cancers among 3067 autopsied LSS participants further documented a significant prevalence of thyroid cancer in female survivors. The relative risk (1.41) in the 50 rad or more group was statistically significant ($p < 0.01$).[97]

In a recent study made by Ezaki et al.,[98] the LSS thyroid cancers during 1958 to 1979 were categorized as 125 cases of clinical cancer (15 males and 110 females) and 155 cases of occult cancer (56 males and 99 females). Clinical cancer increased linearly with increasing dose in females, with a remarkable increase particularly in the age group less than 20 years old ATB. The relative risk of clinical cancer in the 50 rad or more group was 4.2 and the excess risk was $3.4/10^5$ PYR in the age group less than 20 years old ATB. Occult cancer prevalence was 3.5% (155/4425 cases) in autopsied cases and the relative risk in the 50 rad or more group was 1.9 ($p < 0.05$).

10. Cancer in Other Organs

a. Cancer of the Salivary Gland

According to a LSS cohort study made by Belsky et al.,[99, 100] the relative risk of salivary gland cancer was significantly increased in the 300 rad or more group (observed 3, expected 0.40). On the other hand, no evidence of increased benign salivary gland tumors due to radiation was observed.

Further pathological review of salivary gland tumors for an extended study period is awaited to verify the above-described results.

b. Cancers of the Liver, Gallbladder, Bile Duct, and Pancreas

Asano et al.[101] studied primary liver cancer among LSS autopsied samples for 1961 to 1975. No relationship between radiation and incidence of primary liver cancer was observed. Nor was any different histological distribution of liver cancer types noted between the exposed and nonexposed groups.

The mortality study of the LSS-E85 cohort during 1950 to 1982 by Preston et al.[35] suggested a possible correlation of radiation exposure and liver cancer occurrence, as well as intrahepatic bile duct cancer occurrence. When the study period was extended to 1985 and the DS86 dose system was applied, no significantly increased deaths due to these cancers were observed.[27] Also, the dose response of cancers of the gallbladder and the extrahepatic bile duct was not significant. For cancer of the pancreas, no significant dose response was observed in the study periods: 1950 to 1974,[34] 1950 to 1982,[35] and 1950 to 1985.[27]

c. Cancer of the Uterus

No increasing tendency of cervical cancer of the uterus was observed in female survivors in

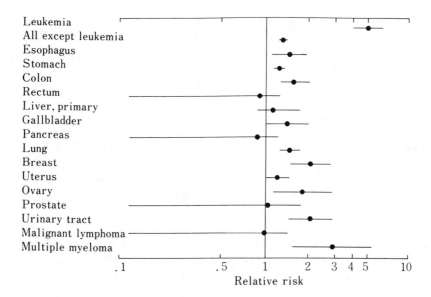

FIGURE 11. Relative risk at 1 Gy (shield kerma) and 90% confidence interval, 1950—1985.[27]

the LSS cohort in the consecutive study periods of either 1950 to 1970,[22] 1950 to 1974,[34] 1950 to 1978,[13] or 1950 to 1982.[35] The relative risk of cervical cancer at the dose level of 100 rad during 1950 to 1985 was 1.43 and was not statistically significant.[27]

d. Tumors of the Brain

No convincing evidence of a relationship between the development of brain tumors and radiation exposure was found in a study based on the histological review of brain tumors in all autopsy and surgical cases during 1973 to 1975 in Nagasaki.[102] Neither was any increasing tendency of intracranial tumor found in the mortality study on the LSS cohort during 1950 to 1978.[13]

However, in the study by Seyama et al.[103] glioma cases (42.2% of all 45 brain tumor cases) from the period 1961 to 1975 in the LSS cohort showed a significantly high standardized relative risk, namely 4.8, in the 100 rad or more group in males. The crude risk of glioma was high in the younger age groups ATB who had been assigned high exposure doses.

No correlation was observed between the prevalence of pituitary adenoma and the magnitude of exposure dose in autopsy cases in the same cohort during 1961 to 1974.[103]

The most important late effect observed in atomic bomb survivors is, as described herein, the increased incidence of malignant neoplasms. Among the survivors in the RERF LSS cohort, the increase in cancer mortality for the period 1950 to 1985 is statistically significant for leukemia, multiple myeloma, cancer of the esophagus, stomach, colon, lung, breast, ovary, and urinary bladder.[26,27]

As mentioned previously, the radiation dosimetry for members of the LSS cohort has changed in 1986 from T65D to DS86. Adoption of DS86, however, does not change the above-described list of radiation-related cancers, although some city differences in dose response based on the T65D doses, such as for leukemia, are no longer significant with the DS86 doses[26,27] (Figure 11).

II. ATOMIC BOMB SURVIVORS AND AGING

The LSS cohort is a large-scale fixed population composed of males and females of all ages, who were exposed to a single incident of whole-body ionizing radiation, plus nonexposed persons (those not present in the city at the time of the atomic bomb detonation) as their controls. As such this cohort can be used to investigate the relationship between radiation and aging.[104] Thus far, consecutive mortality studies of the LSS cohort have shown that a shortening of the life span as a delayed radiation effect is attributable only to deaths resulting from malignant neoplasms.[22,34,104,105]

Other than malignant neoplasms, the following morbid changes are known to be due to radiation exposure in the LSS cohort: intense posterior lenticular opacity, chromosome aberrations in peripheral blood cells, and abnormal growth and development resulting from exposure *in utero* and in infancy.[104]

The lenticular opacities in atomic bomb survivors have been regarded as a unique change resulting from irradiation rather than as a change due to accelerated aging.[104] A few other degenerative changes somewhat similar to the lenticular change are the change of the tissue hexosamine:collagen ratio[106] and the sclerotic change of testicular seminiferous tubules,[107] both of which were found in proximally exposed survivors who were autopsied later. Except for these examples, no other findings suggest a possible correlation to an accelerated aging process.

No significant differences in physiological functions were found between the exposed and the nonexposed in tests of grasping power, skin elasticity, perception of vibration, breathing capacity, or hearing and visual acuities. Nor was any significant difference observed among atomic bomb survivors when categorized by exposure dose.[108, 109] In addition, clinical biochemical tests of the exposed did not reveal any changes associated with exposure dose.[104]

It can be said, therefore, that among the atomic bomb survivors changes correlated with accelerated aging have not been documented as thoroughly as changes related to radiogenic carcinogenicity.

III. SUMMARY

The most important late effect encountered in the atomic bomb survivors since 1945, when they were exposed to ionizing radiation, is the increased incidence of malignant neoplasms including leukemia and cancers in other organs in both Hiroshima and Nagasaki.

Among the survivors, especially in the LSS samples, a fixed RERF study cohort, the increase in cancer morbidity as well as mortality for the period 1950 to 1985 is statistically significant for leukemia, cancer of the esophagus, stomach, colon, lung, breast, ovary, urinary bladder, and multiple myeloma. Increased cancer morbidity has also been noted for the thyroid gland.

The excess risk of radiogenic leukemia began to appear within a few years after the detonation with peak incidence occurring around 1951, continuing for at least 40 years. In contrast, the excess risk of radiogenic cancers other than leukemia began to elevate in around 1960, 15 years after the detonation and is still ongoing.

In comparison to such unequivocal evidence of radiation carcinogenesis among survivors, no evidence exists to indicate that acceleration of aging is a secondary effect of radiation exposure. As yet, no significant difference has been noted between groups of the exposed and the nonexposed in the results of multiple physical tests, such as grasping power, skin elasticity, perception of vibration, breathing capacity, and hearing and visual acuities.

ACKNOWLEDGMENTS

The authors are grateful to Drs. Stuart C. Finch, Hiroo Kato, and Masayoshi Tokunaga, Radiation Effects Research Foundation, and Dr. Charles E. Land, National Cancer Institute, U.S. for giving us their cordial advice and help.

REFERENCES

1. **Finch, S. C. and Moriyama, I. M.**, The Delayed effects of Radiation Exposure among Atomic Bomb Survivors, Hiroshima and Nagasaki, 1945—79. A Brief Summary, *RERF TR16-78*, RERF, Hiroshima, 1978.

2. **Ohkita, T.**, Health effects on individuals and health services of the Hiroshima and Nagasaki bomb, in *Effects of Nuclear War on Health and Health Services: Report of the International Committee of Experts in Medical Sciences and Public Health to Implement Resolution WHA34.38, Annex 4,* World Health Organization, Geneva, 1984, 107.

3. **Court Brown, W. M. and Doll, R.**, Mortality from cancer and other causes after radiotherapy for ankylosing spondylitis, *Br. Med. J.*, 2, 1327, 1965.

4. **Smith, P. G.**, Late effects of X-ray treatment of ankylosing spondylitis, in *Radiation Carcinogenesis: Epidemiology and Biological Significance*, Boice, J. D., Jr. and Fraumeni, J. F., Jr., Eds., Raven Press, New York, 1984, 107.

5. **Boice, J. D., Jr., Blettner, M., Kleinerman, R. A., Stovall, M., Moloney, W. C., Engholm, G., Austin, D. F., Bosch, A., Cookfair, D. L., Krementz, E. T., Latourette, H. B., Peters, L. J., Schulz, M. D., Lundell, M., Pettersson, F., Storm, H. H., Bell, C. M. J., Coleman, M. P., Fraser, P., Palmer, M., Prior, P., Choi, N. W., Hislop, T. G., Koch, M., Robb, D., Robson, D., Spengler, R. F., von Fournier, D., Frischkorn, R., Lochmueller, H., Pompe-Kirn, V., Rimpela, A., Kjorstad, K., Pejovic, M. H., Sigurdsson, K., Pisani, P., Kucera, H., and Hutchison, G. B.**, Radiation dose and leukemia risk in patients treated for cancer of cervix, *JNCI*, 79, 1295, 1987.

6. **Wang, J.-X., Boice, J. D., Jr., Li, B.-X., Zhang, J.-Y., and Fraumeni, J. F., Jr.**, Cancer among medical diagnostic X-ray workers in China, *JNCI*, 80, 344, 1988.

7. **Watanabe, S.**, On the incidence of leukemias in Hiroshima during the past fifteen years from 1946 to 1960, *J. Radiat. Res.*, 2(2), 131, 1961.

8. **Bizzozero, O. J., Jr., Johnson, K. G., and Ciocco, A.**, Distribution, incidence, and appearance time of radiation-related leukemia in Hiroshima and Nagasaki, 1946—64, *N. Engl. J. Med.*, 274, 1095, 1966.

9. **Moloney, W. C. and Kastenbaum, M. A.**, Leukemic effects of ionizing radiation on atomic bomb survivors in Hiroshima City, *Science*, 121, 308, 1955.

10. **Moloney, W. C.**, Leukemia in survivors of atomic bombing, *N. Engl. J. Med.*, 253, 88, 1955.

11. **Tomonaga, M.**, Statistical Investigation of Leukemia in Japan., *RERF TR28-66*, 1966.

12. **Ohkita, T.**, Leukemia in Hiroshima atomic bomb survivors from 1946 to 1975: a summary of the findings and recent trends (in Japanese), *Proc. Hiroshima Univ. RINMB*, 17, 77, 1976.

13. **Kato, H. and Schull, W. J.**, Studies of the mortality of A-bomb survivors. 7. Mortality, 1950—1978. I. Cancer mortality, *Radiat. Res.*, 90, 395, 1982.

14. **Folley, J. H., Borges, W., and Yamawaki, T.**, Incidence of leukemia in survivors of the atomic bomb in Hiroshima and Nagasaki, Japan, *Am. J. Med.*, 3, 311, 1952.

15. **Wald, N.**, Leukemia in Hiroshima City atomic bomb survivors, *Science*, 127, 699, 1958.

16. **Lange, R. D., Moloney, W. C., and Yamawaki T.**, Leukemia in atomic bomb survivors. I. General observations, *Blood*, 9, 574, 1954.

17. **Heyssel, R., Brill, A. B., Woodbury, L. A., Nishimura, E. T., Ghose, T., Hoshino, T., and Yamasaki, M.**, Leukemia in Hiroshima atomic bomb survivors, *Blood*, 15, 313, 1960.

18. **Tomonaga, M., Ichimaru, M., Danno, H., Inoue, A., Okabe, N., Kinoshita, K., Matsumoto, Y., Nonaka, M., Takahashi, Y., Tomiyasu, T., Toyomasu, S., Tamari, K., and Kawamoto, M.**, Leukemia in atomic bomb survivors from 1946 to 1965 and some aspects of epidemiology of leukemia in Japan (English Abstract), *J. Kyu Hem. Soc.*, 17, 375, 1967.

19. **Finch, S. C.**, Leukemia and lymphoma in atomic bomb survivors, in *Radiation Carcinogenesis: Epidemiology and Biological Significance*, Boice, J. D., Jr. and Fraumeni, J. F., Jr., Eds., Raven Press, New York, 1984, 37.

20. **Jablon, S., Ishida, M., and Yamasaki, M.**, Studies of the mortality of A-bomb survivors. III. Description of the sample and mortality, 1950—1960, *Radiat. Res.*, 25, 25, 1965.

21. **Beebe, G. W., Kato, H., and Land, C. E.**, Studies of the mortality of A-bomb survivors. IV. Mortality and radiation dose, 1950—1966, *Radiat. Res.*, 48, 613, 1971.

22. **Jablon, S. and Kato, H.**, Studies of the mortality of A-bomb survivors. V. Radiation dose and mortality, 1950—1970., *Radiat. Res.*, 50, 649, 1972.

23. **Arakawa, E. T.**, Radiation dosimetry in Hiroshima and Nagasaki atomic-bomb survivors, *N. Engl. J. Med.*, 263, 488, 1960.

24. **Milton, R. C. and Shohoji, T.**, Tentative 1965 radiation dose estimation for atomic bomb survivors, Hiroshima-Nagasaki., *RERF TR1-68*, 1968.

25. **Maruyama, T.**, Atomic bomb dosimetry for epidemiological studies of survivors in Hiroshima and Nagasaki, in *Cancer in Atomic Bomb Survivors*, Shigematsu, I. and Kagan, A., Eds., Japan Scientific Societies Press, Tokyo, 1986, 9.

26. **Shimizu, Y., Kato, H., Schull, W. J., Preston, D. L., Fujita, S., and Pierce, D. A.**, Life span study report 11. Part 1. Comparison of risk coefficients for site-specific cancer mortality based on the DS86 and T65DR shielded kerma and organ doses, *RERF TR12-87*, 1987.

27. **Shimizu, Y., Kato, H., and Schull, W. J.**, Life span study report 11. Part 2. Cancer mortality in the years 1950—85 based on the recently revised doses (DS86), *RERF TR5-88*, 1988.

28. **Finch, S. C., Hrubec, Z., Nefzger, M. D., Hoshino, T., and Itoga, T.**, Detection of leukemia and related disorders, Hiroshima and Nagasaki. Research plan, *RERF TR5-65*, 1965.

29. **Matsuo, T., Tomonaga, M., Bennett, J. M., Kuriyama, K., Imanaka, F., Kuramoto, A., Kamada, N., Ichimaru, M., Finch, S. C., Pisciotta, A. V., and Ishimaru, T.**, Reclassification of leukemia among A-bomb survivors by French-American-British (FAB) classification. Part 1. Concordance of diagnosis in Nagasaki cases by RERF members and a member of FAB cooperative group, *RERF TR4-87*, 1987.

30. **Ishimaru, T., Hoshino, T., Ichimaru, M., Okada, H., Tomiyasu, T., Tsuchimoto, T., and Yamamoto, T.**, Leukemia in atomic bomb survivors, Hiroshima and Nagasaki, 1 October 1950—30 September 1966, *Radiat. Res.*, 45, 216, 1971.

31. **Ichimaru, M., Ishimaru, M., Mikami, M., Yamada, Y., and Ohkita, T.**, Incidence of leukemia in a fixed cohort of atomic bomb survivors and controls, Hiroshima and Nagasaki October 1950-December 1978, *RERF TR13-81*, 1981.

32. **Land, C. E. and Tokunaga, M.**, Induction period, in *Radiation Carcinogenesis: Epidemiology and Biological Significance*, Boice, J. D., Jr. and Fraumeni, J. F., Jr., Eds., Raven Press, New York, 1984, 421.

33. **Ichimaru, M., Ishimaru, T., and Belsky, J. L.**, Incidence of leukemia in atomic bomb survivors belonging to a fixed cohort in Hiroshima and Nagasaki, 1950—71. Radiation dose, years after exposure, age at exposure, and type of leukemia, *J. Radiat. Res.*, 19, 262, 1978.

34. **Beebe, G. W., Kato, H., and Land, C. E.**, Studies of the mortality of A-bomb survivors. VI. Mortality and radiation dose, 1950—74, *Radiat. Res.*, 75, 138, 1978.

35. **Preston, D. L., Kato, H., Kopecky, K. J., and Fujita, S.**, Studies of the mortality of A-bomb survivors. VIII. Cancer mortality, 1950—1982, *Radiat. Res.*, 111, 151, 1987.

36. **Watanabe, S.**, Pathology of leukemia in relation to the atomic bomb exposure, with reference to features of leukemic cell proliferation and extension (in Japanese), *J. Hiroshima Med. Assoc.*, 12, 905, 1959.

37. **Anderson, R. E., Yamamoto, T., Yamada, A., and Will, D. W.**, Autopsy study of leukemia in Hiroshima, *Arch. Pathol.*, 78, 618, 1964.

38. **Liu, P. I., Ishimaru, T., Mcgregor, D. H., Okada, M., and Steer, A.**, Autopsy study of granulocytic sarcoma (chloroma) in patients with myelogenous leukemia, Hiroshima-Nagasaki 1949—1969, *Cancer*, 31, 948, 1973.

39. **Liu, P. I., Ishimaru, T., Mcgregor, D. H., Okada, M., and Steer, A.**, Autopsy study of leukemia in atomic bomb survivors, Hiroshima-Nagasaki, 1949—1969, *Cancer*, 31, 1315, 1973.

40. **Liu, P. I., Ishimaru, T., and McGregor, D. H.**, Autopsy study of blast crisis in patients with chronic granulocytic leukemia, Hiroshima and Nagasaki, 1949—1969, *Cancer*, 33, 1062, 1974.

41. **Kirshbaum, J. D., Matsuo, T., Sato, K., Ichimaru, M., Tsuchimoto, T., and Ishimaru, T.**, A study of aplastic anemia in an autopsy series with special reference to atomic bomb survivors in Hiroshima and Nagasaki, *Blood*, 38, 17, 1971.

42. **Amenomori, T., Honda, T., Matsuo, T., Otake, M., Hazama, R., Tomonaga, Y., Tomonaga, M., and Ichimaru, M.**, Proliferation, differentiation, and possible radiation-induced chromosome abnormalities in circulating hemopoietic stem cells, *RERF TR22-85*, 1985.

43. **Kamada, N., Kuramoto, A., Katsuki, T., and Hinuma, Y.**, Chromosome aberrations in B lymphocytes of atomic bomb survivors, *Blood*, 53, 1140, 1979.

44. **Awa, A. A., Sofuni, T., Honda, T., Itoh, M., Neriishi, S., and Otake, M.**, Relationship between the radiation dose and chromosome aberrations in atomic bomb survivors of Hiroshima and Nagasaki, *J. Radiat. Res.*, 19, 126, 1978.

45. **Hakoda, M., Akiyama, M., Kyoizumi, S., Awa, A. A., Yamakido, M., and Otake, A.**, Increased somatic cell mutant frequency in atomic bomb survivors, *RERF TR18-87*, 1987.

46. **Takahashi, H., Ohkita, T., Kamada, N., and Uchino, H.**, Recent trend of leukemia among atomic bomb survivors in Hiroshima (English abstract), *Acta Hematol. Jpn.*, 36, 303, 1973.

47. **Kurihara, M., Munaka, M., Hayakawa, N., Yamamoto, H., Yuzaki, M., Ueoka, H., Ohtaki, M., Ikeuchi, M., Sumida, H., and Kodama, M.**, Cancer mortality among A-bomb survivors in Hiroshima Prefecture. I. Mortality in 1968—1972 (in Japanese), *Nagasaki Med. J.*, 55, 648, 1980.

48. **Hayakawa, N., Kurihara, M., Munaka, M., Yamamoto, H., Ueoka, H., Ohtaki, M., Oride, M., and Matsuura, M.**, Cancer mortality among A-bomb survivors in Hiroshima Prefecture. II. Mortality in 1973—1977 (in Japanese), *J. Hiroshima Med. Assoc.*, 39, 409, 1986.

49. **Kato, H.**, Cancer mortality, in *Cancer in Atomic Bomb Survivors*, Shigematsu, I. and Kagan, A., Eds., Japan Scientific Societies Press, Tokyo, 1986, 53.

50. **Ishimaru, T., Ichimaru, M., and Mikami, M.**, Leukemia incidence among individuals exposed *in utero*, children of atomic bomb survivors, and their controls; Hiroshima and Nagasaki, 1945—79, *RERF TR11-81*, 1981.

51. **Nishiyama, H., Anderson, R. E., Ishimaru, T., Ishida, K., Ii, Y., and Okabe, N.**, The incidence of malignant lymphoma and multiple myeloma in Hiroshima and Nagasaki atomic bomb survivors, 1945—1965, *Cancer*, 32, 1301, 1973.

52. **Anderson, R. E. and Ishida, K.**, Malignant lymphoma in survivors of the atomic bomb in Hiroshima, *Ann. Intern. Med.*, 61, 853, 1964.

53. **Yamamoto, T. and Wakabayashi, T.**, Bone tumors among the atomic bomb survivors of Hiroshima and Nagasaki, *Acta Pathol. Jpn.*, 19, 201, 1969.

54. **Ichimaru, M., Ishimaru, T., Mikami, M., and Matsunaga, M.**, Multiple myeloma among atomic bomb survivors in Hiroshima and Nagasaki, 1950—76: relationship to radiation dose absorbed by marrow, *JNCI*, 69, 323, 1982.

55. **Upton, A. C.**, Biological aspects of radiation carcinogenesis, in *Radiation Carcinogenesis: Epidemiology and Biological Significance*, Boice, J. D., Jr. and Fraumeni, J. F., Jr., Eds., Raven Press, New York, 1984, 9.

56. **Kato, H.**, personal communication, 1988.

57. **Kato, H. and Schull, W. J.**, Cancer mortality among atomic bomb survivors, 1950—78, *RERF TR12-80*, 1980.

58. **Obo, G.**, Statistical observations of cancer mortality in atomic bomb survivors (in Japanese), *Jpn. Med. J.*, 1986, 8, 1956.

59. **Harada, T. and Ishida, M.**, Neoplasms among A-bomb survivors in Hiroshima: first report of the research committee on tumor statistics, Hiroshima City Medical Association, Hiroshima, Japan, *JNCI*, 25, 1253, 1960.

60. **Murphy, E. S. and Yasuda, A.**, Carcinoma of the stomach in Hiroshima, Japan, *Am. J. Pathol.*, 34, 531, 1958.

61. **Uraki, J.**, Summary of malignant neoplasms: the digestive tract, especially the stomach (in Japanese), *J. Hiroshima Med. Assoc.*, 20(Suppl.), 378, 1967.

62. **Ito, C., Hasegawa, K., and Kumasawa, T.**, Investigation of stomach diseases in atomic bomb survivors. V: Prevalence of gastric cancer by dose (in Japanese), *J. Hiroshima Med. Assoc.*, 37, 457, 1984.

63. **Nakamura, K.**, Stomach cancer in atomic bomb survivors, *Lancet*, 2, 866, 1977.

64. **Yamamoto, T., Kato, H., Ishida, K., Tahara, E., and McGregor, D. H.**, Gastric carcinoma in a fixed population: Hiroshima and Nagasaki, *Jpn. J. Cancer Res. (Gann)*, 61, 473, 1970.

65. **Matsuura, H., Yamamoto, T., Sekine, I., Ochi, Y., and Otake, M.**, Pathological and epidemiologic study of gastric cancer in atomic bomb survivors, Hiroshima and Nagasaki, 1950—77, *J. Radiat. Res.*, 25, 111, 1984.

66. **Nakatsuka, H., Yamamoto, T., Shimizu, Y., Takahashi, M., Ezaki, H., Tahara, E., Sekine, I., Shimoyama, T., Mochinaga, N., Tomita, M., and Tsuchiya, R.**, Colorectal cancer among atomic bomb survivors in Hiroshima and Nagasaki, 1950—80, *Nagasaki Med. J.*, 59, 473, 1984.

67. **Nakatsuka, H. and Ezaki, H.**, Colorectal cancer among atomic bomb survivors, in *Cancer in Atomic Bomb Survivors*, Shigematsu, I. and Kagan, A., Eds., Japan Scientific Societies Press, Tokyo, 1986, 155.

68. **Beebe, G. W. and Kato, H.**, A review of thirty years study of Hiroshima and Nagasaki atomic bomb survivors. E. Cancer other than leukemia, *J. Radiat. Res.*, 16(Suppl.), 97, 1975.

69. **Wanebo, C. K., Johnson, K. G., Sato, K., and Thorslund, T. W.**, Lung cancer following atomic radiation, *Am. Rev. Resp. Dis.*, 98, 778, 1968.

70. **Mansur, G. P., Keehn, R. J., Hiramoto, T., and Will, D. W.**, Lung carcinoma among atomic bomb survivors Hiroshima-Nagasaki, 1950—64, *RERF TR19-68*, 1968.

71. **Cihak, R. W., Ishimaru, T., Steer, A., and Yamada, A.**, Lung cancer at autopsy in A-bomb survivors and controls, Hiroshima and Nagasaki, 1961—1970. I. Autopsy findings and relation to radiation, *Cancer*, 33, 1580, 1974.

72. **Ishimaru, T., Cihak, R. W., Land, C. E., Steer, A., and Yamada, A.**, Lung cancer at autopsy in A-bomb survivors and controls, Hiroshima and Nagasaki, 1961—1970. II. Smoking, occupation, and A-bomb exposure., *Cancer*, 36, 1723, 1975.

73. **Yamamoto, T., Kopecky, K. J., Fujikura, T., Tokuoka, S., Monzen, T., Nishimori, I., Nakashima, E., and Kato, H.**, Lung cancer incidence among Japanese A-bomb survivors, 1950—80, *J. Radiat. Res.*, 28, 156, 1987.

74. **Saccomanno, G., Archer, V. E., Saunders, R. P., James, L. A., and Beckler, P. A.**, Lung cancer of uranium miners on the Colorado plateau., *Health Phys.*, 10, 1195, 1964.

75. **Miller, R. W.**, Some contributions to science by the Radiation Effects Research Foundation (formely the Atomic Bomb Casualty Commission), *Jpn. J. Cancer Res. (Gann)*, 77, 1050, 1986.

76. **Pinkston, J. A., Wakabayashi, T., Yamamoto, T., Asano, M., Harada, Y., Kumagami, H., and Takeuchi, M.**, Cancer of the head and neck in atomic bomb survivors: Hiroshima and Nagasaki, 1957—1976, *Cancer*, 48, 2172, 1981.

77. **Wanebo, C. K., Johnson, K. G., Sato, K., and Thorslund, T. W.**, Breast cancer after exposure to the atomic bombings of Hiroshima and Nagasaki, *N. Engl. J. Med.*, 279, 667, 1968.

78. **McGregor, D. H., Land, C. E., Choi, K., Tokuoka, S., Liu, P. I., Wakabayashi, T., and Beebe, G. W.**, Breast cancer incidence among atomic bomb survivors. Hiroshima and Nagasaki, 1950—69, *JNCI*, 59, 799, 1977.

79. **McGregor, D. H., Land, C. E., Choi, K., Tokuoka, S., Liu, P. I., Wakabayashi, T., and Beebe, G. W.**, Breast cancer among atomic bomb survivors Hiroshima and Nagasaki, 1950—69. Pathologic features, *RERF TR33-71*, 1971.

80. **Tokunaga, M., Norman, J. E., Jr., Asano, M., Tokuoka, S., Ezaki, H., Nishimori, I., and Tsuji, Y.,** Malignant breast tumors among atomic bomb survivors, Hiroshima and Nagasaki, 1950—74, *JNCI*, 62, 1347, 1979.

81. **Tokuoka, S., Asano, M., Yamamoto, T., Tokunaga, M., Sakamoto, G., Hartmann, W. H., Hutter, R. V. P., Land, C. E., and Henson, D. E.,** Histologic review of breast cancer cases in survivors of atomic bombs in Hiroshima and Nagasaki, Japan, *Cancer*, 54, 849, 1984.

82. **Tokunaga, M., Land, C. E., Yamamoto, T., Asano, M., Tokuoka, S., Ezaki, H., and Nishimori, I.,** Incidence of female breast cancer among atomic bomb survivors, Hiroshima and Nagasaki, 1950—1980, *Radiat. Res.*, 112, 243, 1987.

83. **Tokunaga, M., Land, C. E., Yamamoto, T., Asano, M., Tokuoka, S., Ezaki, H., Nishimori, I., and Fujikura, T.,** Breast cancer among atomic bomb survivors, in *Radiation Carcinogenesis: Epidemiology and Biological Significance*, Boice, J. D., Jr. and Fraumeni, J. F., Jr., Eds., Raven Press, New York, 1984, 45.

84. **Boice, J. D., Jr. and Monson, R. R.,** Breast cancer in women after repeated fluoroscopic examinations of the chest, *JNCI*, 59, 823, 1977.

85. **Shore, R. E., Hempelmann, L. H., Kowaluk, E., Mansur, P. S., Pasternack, B. S., Albert, R. E., and Haughie, G. E.,** Breast neoplasms in women treated with x-rays for acute postpartum mastitis, *JNCI*, 59, 813, 1977.

86. **Land, C. E., Boice, J. D., Jr., Shore, R. E., Norman, J. E., and Tokunaga, M.,** Breast cancer risk from low-dose exposure to ionizing radiation: results of parallel analysis of three exposed population of women, *JNCI*, 65, 353, 1980.

87. **Kinutani, K.,** Two cases of an ovarian tumor developed in a female exposed to the atomic bomb explosion (in Japanese), *J. Hiroshima Med. Assoc.*, 11, 892, 1958.

88. **Obo, G.,** Statistical studies on cancer mortality in atomic bomb survivors. 2nd report (in Japanese), *Jpn. Med. J.*, 1839, 27, 1959.

89. **Mitani, Y. and Mori, S.,** Cancer mortality among atomic bomb survivors in Nagasaki, (in Japanese), *Nagasaki Med. J.*, 36, 724, 1961.

90. **Preston, D. L., Kato, H., Kopecky, K. J., and Fujita, S.,** Life span study report 10. Part 1., Cancer mortality among A-bomb survivors in Hiroshima and Nagasaki, 1950—82, *RERF TR1-86*, 1986.

91. **Tokuoka, S., Kawai, K., Shimizu, Y., Inai, K., Ohe, K., Fujikura, T., and Kato, H.,** Malignant and benign ovarian neoplasms among atomic bomb survivors, Hiroshima and Nagasaki, 1950—80, *JNCI*, 79, 47, 1987.

92. **Sanefuji, H. and Ishimaru, T.,** Urinary bladder tumors among atomic bomb survivors Hiroshima and Nagasaki, 1961—72, *RERF TR18-79*, 1979.

93. **Bean, M. A., Yatani, R., Liu, P. I., Fukazawa, K., Ashley, F. W., and Fujita, S.,** Prostatic carcinoma at autopsy in Hiroshima and Nagasaki Japanese, *Cancer*, 32, 498, 1973.

94. **Socolow, E. L., Hashizume, A., Neriishi, S., and Niitani, R.,** Thyroid carcinoma in man after exposure to ionizing radiation: a summary of the findings in Hiroshima and Nagasaki, *N. Engl. J. Med.*, 268, 406, 1963.

95. **Wood, J. W., Tamagaki, H., Neriishi, S., Sato, T., Sheldon, W. F., Archer, P. G., Hamilton, H. B., and Johnson, K. G.,** Thyroid carcinoma in atomic bomb survivors Hiroshima and Nagasaki, *Am. J. Epidemiol.*, 89, 4, 1969.

96. **Parker, L. N., Belsky, J. L., Yamamoto, T., Kawamoto, S., and Keehn, R. J.,** Thyroid carcinoma after exposure to atomic radiation: a continuing survey of a fixed population, Hiroshima and Nagasaki, 1958—1971, *Ann. Intern. Med.*, 80, 600, 1974.

97. **Sampson, R. J., Key, C. R., Buncher, C. R., and Iijima, S.,** Thyroid carcinoma in Hiroshima and Nagasaki. I. Prevalence of thyroid carcinoma at autopsy, *JAMA*, 209, 65, 1969.

98. **Ezaki, H., Ishimaru, T., Hayashi, Y., and Takeichi, N.,** Cancer of the thyroid and salivary glands, in *Cancer in Atomic Bomb Survivors*, Shigematsu, I. and Kagan, A., Eds., Japan Scientific Societies Press, Tokyo, 1986, 129.

99. **Belsky, J. L., Tachikawa, K., Cihak, R. W., and Yamamoto, T.,** Salivary gland tumors in atomic bomb survivors, Hiroshima- Nagasaki, 1957 to 1970, *JAMA*, 219, 864, 1972.

100. **Belsky, J. L., Takeichi, N., Yamamoto, T., Cihak, R. W., Hirose, F., Ezaki, H., Inoue, S., and Blot, W. J.,** Salivary gland neoplasms following atomic radiation: additional cases and reanalysis of combined data in a fixed population, 1957—1970, *Cancer*, 35, 555, 1975.

101. **Asano, M., Kato, H., Yoshimoto, K., Seyama, S., Itakura, H., Hamada, T., and Iijima, S.,** Primary liver carcinoma and liver cirrhosis in atomic bomb survivors, Hiroshima and Nagasaki, 1961—75, with special reference to hepatitis B surface antigen, *JNCI*, 69, 1221, 1982.

102. **Kishikawa, M., Yushita, Y., Toda, T., Ito, M., Iseki, M., Shimizu, K., Takiguchi, K., Takaki, Y., Araki, J., Takahira, R., Sekine, I., Nishimori, I., Kondo, H., Matsuo, T., and Ikeda, T.,** Pathology study of brain tumors among atomic bomb survivors in Nagasaki (in Japanese), *J. Hiroshima Med. Assoc.*, 35, 428, 1982.

103. **Seyama, S., Ishimaru, T., Iijima, S., and Mori, K.,** Primary intracranial tumors among atomic bomb survivors and controls, Hiroshima and Nagasaki, 1961—75, RERF TR15-79, 1979.

104. **Finch, S. C. and Beebe, G. W.,** A review of thirty years study of Hiroshima and Nagasaki atomic bomb survivors. II. Biological effects. F. Aging, *J. Radiat. Res.*, 16(Suppl.), 108, 1975.

105. **Beebe, G. W. and Hamilton, H. B.,** A review of thirty years study of Hiroshima and Nagasaki atomic bomb survivors. B. Future research, *J. Radiat. Res.,* 16(Suppl.), 149, 1975.

106. **Anderson, R. E.,** Aging in Hiroshima atomic bomb survivors, *Arch Pathol.,* 79, 1, 1965.

107. **Jordan, S. W., Hasegawa, C. M., and Keehn, R.,** Testicular changes in atomic bomb survivors, *Arch. Pathol.,* 82, 542, 1966.

108. **Belsky, J. L., Moriyama, I. M., Fujita, S., and Kawamoto, S.,** Aging studies in atomic bomb survivors, RERF TR11-78, 1978.

109. **Okajima, S., Miyajima, J., Ichimaru, M., Koike, Y., Yamashita, K., Shiomi, T., Nakamura, T., and Mori, H.,** Studies on aging in atomic bomb survivors (in Japanese), *J. Hiroshima Med. Assoc.,* 35, 389, 1982.

Chapter 11

GEOGRAPHICAL PATTERNS OF CANCER: ROLE OF ENVIRONMENT

C. S. Muir

TABLE OF CONTENTS

I. INTRODUCTION

Here we examine the global burden of cancer in selected demographic regions of the world. The proportion of the global burden that can be attributed to known or likely risk factors is considered. The significance of these findings in relation to aging populations is discussed in terms of future cancer burden, reliability of diagnosis of cancer in older persons, the results of treatment, and prevention.

While the existence of differing patterns of cancer occurrence throughout the world has been known for many years,[11] it was not until 1984 that an estimate was made of the world cancer burden.[25] This estimate, for the year 1975, not only assessed the global burden but did so for each of the 24 demographic regions recognized by the United Nations. Comparable estimates were recently produced for 1980[27]; the top ten cancers are given in Table 1. The global total number of new cancers was considered to be 6.35 million, almost exactly divided between the sexes and between developed and developing countries, although two thirds of the world population dwells in the latter.

Lung cancer is by far the most common malignancy in males, as is breast in females. When the two sexes are combined, however, stomach cancer, though declining in incidence, is ranked first. The high proportion of mouth/pharynx cancer in males is a reflection of the frequency of these cancers in the Indian subcontinent.

The data for northern America presented in Figure 1 emphasize the relative importance of prostatic and large bowel cancers in males. Lung is in third place in females following breast and large bowel. It should be emphasized that given the poor prognosis of lung cancer, there are currently more deaths from lung cancer than from breast cancer in women in the U.S. (and in other populations such as Scotland).

In western Europe (Figure 2), stomach cancer is still among the first five ranking sites in both sexes; lung cancer, however, is not among the first five in females. Although the rank order differs slightly and incidence levels are, in general, lower for many forms of cancer, stomach excepted, the pattern in eastern Europe (Figure 3) is substantially the same as in the West. In contrast, the data for Japan (Figure 4) show the overwhelming preponderance of gastric cancer in both sexes. Primary liver cancer is in fourth rank in females and lung in fifth place.

The patterns for China (Figure 5), where one fifth of the world's population lives, show that esophageal and liver cancer occupy 2nd and 3rd ranks, respectively, in males. While cervix uteri is in first place in females, cancers of the stomach, esophagus, large bowel, and liver are more common than those of the breast, in contrast to occidental populations.

In S.E. Southeast Asia (Figure 6), which excludes the Indian subcontinent, cancers of the mouth and pharynx are nearly as common as those of the lung in males and occupy third rank in females.

The estimates for western Africa (Figure 7) show a preponderance of liver cancer in males and very high levels of malignant lymphoma, mainly Burkitt's lymphoma in children. In females, cervical cancer is by far the most common site. Many of the forms of malignancy common in other parts of the world such as lung, stomach, and large bowel are rare.

These estimates are, regrettably, not all based on incidence data collected by cancer registries but depend on a variety of sources of information, including cancer incidence, extrapolation of incidence from mortality, and in large areas of the world, from relative frequency data largely obtained from the monograph *Cancer Occurrence in Developing Countries*.[26] With such varied source materials it must be stressed that the figures presented are estimates. The methods used, notable for the developing countries, are discussed in the original articles. Despite the caveats appearing in these papers, the information presented probably reflects reasonably well the relative burden and site pattern in many parts of the world. Regrettably, the calculation of age-specific and age-standardized incidence rates, which provide a measure of the differences in risk

TABLE 1
The Most Frequent Cancers Worldwide, 1980[27]

	Males	Number[a]	%		Females	Number[a]	%
1.	Lung	513.6	(15.8)	1.	Breast	572.1	(18.4)
2.	Stomach	408.8	(12.6)	2.	Cervix	465.6	(15.0)
3.	Colon/rectum	286.2	(8.8)	3.	Colon/rectum	285.9	(9.2)
4.	Mouth/pharynx	257.3	(7.9)	4.	Stomach	260.6	(8.4)
5.	Prostate	235.8	(7.3)	5.	Corpus uteri	148.8	(4.8)
6.	Esophagus	202.1	(6.2)	6.	Lung	146.9	(4.7)
7.	Liver	171.7	(5.3)	7.	Ovary	137.6	(4.4)
8.	Bladder	167.7	(5.2)	8.	Mouth/pharynx	121.2	(3.9)
9.	Lymphoma	139.9	(4.3)	9.	Esophagus	108.2	(3.5)
10.	Leukemia	106.9	(3.3)	10.	Lymphoma	98.0	(3.2)

[a]   In thousands.

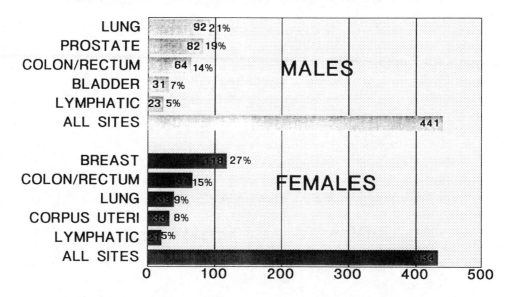

FIGURE 1. The figure for northern America reveals the importance of prostatic and large bowel cancers in males; lung is in third place in females, following breast and large bowel. The numbers within the bars of the histogram give the estimated number of incident cases in thousands.

between populations was not possible. A further disadvantage is that the patterns of malignant disease in the elderly cannot be examined in any detail. However, in much of the world there are relatively few persons in the upper age groups and hence the numbers of cancers is low. The reliability of the diagnosis of cancer in older people is discussed below.

II. THE CAUSES OF CANCER

Haviland, the first to map cancer, noted in 1875 that the distribution of cancer in females, notably that of the breast, in England and Wales, was not uniform and concluded that this must in some way be related to the environment. A recent series of atlases portraying the mortality and, less frequently, the incidence of cancer within countries have again uncovered a remarkable diversity of risk for many, but not all, cancers. Atlases covering more than one country, such as that for cancer mortality in the countries of the European Economic Community, again reveal

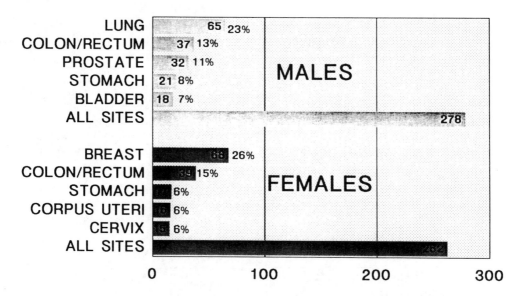

FIGURE 2. In western Europe, stomach cancer is still among the first five ranking sites in both sexes. Lung cancer, however, is not among the first five sites in females.

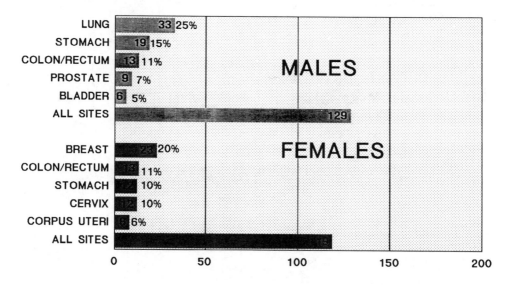

FIGURE 3. Although the order differs slightly, the pattern in eastern Europe is substantially the same as in western Europe.

very large differences.[29] That these differences cannot be entirely due to genetic factors seems likely when it can be shown that migrants moving from a country with a given pattern of risk for a series of cancers, are found to gradually acquire the levels of risk characteristic of the host country.[2,8,17] The fact that cancer incidence may vary quite substantially in relatively short periods of time in either direction within a population (e.g., malignant melanoma of skin is increasing in some fair-skinned populations at some 3 to 5%/year and stomach and cervix uteri are decreasing virtually everywhere) again lends credence to the belief that external factors must be of importance, a conclusion endorsed by the World Health Organization, which in 1964 stated that up to 80% of human cancers were environmentally induced.[31]

Unfortunately, many like Humpty Dumpty in *Alice Through the Looking Glass* who stated,

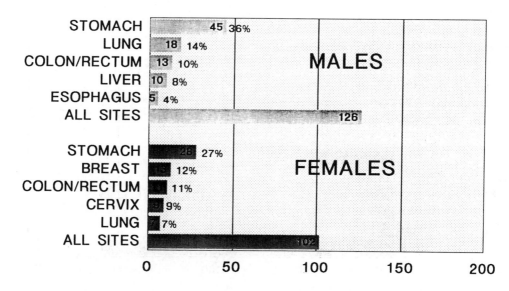

FIGURE 4. The data for Japan show the overwhelming preponderance of gastic cancer in both sexes. Primary liver cancer is in fourth rank in males and lung in fifth in females.

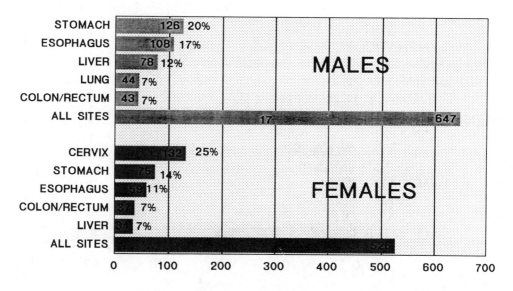

FIGURE 5. In contrast, in China, esophageal and liver cancer occupy second and third ranks in males. While cervix is in first rank in females, cancers of the stomach, esophagus, large bowel, and liver are more common than those of the breast.

"When I use a word it means what I choose it to mean — neither more nor less", have taken their own meaning for the word environment, frequently restricting it to exposure to man-made chemicals. In this chapter, the word environment means not only the air we breathe, the water we drink, the food we eat, and exposures at work, but also personal habits such as use of tobacco and alcoholic beverages, the nature and the quantity of food consumed, and culturally influenced habits such as age of first coitus and full-term pregnancy. In other words, all factors impinging on the human organism.

Around 1980, several estimates were made of the probable relative importance of these various aspects of the environment for the U.S.[4,33] and for Birmingham, England and Bombay,

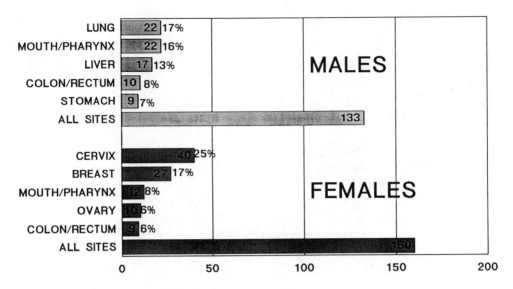

FIGURE 6. In S.E. Southeast Asia, cancers of the mouth and pharynx are nearly as comon as those of the lung in males and occupy third rank in females, cervix cancers being more frequent than those of the breast.

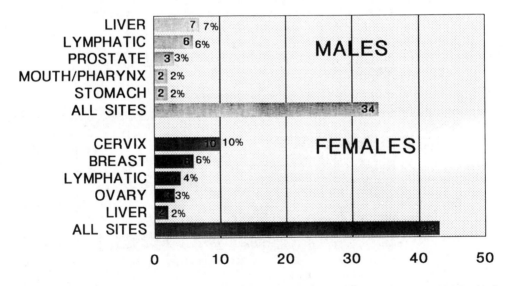

FIGURE 7. The estimates for West Africa show a preponderance of liver cancer in males and very high levels of malignant lymphoma, e.g., Burkitt's lymphoma. In females, cervix is by far the most common form of cancer.

India[10] (Figure 8). Although Doll and Peto gave a wide range of possible values for each element of the environment, the various independent estimates were remarkably close.

Higginson and Muir,[10] Wynder and Gori,[33] and Doll and Peto[4] based their estimates of the proportion of the cancer burden due to specific causes on evidence from many sources. These included the results of case-control studies which permitted the calculation of population attributable risk (see below), the increase in incidence observed in exposed persons in a variety of cohort studies, changes in risk on migration, changes over time, etc. While such methods may be acceptable for a given population, they may not be extrapolatable from one country to another, or from one time period to the next. The ensuing paragraphs, which follow the order of the neoplasm chapter of the International Classification of Diseases, briefly outline the major

193

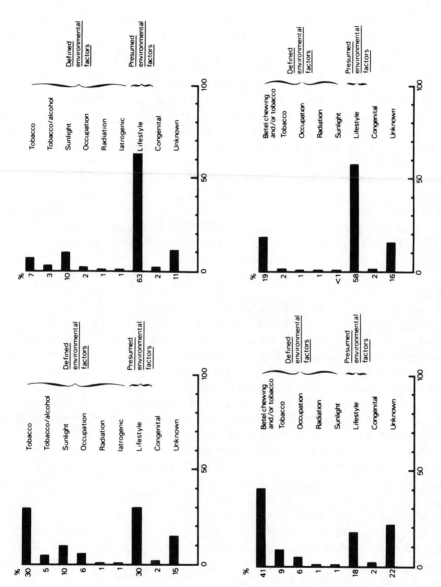

FIGURE 8.   The proportion of cancers attributed to the causes listed in Birmingham and the West Midlands region of England and Greater Bombay, India.

known causes of cancer. It is, of course, impossible to summarize all that is known about the causation of cancer in one chapter, so discussion is confined to the first six ranking sites in Table 1. The relative importance of a particular exposure may be calculated for a given cancer from case-control studies by computation of the population attributable risk. Thus, most investigations show that 85% of lung cancer is attributable to cigarette smoking, while bladder cancer risk is frequently shown to have an occupational component on the order of 20%[3] as well as that due to tobacco. Such results are, however, normally calculated for the age span covered by the subjects in the study, many of which are restricted to persons below a certain age, frequently 70 years, as it may be difficult to obtain appropriate controls. Further, some exposures are characteristic for a given country or region. There have been few studies of risk factors in older persons and in the following it is assumed that causes affecting younger ages also exert their effects later in life.

Cancers of the mouth and pharynx are particularly common in the Indian subcontinent where they are due to chewing of tobacco in the form of the betel quid. This habit, increasingly combined with smoking either of bidi (handrolled cigarettes made of sun-dried Indian tobacco, rolled in the leaf of the temburni tree) or Western-style cigarettes, is very widespread.[18] Elsewhere, many are linked to consumption of tobacco and alcohol,[14] notably in the so-called "Latin" countries of Europe.

Esophageal cancers, twice as common in U.S. blacks as in whites, are very common in parts of France where, indeed, these cancers are almost as frequent as those of the lung; in parts of Spain and Italy, they are due to the combined habit of tobacco and alcohol consumption. In contrast, the exceedingly high rates in the Caspian Littoral of Iran and in northern China are likely to be due to other carcinogens, acting on populations with diets poor in riboflavin and vitamin A for substantial portions of the year.[21]

While comparatively little is known about the risk factors for stomach cancer, numerous studies have consistently shown that risk is diminished in those consuming diets containing adequate amounts of fresh fruits and vegetables. Nearly everywhere, gastric cancer incidence is falling, even in high incidence areas such as Japan. Such changes in risk are usually observed in younger age cohorts, as it is usually more recent cohorts which adopt new habits. Thus, at a time when overall gastric cancer mortality was rising in Japan, a fall could be detected in those aged 40 to 44.[20] The increasing availability of fresh fruit and vegetables throughout the year in many parts of the world due to refrigeration and better food distribution, with a decline in the use of smoked and salt-preserved foodstuffs, is clearly of significance. There is increasing evidence that this cancer may be influenced by endogenous nitrosation, N-nitroso compounds being formed in the stomach from normal dietary constituents, nitrates and secondary amines. This reaction is inhibited by vitamin C providing a possible mechanistic explanation for the risk reduction accompanying consumption of fresh fruit and vegetables.

Cancers of the large bowel, particularly the colon, have been increasing in many populations in which they have hitherto been unusual. Such changes of risk are often accelerated on migration, for example, the Japanese to the U.S., southern Italians and Greeks to Australia.[17] This phenomenon has been attributed to an increasing proportion of dietary calories from animal fat sources in many populations and concurrent diminution in the intake of dietary fiber. The underlying mechanistic hypothesis is that the carcinogenic bile acids, which are produced following the metabolism of fatty acids, are diluted in the intestine by the increased fecal bulk resulting from fiber intake. A low fat high fiber diet is thus characteristic of low risk populations. It is possible that the sources of dietary fiber, such as cabbage, also contain protective chemicals such as flavenoids.

While in 7th rank in global terms, primary liver cancer is in first place in males in West Africa and in third (males) and fifth rank (females) in China. The vast majority of these cancers occur in hepatitis B carriers (in whom the relative risk, over 100, is much higher than that of lung cancer in heavy smokers) and thus should be preventible by vaccination at or shortly after birth. Such campaigns are underway in The Gambia, West Africa[6] and in East China and Southeast Asia.

The causes of cancer of the prostate, like those of cancer of the breast, remain somewhat of an enigma. The incidence rates in American blacks are double those in American whites, which are in turn twice those in most European populations, the incidence in Japanese being again about half that in Europe. Consumption of animal fats has been suggested as being responsible. There is evidence that with advancing age the frequency of small, so-called "latent" cancers of the prostate increases at a given age. The frequency, however, of small lesions probably does not vary between populations, although that of larger and clinically evident prostate cancer does, a finding which suggests that there are factors which induce the malignant change and perhaps others which cause the small "latent" lesions to progress. The frequency of autopsy and the care with which the prostate is examined at autopsy can have considerable influence on the incidence of this form of cancer. Thus, in Malmö, Sweden, in 1981, the incidence was 151.1/100,000/year, a figure some 50% greater than that of the Swedish national average. However, nationwide, 298 cases were discovered at autopsy (7.6%), in contrast to Malmö where 61 of 177 registered cases were discovered (34.5%) after autopsy.[22] Given that this cancer is very rare before the age of 50, increasing rapidly after 70, an increase in the average age of a population will increase the frequency of the disease on demographic grounds alone.

Some 85% of lung cancers are due to smoking. Some of those in nonsmokers are likely to be due to so-called passive or involuntary smoking[12] and, for those dwelling in houses with high radon exposure, the risk is also likely to be increased.[13] A certain number have been caused by occupational exposures such as bis-chloromethyl ether and, in some Chinese nonsmoking women, exposure to cooking oil fumes has been implicated.[7] While tobacco consumption is falling in males in a few European countries and in North America, with an observable decline in lung cancer incidence in, for example, Finland, England, and Wales, the increasing consumption of tobacco by some 2%/year in developing countries and by women in the developed world must result in substantial increases in the lung cancer burden. This is clearly foreshadowed in birth cohort analysis (Figure 9) with successive generations on reaching a given age having higher age-specific incidence rates than those born earlier.

The earlier onset on menarche, delay of the menopause, and the increasing average age of first full-term pregnancy in many parts of the world has resulted in an increasing risk for breast cancer. It will be recalled that a first pregnancy before the age of 23 halves the risk of breast cancer compared to the nulliparous. The increasing consumption of animal fat has also been shown in several studies to be important. Yet, an approximately equal number of case-control investigations carried out by equally competent investigators did not find such an association. Breast cancer risk is currently low in China (an age-standardized risk of less than 20/100,000/ year); in California Chinese the rates are around 40 and in Hawaii Chinese the rates are close to 60, as in the U.K. or Sweden. If the risk factors become widespread in China, breast cancer will become an even larger problem than it is currently. Current social pressures in that country tend to increase the age at first pregnancy.

There is now evidence that cancer of the cervix uteri, which is diminishing nearly worldwide (although far more common than breast cancer in the developing world), is a venereal disease induced by exposure to the human papillomavirus types 16 and 18. Cancer of the corpus uteri is common in obese, tall, nulliparous women and frequently parallels the incidence of breast cancer. The widespread use, notable in California, of conjugated estrogen by postmenopausal women, was accompanied by a very rapid rise in the incidence of endometrial cancer. When this became known and the use of these products virtually ceased, incidence rates fell over the next 5 years close to where they had been some 10 years previously. This rapid appearance and disappearance argue strongly for a promoting effect for these hormones.

The patterns of the developing world are currently different from those of the more prosperous regions, yet it is likely that in time these variegated patterns will blur into a kind of "globocancer". When patterns are uniform it becomes more difficult to investigate the causes, hence, the need to mount etiological studies now.

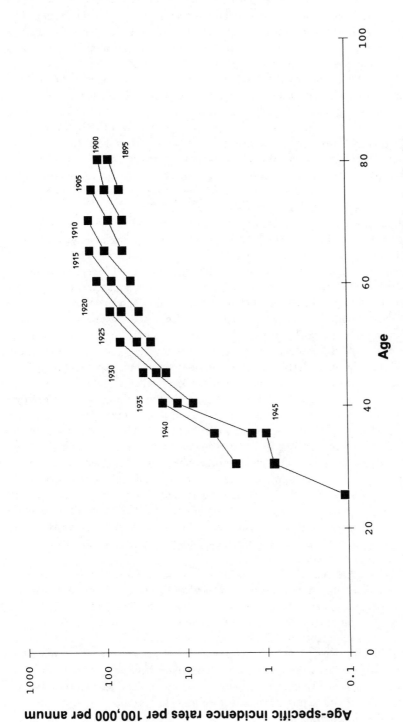

FIGURE 9. The incidence of lung cancer in Detroit, MI, 1969—1982, is shown by birth cohort (females).

III. RELIABILITY OF CANCER DIAGNOSIS IN OLDER PERSONS

It is frequently held that the quality of diagnosis in elderly persons is not as good as in the younger. Volume V of the monograph series *Cancer Incidence in Five Continents*[16] provides information for several indices of data reliability by broad age group. These indices include:

1. The proportion of notifications with age unknown (which should normally be very low other than for nonmelanoma skin cancer)
2. The proportion of diagnoses with histological verification (HV%); this may vary by site as other reliable methods of diagnosis exist, e.g., radiology for cancer of the esophagus, serum fetoprotein levels for primary liver cancer, etc.
3. DCO%, the proportion of all notifications for which the only information available to the cancer registry was a statement on a death certificate that a deceased person had cancer, usually less than 5% in most registries
4. The relationship between mortality and incidence for a given cancer in the registration area at a particular time (M/I%). This ratio varies considerably from site to site, being close to unity for rapidly fatal forms of malignancy such as those of the esophagus and very low for nonmelanoma skin cancer

Data for older persons in selected populations are presented in Tables 2 to 4.

The SEER (Surveillance, Epidemiology and End Results) registries of the U.S., whose work is coordinated by the U.S. National Cancer Institute, maintain very complete records on the basis of diagnosis. These are given for selected sites in Table 2 by age and sex. Although the proportion of histological verification at 65 to 69 and 70 to 74 is much the same for the sites listed, after 75 there is a gradual diminution in the proportion with histological verification, a rise in the proportion diagnosed on clinical grounds, and an increase in the proportion registered on the basis of a death certificate only.

Table 3 compares HV%, DCO%, and M/I% for males in Connecticut and in Miyagi Prefecture in Japan for gastric cancer. The proportion with histological verification is substantially higher at all ages in Connecticut and the proportion registered on the basis of a death certificate only very low, whereas in the 85-plus age group in Japan over half of the cases in the Miyagi cancer registry had not been reported to the registry before death. By definition, a DCO case cannot have histological verification of diagnosis. Nonetheless, when the mortality/incidence ratios are compared (Table 4), up to the age of 79 these are remarkably similar in both areas, suggesting that despite the high level of DCO, most cases in Japan were in fact recognized although not reported to the cancer registry before death. Comparison in the same table of similar data for males in the German Democratic Republic reveals a very low percentage of DCO and a somewhat greater proportion with histological verification of diagnosis than in Japan, which should indicate more reliable data than in Japan. Yet, in the older age groups in the German Democratic Republic, there are more deaths stated to be due to gastric cancer than there were incident cases, reflecting either underregistration or poor death certification.

Fujimoto and Hanai[5] discuss the reasons for the very high proportion of death certificate only cases in registries in Japan and demonstrate that the diagnosis of cancer for DCO cases there is highly reliable. Thus, while the overall proportion of HV in male Japanese in Miyagi and in Los Angeles was 66.8% and 95.2%, respectively, the overall M/I ratios were 0.67 and 0.61, respectively, i.e., survival was fairly close in both groups. Comparison of these indicators of data quality in Miyagi, by sex, revealed a comparable proportion of HV, 68%, and death certificates only, 15%, and somewhat better survival for females, the M/I ratios being 0.66 and 0.59. Comparing male lung cancer and female breast cancer in Connecticut and Miyagi, survival at any age tends to be slightly better in Connecticut for the former and in Miyagi for the latter tumor, the M/I ratios for lung being 0.78 and 0.83 and for breast, 0.34 and 0.25, respectively.

While these indices of reliability are useful guides to data quality, they cannot be used without

TABLE 2
SEER Registries 1983—1966 — Indices of Data Reliability[a]

Age Group / Mode of Diagnosis		65—69				70—74				75—79				80—84				85 +			
		HV	A	C	DCO	HV	A	C	DCO	HV	A	C	DCO	HV	A	C	DCO	HV	A	C	DCO
Esophagus	M	97.5	0.2	1.6	0.2	93.9	0.5	4.3	0.5	92.5	1.6	4.0	2.0	91.8	0.8	5.2	1.5	80.6	1.0	15.3	3.1
	F	98.8	—	—	0.6	95.6	0.6	1.9	1.2	92.7	0.7	2.9	3.7	93.0	—	7.5	3.5	79.1	—	16.3	4.7
Stomach	M	97.6	0.4	0.9	0.9	96.5	1.0	1.0	1.0	94.5	0.6	3.9	0.5	92.8	1.2	4.0	1.4	84.6	1.3	11.2	2.4
	F	98.5	—	—	0.5	94.4	0.4	3.3	2.0	92.8	0.6	4.2	2.0	90.0	1.6	7.5	0.7	70.9	1.8	20.4	5.7
Liver	M	73.9	5.1	17.1	2.3	72.5	8.2	13.0	4.8	71.5	7.8	16.8	3.4	69.0	6.0	18.1	6.9	58.6	8.6	20.7	
10.3	F	81.1	2.1	12.6	4.2	76.7	1.9	13.6	4.9	71.1	4.4	18.9	5.6	72.6	5.5	19.2	2.7	52.9	2.9	25.7	
11.4																					
Pancreas	M	80.5	1.7	14.3	2.2	77.8	1.7	17.7	1.8	69.9	2.0	23.6	3.3	54.6	1.2	39.8	3.6	43.1	1.5	45.2	7.5
	F	83.4	1.1	13.8	1.1	77.3	0.9	19.2	1.9	69.7	1.0	24.5	4.1	57.7	1.1	36.7	3.9	34.7	1.7	55.5	6.8
Lung	M	93.8	0.9	3.8	1.0	91.3	1.0	6.2	1.1	86.8	1.4	9.4	1.9	77.1	1.0	18.1	3.1	58.5	2.0	31.8	6.8
	F	93.3	0.7	4.3	1.1	90.8	0.8	6.2	1.7	85.6	1.1	10.6	2.0	70.3	2.0	23.7	3.5	54.8	1.3	32.9	4.1
Breast	F	99.3	—	0.4	0.2	98.3	0.1	1.0	0.5	97.5	0.1	1.5	0.7	94.7	0.2	3.6	1.5	85.8	0.1	9.4	8.9
Prostate	M	97.5	1.4	0.9	0.2	97.1	1.4	1.2	0.2	95.2	1.4	2.5	0.5	92.2	1.8	4.6	0.9	83.6	2.6	10.6	2.4
Brain	M	90.2	0.3	8.3	0.9	82.1	—	14.9	3.1	69.9	2.9	28.3	1.7	56.1	—	36.6	6.1	42.9	—	47.6	7.1
	F	83.3	—	15.7	0.4	80.5	—	17.5	1.6	71.4	0.5	22.9	3.7	44.1	2.5	46.9	5.9	35.3	—	52.9	5.9
All sites	M	95.5	0.9	2.6	0.9	94.0	1.0	1.9	0.8	91.6	1.2	5.6	1.1	87.4	1.3	8.8	1.9	79.2	1.7	14.5	3.7
	F	96.6	0.3	2.2	0.6	94.6	0.4	3.7	1.0	92.3	0.6	5.3	1.4	87.2	0.7	9.4	2.2	76.6	0.7	16.7	4.9

[a] All figures are percentages.

Note: Totals are less than 100% due to small numbers of cases diagnosed in hospital for which the record did indicate one way or another whether diagnosis was histologically confirmed or not. HV - histological verification, DCO - death certificate only, A - diagnosed at autopsy, and C - clinical diagnosis only.

Basic data were kindly provided by Ms. V. Van Holten and Mrs. C. Percy of the U.S. National Cancer Institute.

TABLE 3
Indicators of Incidence Data Quality — Stomach Cancer in
Selected Cancer Registries 1978—1982[16]

	0—34	35—64	65—69	70—74	75—79	80—85	85 +
			Connecticut Whites - Males				
HV%	100.0	98.3	94.3	96.2	93.3	88.8	70.2
DCO%	—	1.1	1.7	—	1.5	2.0	4.8
M/I	0.80	0.59	0.66	0.65	0.80	0.70	0.75
			Japan, Miyagi - Males				
HV%	89.9	85.3	78.6	69.2	50.0	30.8	(17.3)
DCO%	5.1	6.8	11.0	18.4	29.9	41.4	(59.7)
M/I	0.46	0.47	0.62	0.70	0.82	0.91	(0.98)
			German Democratic Republic - Males				
HV%	97.9	89.0	82.3	75.8	68.1	58.7	(55.1)
DCO%	—	0.1	0.3	0.7	1.0	2.1	(0.8)
M/I	0.77	0.80	0.88	0.92	1.01	1.05	(1.14)

Note: ( ) = data available for age groups up to 95+.

TABLE 4
Mortality/Incidence Ratios 1978—1982[16]

	0—34	35—64	65—69	70—74	75—79	80—85	85 +	All
				Lung - Males				
Connecticut	0.65	0.72	0.76	0.83	0.84	0.92	0.92	0.78
Miyagi	0.86	0.72	0.86	0.82	0.92	0.99	(1.00)	0.83
				Breast - Females				
Connecticut	0.15	0.31	0.36	0.36	0.38	0.44	0.50	0.34
Miyagi	0.17	0.24	0.28	0.28	0.63	0.41	(0.50)	0.25

some knowledge of local circumstances. A high proportion of HV may reflect complete reporting by pathologists and lesser degrees by other sources. A low proportion of histological verification may reflect an unwillingness to investigate elderly persons exhaustively. A high proportion of DCO may, as in Japan, reflect the inability of cancer registration systems to link hospital records with death certificates. The M/I ratio may be distorted by poor or imprecise death certification, e.g., there are usually more deaths attributed to unspecified leukemias than there are incident cases, as the more precise data on cell type available to the clinician and cancer registry do not appear on the death certificate.

IV. RESULTS OF TREATMENT

Unfortunately in many countries it is not possible to estimate cancer survival for the population as a whole, as to do so requires knowledge of all persons with newly diagnosed cancer, their date of diagnosis, and their date of death. This implies either national cancer registration, or, if registration covers only part of the country, the ability to determine whether registered cancer patients are alive or dead, no matter where they happen to reside at the time

TABLE 5
Trends in Relative 5-Year Survival for Common Cancers in the U.S.[a]
(cases diagnosed in 1979—1984), and Geneva[b]
(cases diagnosed in 1978—1982)

Site and ICD no.	U.S. (whites)[c] both sexes	Geneva Males	Geneva Females
151 Stomach	15.7	27	21
153 Colon	54.1	49	51
154 Rectum	51.5	52	55
157 Pancreas	2.7	d	d
162 Lung	12.9	10	20
172 Malignant melanoma	80.3	91	94
174 Breast	75.0	—	73
180 Cervix uteri	66.7	—	65
182 Corpus uteri	83.3	—	74
183 Ovary	37.3	—	37
185 Prostate	72.6	54	—
201 Hodgkin's disease	73.8	78	80

[a] National Cancer Institute, 1988.[23]
[b] Registre Genevois des Tumeurs, 1989.[28]
[c] For blacks, survival for most sites is poorer.
[d] No 5-year survivors.

of death. Unfortunately in several western European countries consideration of so-called confidentiality prevents such matches being made (see below). It must be stressed that the survival figures emerging from controlled clinical trials are in no way representative of the cancer survival of a given population, in that patients entered in these trials are rightly highly selected so that valid comparisons can be made between treatment regimes.

Five-year relative survival rates for some common cancers are given in Table 5 for selected areas of the U.S.[23] and Geneva.[28] The information for the U.S. covers the period 1979 to 1984 and that for Geneva 1978 to 1982. From Figure 10 it is seen that for several major cancer sites there has been very little change in the 5-year relative survival rate. It is always possible that when the results for the next 5 years become available there will have been significant improvement, but this currently would appear unlikely. There have, of course, been very substantial improvements in survival for Hodgkin's disease, acute lymphocytic leukemia in childhood, choriocarcinoma, and testis cancer — all rather uncommon forms of malignancy.

Survival, or lack thereof, can be presented in other ways. While the disappearance of cancer would extend average expectation of life by 2 to 3 years, for those dying from the disease the picture is quite different, cancer being responsible on average for loss of 10 years of life. In terms of years of life lost in Geneva, cancer as a whole was responsible for 27% of the years of life lost in males and nearly 35% in females. (For these analyses the natural life span was assumed to end at 75 years.) For males dying from cancer 29.3% of the years of life lost were due to lung cancer; for females 9.9%. Breast cancer was responsible for 30.1% of the years of life lost from cancer in women; cancer of the prostate was responsible for the loss of 3.0% of the years in men. Death at an early age, e.g., from childhood leukemia, contributes more to this statistic than death from prostatic cancer at age 70.

V. TREATMENT OF CANCER IN ELDERLY PERSONS

The precision of cancer diagnosis may depend on the attitude of physicians to treatment of

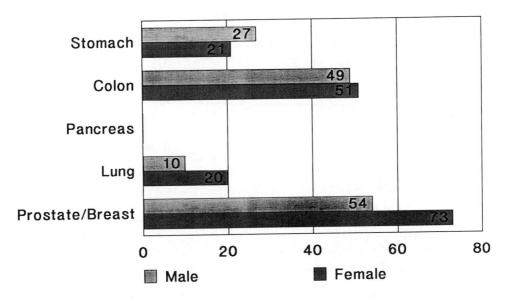

FIGURE 10. The 5-year relative survival (percentage) in Geneva for selected common cancers is shown by sex, 1978—1982. Note that there were no 5-year survivors for pancreatic cancers.

older persons. While there is no reason why the elderly person with cancer should not be treated as energetically as those who are younger (and indeed, as the neoplasms often grow more slowly, with success), physicians are often reluctant to submit elderly patients to the discomfort of invasive diagnostic procedures and aggressive therapy. For a proportion of the elderly the presence of concomitant cardiovascular, cardiorespiratory, or other disease may in effect rule out therapy for the cancer. Nonetheless, results are often better than might be imagined, although not as favorable as in younger patients. This type of information is rarely available, but has been published by the Norwegian Cancer Registry[24] (1980) (Table 6). At any age, stage at diagnosis is a more important prognostic factor than age per se. The use of the relative survival rate takes the effect of weight of other causes of death into account.

VI. THE FUTURE: REDUCING THE CANCER BURDEN IN THE ELDERLY

The increasing average age of many populations means that should present cancer patterns and levels of risk be "frozen", there would nontheless be substantial increases in the total cancer burden. Thus, in southern Europe the U.N. (1986) calculated that there would be a 15% increase in total population between the years 1975 and 2000. Further, the proportion of the population aged over 60 would increase by 24% in males and 27% in females in contrast to northern Europe where population size and age structure were considered to be virtually stable. The ratio of the cancer burden in the year 2000 compared to that in 1975, has been assessed assuming that the projected population rises and change in age structure takes place and taking into account likely secular trends in cancer risk.[15] While the numbers of northern Europe would show little change, there would be increases of between 60 and 80% in eastern and southern Europe, and between 10 and 30% in western Europe.

As noted above changes in the level of cancer in either direction are often first observed in younger age groups as change in exposures is often the reflection of changes in the habits of a particular generation or birth cohort. As most cancers are the result of life-long exposures, the risk of developing malignant disease after the age of 65, and it will be recalled that there are normally as many cancers between 65 and 74 as there are from birth to 64, is probably largely

TABLE 6
Five-Year Relative Survival in Colon Cancer by
Stage and Sex in Norway 1968—1975[24]

Stage		<54 years	55—74 years	75+ years
Localized	M	0.77	0.69	0.60
	F	0.79	0.71	0.56
Regional	M	0.48	0.42	0.35
Spread	F	0.45	0.42	0.36
Distant	M	0.05	0.04	0.08
Spread	F	0.08	0.06	0.05

already determined on reaching the age of 65 and is frequently characteristic for a given birth cohort. Thus, successive birth cohorts, on reaching age 65 in many fair-skinned populations, have higher age-specific incidence rates for malignant melanoma than those born previously, rates which are in turn lower at the same age in those born subsequently. While it would currently appear very difficult to undo or reverse the cellular damage already sustained on reaching older ages, nonetheless, for the initiated cells to be transformed, it is believed that prolonged exposure to promoting agents is needed. If exposure to promoters can be avoided or reduced and indeed antipromoters given, then the malignant transformation may not take place or be delayed. Although Berenblum[1] stated, "interference with the promoting phase of carcinogenesis would seem to offer the best prospects for cancer prevention, if only because the promoting phase covers most of the latent period of carcinogenesis (which, in humans, may be 30 years or more)...", it is only recently that extensive work, including search for short-term tests of promoting activity, has begun on this topic. It is currently believed that fresh fruit and vegetables may contain antipromoters and their use by elderly persons should be encouraged. Unfortunately, dietary habits are often set at a much younger age and it may not be easy to persuade older persons of the need to change. In terms of lung cancer risk, it is probable that ceasing to smoke would be beneficial at any age. The beneficial effect of small quantities of alcohol need not be abandoned.

VII. SUMMARY

In the absence of change in cancer risk, demographic trends alone are bound to increase the world cancer burden. Increasing longevity alone will result in many more cancers in elderly persons to be diagnosed and treated. The results of therapy for common cancers such as lung and stomach show little improvement. The burden of medical care budgets with an ever-decreasing productive population base is likely to be such that no nation, however prosperous, will be able to cope. Prevention is surely to be preferred. Tobacco is responsible for at least 10% of the global cancer burden and viruses (liver and cervix uteri) for another 10%.[19] The major enigma remains the etiology of cancers of breast, large bowel, and prostate; it is here that research effort should be concentrated. Rational prevention demands a knowledge of cause.

REFERENCES

1. **Berenblum, I.,** Cancer prevention as a realizable goal, in *Accomplishments in Cancer Research 1980,* Fortner, J. G. and Rhoads, J. E., Eds., General Motors Cancer Research Foundation, Lippincott, Philadelphia, 1980, 101.
2. **Bonett, A. and Roder, D.,** Epidemiology of Cancer in South Australia. Incidence, Mortality and Survival 1977 to 1986 Analysed by Type, Country of Birth and Geographical Location, South Australia Health Commission, Adelaide, 1988.

3. **Cole, P.,** A population-based study of bladder cancer, in *Host Environment Interactions in the Etiology of Cancer in Man,* Doll, R. and Vodopija, I., Eds., International Agency for Research on Cancer, Lyon, 1973, 83.

4. **Doll, R. and Peto, R.,** The causes of cancer: quantitative estimates of avoidable risks of cancer in the United States today, *J. Natl. Cancer Inst.,* 66, 1191, 1981.

5. **Fujimoto, I. and Hanai, A.,** Japan, Osaka Prefecture, in *Cancer Incidence in Five Continents,* Muir, C. S., Waterhouse, J., Mack, T., Powell, J., and Whelan, S., Eds., Vol. 5, IARC Sci. Publ. No. 88, International Agency for Research on Cancer, Lyon, 1987.

6. The Gambia Hepatitis Study Group, The Gambia Hepatitis Intervention Study, *Cancer Res.,* 47, 5782, 1987.

7. **Gao, Yu-Tang, Blot, W. J., et al.,** Lung cancer among Chinese women, *Int. J. Cancer,* 40, 604, 1987.

8. **Haenszel, W. and Kurihara, M.,** Studies of Japanese migrants. I. Mortality from cancer and other diseases among Japanese in the United States, *J. Natl. Cancer Inst.,* 40, 43, 1968.

9. **Haviland, A.,** *The Geographical Distribution of Diseases in Great Britain,* Smith, Elder & Co., London, 1875.

10. **Higginson, J. and Muir, C. S.,** Environmental carcinogenesis: misconceptions and limitations to cancer control — a review, *J. Natl. Cancer Inst.,* 63, 1291, 1979.

11. **Hoffman, F. L.,** *The Mortality from Cancer Throughout the World,* Prudential Press, Newark, 1915.

12. International Agency for Research on Cancer, *IARC Monographs on the Evaluation of Carcinogenic Risks to Humans,* Vol. 38, *Tobacco Smoking,* IARC, Lyon, 1986.

13. International Agency for Research on Cancer, *IARC Monographs on the Evaluation of Carcinogenic Risks to Humans,* Vol. 43, *Man-Made Mineral Fibres and Radon,* IARC, Lyon, 1988.

14. International Agency for Research on Cancer, *IARC Monographs on the Evaluation of Carcinogenic Risks to Humans,* Vol. 44, *Alcohol Drinking,* IARC, Lyon, 1988.

15. **Muir, C. S.,** Changing international patterns of cancer incidence, in *Accomplishments in Cancer Research 1988,* Fortner, J. G. and Rhoads, J. E., Eds., General Motors Cancer Research Foundation, Lippincott, Philadelphia, 1989, 126.

16. **Muir, C. S., Waterhouse, J., Mack, T., Powell, J., and Whelan, S., Eds.,** *Cancer Incidence in Five Continents,* Vol. 5, IARC Sci. Publ. No. 88, International Agency for Research on Cancer, Lyon, 1987.

17. **Muir, C. S. and Staszewski, J.,** Geographical epidemiology and migrant studies, in *Biochemical and Molecular Epidemiology of Cancer,* Harris, C., Ed., Alan R. Liss, New York, 1986, 135.

18. **Muir, C. S. and Zaridze, D.,** Smokeless tobacco and cancer: an overview, in *Tobacco, A Major International Health Hazard,* IARC Sci. Publ. No. 74, Zaridze, D. G., and Peto, R., Eds., International Agency for Research on Cancer, Lyon, 1986, 34.

19. **Muir, C. S. and Parkin, D. M.,** The world cancer burden: prevent or perish, *Br. Med. J.,* 290, 5, 1985.

20. **Muir, C. S., Choi, N. W., and Schifflers, E.,** Time trends in cancer mortality in some countries: their possible causes and significance, in *Proceedings of the Skandia International Symposium,* Stockholm, 1981, 269.

21. **Munoz, N., Wahrendorf, J., Lu, J. B., Crespi, M., Day, N. E., Thurnham, D. I., Zheng, H. J., Li, B., Li, W. Y., Lin, G. L., Lan, X. Z., Correa, P., Grassi, A., O'Conor, G. T., and Bosch, F. X.,** No effect of riboflavin, retinol and zinc on precancerous lesions of the oesophagus. A randomized double-blind intervention study in a high risk population of China, *Lancet,* 2, 111, 1985.

22. National Board of Health and Welfare, The Cancer Registry, Cancer Incidence in Sweden, 1981, Stockholm Socialstyrelsen, 1984.

23. National Cancer Institute, 1987 Annual Cancer Statistics Review Including Cancer Trends, 1950—1985, NIH Publ. No. 88-2789, National Institutes of Health, Bethesda, MD, 1988.

24. The Cancer Registry of Norway, Survival of Cancer Patients: Cases Diagnosed in Norway 1968—1975, Norwegian Cancer Registry, Oslo, 1980.

25. **Parkin, D. M., Stjernsward, J., and Muir, C. S.,** Estimates of the world-wide frequency of twelve major cancers, *Bull. WHO,* 62, 163, 1984.

26. **Parkin, D. M., Ed.,** *Cancer Occurrence in Developing Countries,* IARC Sci. Publ. No. 75, International Agency for Research on Cancer, Lyon, 1986.

27. **Parkin, D. M., Läärä, E., and Muir, C. S.,** Estimates of the worldwide frequency of sixteen major cancers in 1980, *Int. J. Cancer,* 41, 184, 1988.

28. *Cancer à Genève: Incidence, Mortalité et Survie 1970—1986,* Registre Genevois des Tumeurs, Geneva, 1988.

29. **Smans, M., Boyle, P., and Muir, C. S.,** Cancer mortality atlas of the European community, in *Recent Results in Cancer Research,* Vol. 114, *Cancer Mapping,* Boyle, P., Muir, C. S., and Grundmann, E., Eds., Springer-Verlag, Heidelberg, 1989.

30. *Demographic Indicators of Countries: Estimates and Projections as Assessed in 1984,* United Nations Organization, New York, 1986.

31. Prevention of Cancer, Report of a WHO Expert Committee (Geneva 1963), Tech. Rep. Ser. No. 276, World Health Organization, Geneva, 1964.

32. *WHO International Statistical Classification of Diseases, Injuries and Causes of Death Based on the Recommendations of the 9th Revision Conference, 1975,* Vol. 1 and 2, World Health Organization, Geneva, 1977.

33. **Wynder, E. L. and Gori, G. B.,** Contribution of the environment to cancer incidence: an epidemiologic exercise, *JNCI,* 58, 825, 1977.

Part II:
Cancer Incidence
and Progression

Chapter 12

CHILDHOOD CANCER — INCIDENCE AND ETIOLOGICAL CONSIDERATIONS

Lyly Teppo

TABLE OF CONTENTS

Malignant neoplasms in childhood differ greatly from those occurring in adults. The affected organs are different, and the histological types often unique. Intrauterine exposures, short latent periods, and the role of hereditary factors characterize the etiology and pathogenesis of cancer among children.

In many countries, cancer is second to accidents among the leading causes of death among children under 15 years of age. Thus, even though childhood cancers are rare they constitute an important group when mortality is concerned. In general, some 20% of all deaths in the age group of 1 to 14 years are caused by malignant neoplasms in many developed countries.

In this chapter, the occurrence of childhood cancer in the Nordic countries, and especially in Finland, is outlined, and a description is given of the histological features of certain types of childhood cancer. In addition, the etiology of childhood cancer is considered to some extent.

I. FINNISH CANCER REGISTRY

In each of the five Nordic countries, i.e., Denmark, Finland, Iceland, Norway, and Sweden, there is a countrywide population-based cancer registry. Incidence data on childhood cancer from these countries is considered to be reliable.[1]

The Finnish Cancer Registry was established in 1952. It receives notifications on cancer patients from hospitals, pathological laboratories, and practicing physicians. In addition, death certificate information is obtained from the Central Statistical Office of Finland. The coverage of the Finnish Cancer Registry as to cancers diagnosed in the country has been shown to be high.[2]

In the Finnish Cancer Registry, data on each individual primary tumor are evaluated, coded, and stored for data processing. Special emphasis is paid to the correctness of the code of the primary site. All stages of the registration process are supervised by a physician who finally checks the coding. In addition, inquiries are often sent to clinicians in order to obtain additional information. All this is likely to improve accuracy and minimize erroneous inclusion of benign lesions in the Registry files. However, one has to notice that according to the worldwide practice, all benign intracranial neoplasms are included (hence, the term "brain tumors"). Skin cancers with same histology located at the same anatomical area (e.g., face) within 20 years are coded only once. Otherwise, each lesion is counted separately.

Here the trends in the incidence of childhood cancer in Finland are given for a 32-year period, 1955 to 1986. Cases diagnosed during a 14-year period, 1971 to 1984, were analyzed in more detail and referred to when data on age distributions and histological types of childhood cancer are discussed.[3]

The mean population 0 to 14 years of age in Finland in 1971 to 1984 was 516,000 boys and 494,000 girls. In Denmark, the sizes of the populations were about the same, in Norway somewhat smaller, and in Sweden about 50% larger than in Finland.

Age-specific data were produced in three age groups: 0 to 4, 5 to 9, and 10 to 14 years. Incidence rates were adjusted for age to the "world standard population" (truncated incidence rates), and reported here per 1 million person-years. Histological diagnoses are those given on the pathologists' reports to the Registry, i.e., no review of the slides was made.

II. INCIDENCE OF CHILDHOOD CANCER

A. ALL SITES

In the Nordic countries, which are rather similar in terms of way of life and standard of living, the incidence rates of childhood cancer (all sites taken together) did not show much variation in the late 1970s (Table 1). Due to small numbers, data from Iceland are not presented. Boys experience a consistently higher risk of cancer than girls.

In 1971 to 1984, the average annual number of new cases of childhood cancer in Finland was about 75 in boys and 55 in girls. Childhood cancer constituted less than 1% of cancers diagnosed at all ages.

TABLE 1
Mean Annual Age-Adjusted ("World Standard Population") Incidence Rates per 1 Million Person-Years of Selected Cancers Among Children Aged 0—14 Years in the Nordic Countries in 1976—1980, by Sex[1a]

Cancer	Denmark M	Denmark F	Finland M	Finland F	Norway M	Norway F	Sweden M	Sweden F
All sites[a]	143	109	151	103	141	107	155	135
Acute leukemia	37	33	37	36	49	37	46	45
NHL	11	4	15	5	8	6	13	4
Kidney	10	12	14	7	8	8	9	8
Testis	4	—	2	—	6	—	4	—

[a] Excludes basal cell carcinomas of the skin.

TABLE 2
Age-Specific Numbers of Cases and Incidence Rates per 1 Million Person-Years of Cancer at All Sites[a] Among Children Aged 0—14 Years in Finland in 1971—1984, by Sex [3]

Age group (years)	Males No. of cases	Males Incidence rate	Females No. of cases	Females Incidence rate
<1	104	227	60	138
1—4	356	196	251	145
5—9	269	111	211	91
10—14	186	112	247	100

[a] Includes basal cell carcinomas of the skin.

The risk of cancer was highest in the age group 0 to 4 years (Table 2). In boys aged less than 1 year the risk was somewhat higher than that in the age group of 1 to 4 years, whereas in girls no such excess risk during the first year of life was observable.

In 1955 to 1986, the age-adjusted incidence of childhood cancer, all types taken together, remained almost unchanged in girls, and only a very slight increase in the rate was observable in boys (Figure 1). Analysis by age groups showed that a slow increase took place in boys 0 to 4 years of age, but not in girls (Figure 2). In the two other age groups the rates have remained stable throughout the whole 32 year period of observation.

Table 3 lists the relative frequencies of the most common cancers among boys and girls 0 to 14 years of age. Leukemia was the leading type comprising almost one third of all cases in both sexes. The second position was occupied by tumors of the central nervous system. These two sites constituted more than 50% of all malignant neoplasms in children. Other types were far less common. The tumors occurring most frequently in Finland are the same as those in other developed countries.[4]

B. LEUKEMIA
In the late 1970s, the incidence of acute leukemia in the Nordic countries was on the same level in boys and girls except in Norway where the risk among boys was higher (Table 1). The rate among girls was highest in Sweden.

Leukemia constituted almost one third of all malignant neoplasms in children in Finland

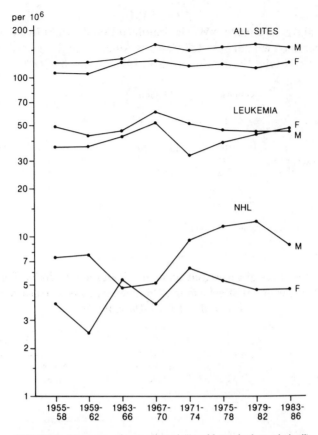

FIGURE 1. Mean annual age-adjusted ("world standard population") incidence rates per 1 million person-years of cancer at all sites (excluding basal cell carcinomas of the skin), leukemia and non-Hodgkin's lymphoma (NHL) among children aged 0—14 years in Finland in eight 4-year periods in 1955—1986, by sex. (Data courtesy of the Finnish Cancer Registry.)

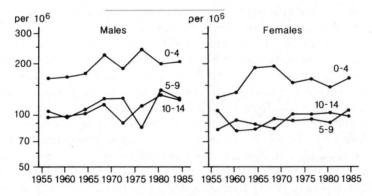

FIGURE 2. Age-specific incidence rates per 1 million person-years of cancer at all sites in Finland in eight 4-year periods in 1955—1986, by sex. Basal cell carcinomas of the skin are excluded. (Data courtesy of the Finnish Cancer Registry.)

(Table 3). Almost one half of all childhood leukemia patients in 1971 to 1984 were 0 to 4 years of age at the time of diagnosis (Table 4).

No apparent change has taken place in Finland in the age-adjusted incidence of leukemia

TABLE 3

Numbers of Cases and Percentage Distribution of the Most Common Cancers Among Children Aged 0 to 14 Years in Finland in 1971—1984, by Sex.[3]

Primary site	Males No. of cases	Males %	Females No. of cases	Females %
Leukemia	316	31.1	247	32.1
Central nervous system	228	22.4	185	24.1
Sympathic nervous system	66	6.5	52	6.8
Kidney	65	6.4	52	6.8
Non-Hodgkin's lymphoma	77	7.6	33	4.3
Bone	58	5.7	34	4.4
Soft tissues	33	3.2	26	3.4
Eye	34	3.3	19	2.5
Hodgkin's disease	28	2.8	20	2.6
Skin[a]	21	2.1	22	2.9
Liver	12	1.2	7	0.9
Colon	4	0.4	14	1.8
Testis	18	1.8	—	—
Ovary	—	—	13	1.7
Thyroid gland	4	0.5	7	0.9
Peripheral nerves	5	0.5	5	0.7
Pineal body	8	0.8	1	0.1
Urinary bladder	7	0.7	2	0.3
Other	27	2.7	26	3.4
Unknown	5	0.5	4	0.5
Total	1016	100	769	100

[a] Includes basal cell carcinomas.

TABLE 4

Age Distribution of Selected Cancers Among Children Aged 0—14 Years in Finland in 1971—1984, by Sex[3]

Primary site	Males 0—4	Males 5—9	Males 10—14	Males Total	Females 0—4	Females 5—9	Females 10—14	Females Total
All sites[a]	460	269	286	1016	311	211	247	769
Leukemia	154	93	69	316	113	84	50	247
Non-Hodgkin's lymphoma	25	26	26	77	14	11	8	33
Hodgkin's disease	2	6	20	28	—	3	17	20
Central nervous system	84	73	71	228	65	56	64	185
Glioma	28	37	38	103	32	32	41	105
Medulloblastoma	21	17	6	44	9	5	4	18
Ependymoma	14	4	3	21	10	5	8	23
Kidney	49	15	1	65	34	16	2	52
Sympathic nervous system	52	11	3	66	43	6	3	52
Bone	4	15	39	58	2	9	23	34
Osteogenic sarcoma	—	10	24	34	1	6	15	22
Ewing's sarcoma	—	3	13	16	1	3	6	10
Eye	32	1	1	34	13	2	4	19
Soft tissues	14	6	13	33	10	4	12	26

[a] Includes basal cell carcinomas of the skin.

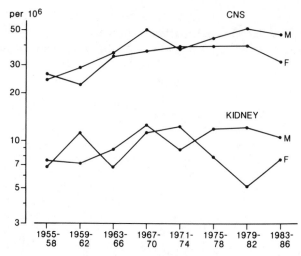

FIGURE 3.   Mean annual age-adjusted ("world standard population") incidence rates per 1 million person-years of tumors of the central nervous system (CNS) and kidney cancer among children aged 0—14 years in Finland in eight 4-year periods in 1955—1986, by sex. (Data courtesy of the Finnish Cancer Registry.)

since the mid-1950s (Figure 1). Both the incidence rates of acute childhood leukemia and their trends have been quite similar in the five Nordic countries (Denmark, Finland, Iceland, Norway, and Sweden).[1] More than 90% of all childhood leukemias in Finland were acute lymphatic leukemias (ALL), the rest being of other or unknown cell type.

C. LYMPHOMAS

The incidence of non-Hodgkin's lymphoma (NHL) in boys was distinctly higher than that in girls in all the Nordic countries (Table 1). There were almost equal numbers of new cases of NHL in 1971 to 1984 in age groups 0 to 4, 5 to 9, and 10 to 14 years in Finland, whereas most of the patients with Hodgkin's disease were 10 to 14 years of age (Table 4). The most common type of NHL was lymphosarcoma or a related disorder (61% of all cases); data according to a more modern histological classification are not available in the Cancer Registry. The incidence of NHL among boys in the 1970s and 1980s was somewhat higher than that observed earlier, while no such increasing trend was observable among girls (Figure 1). It is noteworthy that among the extranodal NHL (not included in the lymphoma figures given above) there were six tumors in the ileum in boys but only one in girls. Burkitt's lymphomas of the jaws, typical in Africa, do not occur in Finland.

D. TUMORS OF THE CENTRAL NERVOUS SYSTEM (CNS)

Almost one fourth of all childhood cancers originated in the CNS, i.e., the brain and spinal cord (Table 3). There was no marked difference between boys and girls in the incidence of CNS tumors. A slight increase in the incidence of CNS tumors has taken place in boys, while the trend curve for girls has run a rather stable course (Figure 3).

Under the age of 1 year, CNS tumors were rare constituting only 8% of all childhood CNS tumors in boys, and 4% in girls. The incidence was highest in the age group of 1 to 4 years. It is possible that due to new diagnostic techniques, e.g., computerized tomography, the age incidence pattern of brain tumors has changed, part of the tumors being now diagnosed at younger age groups than in the 1970s.

A variety of histological types of CNS tumors were reported to the Finnish Cancer Registry. Glioma (including astrocytoma) was the largest group (49% of all), followed by medulloblastoma (15%), ependymoma (10%), and craniopharyngeoma (4%). It should be noticed that for

9% of the tumors of the central nervous system no histological diagnosis was obtained, and for a further 3% the histology code at the Cancer Registry was "malignant tumor, unspecified". Patients with ependymoma or medulloblastoma were younger than those with glioma (Table 4).

It is interesting that six out of seven patients with meningioma were boys. Similarly, eight out of nine tumors in the pineal body (included in cancers of the endocrine organs although being intracranial) were diagnosed in boys.

E. TUMORS OF THE SYMPATHIC NERVOUS SYSTEM

About 7% of all childhood cancers originated in the sympathic nervous system in Finland. The risk was slightly higher in boys. Some 90% of the tumors were neuroblastomas, the rest being ganglioneuroblastomas. More than 80% of the cases were 0 to 4 years of age at the time of diagnosis (Table 3).

F. CANCERS OF THE KIDNEY

In the Nordic countries, the incidence of kidney cancer among boys was highest in Finland and among girls in Denmark (Table 1). No trend was observable in Finland in the incidence of kidney cancer among children (Figure 3).

Kidney tumors constituted some 7% of all childhood cancers in Finland (Table 3). In the 1980s, the risk has been somewhat higher in boys. A great majority of tumors were nephroblastomas (Wilms' tumors), but two adenocarcinomas were also diagnosed, both in girls. A majority of kidney cancers occurred in children under 5 years of age (Table 4).

G. OTHER CANCERS

The risk of bone cancer was equal among boys and girls. Osteogenic sarcoma was the most common type of childhood bone cancer (61%) followed by Ewing's sarcoma (28%). A majority of patients with these tumor types were 10 to 14 years of age at the time of diagnosis (Table 4).

Among soft tissue cancers a variety of different histological diagnoses were made, rhabdomyosarcoma being the most common type in this material. Only few cases occurred in the age group of 5 to 9 years, both other 5 year age groups having almost equal numbers of cases (Table 4). No difference was found between boys and girls.

Retinoblastoma was the leading type of eye cancer in children in Finland. There was a distinct male preponderance, 34 tumors being found in boys, 19 in girls. Only few patients with eye cancer were older than 5 years of age at the time of diagnosis (Table 4).

Almost one half of all skin cancers were basal cell carcinomas (19 of 43). There were 12 melanomas, 7 dermatofibrosarcomas and 1 Kaposi's sarcoma. The skin cancer pattern was similar in boys and girls.

Sixteen of the 18 colon cancers were carcinoid tumors, and only one adenocarcinoma was diagnosed. Not a single case of colon cancer occurred in children 0 to 4 years of age. A great majority (14 of 18) of the patients were girls.

Testis cancer is rare. The incidence rate was lowest in Finland and highest in Denmark (Table 1). It is interesting that the rate in Finland is exceptionally low also among adults whereas Denmark and Norway belong to high-risk countries.[5] Almost 80% of testis cancers occurred in boys under 5 years of age. Yolk sac tumors constituted the largest histological group (11 of 18).

III. MULTIPLE CANCER

A study was undertaken in the Finnish Cancer Registry in which the risk of a subsequent new primary cancer among childhood cancer patients was evaluated.[6] All cancer patients who at the time of diagnosis in 1953 to 1979 were 0 to 14 years of age were followed up through the files of the Cancer Registry in order to identify new primary malignant neoplasms. There were five new cancers among males and also five cases among females.

The expected number of cancers among a group of children similar as to the size and age distribution during a similar follow-up period would have been 1.11 for boys and 0.95 for girls. The standardized incidence ratio was thus 5/1.11 = 4.49 for boys and 5/0.95 = 5.25 for girls. In other words, a distinct excess risk of cancer was observed among childhood cancer patients.

Two explanations are readily available for this observed excess risk. One is the effect of treatment, either radiation or cytostatic drugs. It is well known that a malignant tumor may develop in areas exposed to ionizing radiation during cancer therapy, and cytostatic drugs are known to possess carcinogenic properties. This problem is becoming more important when the average survival time of childhood cancer patients increases and the long-term adverse effects of the treatment become apparent. For example, many patients with Hodgkin's disease are going to contract leukemia after a follow-up of 5 years or more.

Another explanation is the general susceptibility of childhood cancer patients toward carcinogenesis, at least partly due to hereditary factors, such as those operating in xeroderma pigmentosum and some other syndromes in which different malignant (and also benign) neoplasms are common.[7]

IV. ETIOLOGICAL CONSIDERATIONS

The length of the latent period of cancer among children is much shorter than that observable in adults. Even newborns can have malignant tumors, and for many cancers it is clear that the process leading to clinical cancer has started already *in utero*. The short latent period is an interesting special feature of childhood carcinogenesis to be taken into account in experimental and cell biological research.

Genetic determinants can be found in only few adult cancer patients, while a large proportion of childhood cancers are associated with inherited syndromes or conditions. In addition, chromosomal aberrations without any genetic background can lead to an excess risk of cancer. A well-known example is Down syndrome (trisomy-21) in which the risk of leukemia is markedly increased.

Certain syndromes with autosomal recessive inheritance led to an increased risk of cancer. For instance, many patients with Fanconi's anemia have leukemia and also other tumors, and in xeroderma pigmentosum multiple cutaneous cancers, both carcinomas and melanomas, develop in early life in skin areas exposed to sunlight. In xeroderma pigmentosum the basic cell biological defect is known: the mechanism to repair UV radiation induced DNA damage is defective. Xeroderma pigmentosum is a good example of genetic-environmental interactions which are possibly more important in carcinogenesis than is so far generally recognized.

There are also syndromes with autosomal dominant inheritance in which cancers occur in childhood. Patients with neurofibromatosis develop several types of cancer (e.g., nephroblastoma, melanoma, and myeloid leukemia). Basal cell nevus syndrome is associated with basal cell carcinomas of the skin and medulloblastoma of the brain.

Bilateral retinoblastoma is an inherited disease. In addition, the patients are exceptionally susceptible toward irradiation bone and soft tissue carcinogenesis, probably due to a chromosomal alteration present in the cells of these individuals.

Irradiation *in utero* increases the risk of childhood leukemia in the offspring.[8,9] In addition, children who have received radiation treatment due to noncancerous illnesses, such as tinea capitis or enlarged thymus, have later in life experienced an increased risk of NHL.

Another example of transplacental intrauterine carcinogenic exposures is provided by the increased risk of testis cancer among boys whose mothers were exposed to an excess of estrogens during pregnancy, either through medication for threatening abortion or by means of endogenic hyperestrogenism resulting in symptoms, such as vomiting.[5] Similarly administration of diethylstilbestrol to pregnant women resulted in clear cell carcinomas of the vagina in female offspring. In addition to being carcinogenic, transplacental exposure to estrogens is likely to be also teratogenic leading to congenital defects of the genitourinary tract in both boys and girls.

Epstein-Barr virus is considered to play an important role in the etiology of Burkitt's lymphoma. The pandemic of the "Asian influenza" in 1956 in Finland was followed by an increase in the incidence of leukemia among children whose mothers had been pregnant at the time of that epidemic.[10] No such increase was observable after the later influenza epidemics in the 1960s. The role of viruses in the etiology of childhood Hodgkin's disease is still unclear.

A great number of chemicals and dusts are known to be carcinogenic, but exposure to them increases the risk of cancer almost exclusively in adults. Hypotheses on the increased risk of brain tumors among children after occupational exposure to hydrocarbons of their fathers have not been confirmed.[11]

V. CONCLUDING REMARKS

It is interesting, and probably important, that no major increase in the risk of childhood cancer has taken place in Finland during the 30 year period since the mid-1950s. The stability of the trend curves could indicate that the environmental exposures leading specifically to childhood cancer are of lesser importance compared to genetic and related mechanisms, or at least have not changed very much with time. On the other hand, it is clear that large-scale prevention of childhood cancer is not yet likely to be successful through elimination of environmental risk factors. Thus, in addition to strengthening the research on risk factors of childhood cancer, great attention should be paid on identification of high-risk individuals (genetic disposition), methods of early diagnosis, and development of treatment.

The general pattern of childhood cancer in Finland corresponds to that found in many other western countries, leukemia and tumors of the central nervous system being the leading types.[4] The most common cell type of childhood leukemia (ALL) is rare in adults, and many histological subtypes, such as nephroblastoma, neuroblastoma, retinoblastoma, and hepatoblastoma, are found almost exclusively in children. On the other hand, adult-type cancers (carcinomas) may appear earlier than usually, and even in childhood, in connection with different inherited syndromes.

Although no new childhood tumor types are emerging in the Finnish population, continuous monitoring of the occurrence of childhood cancer is warranted. This is effected in the most feasible way through a cancer registration system which must be organized so that the incidence of each cancer type and age group can be monitored separately. An example of this kind of activity is provided by an international project that has been launched recently in which the long-term effects of the irradiation exposure after the Chernobyl accident will be evaluated by monitoring the incidence of childhood leukemia in areas with different exposure levels.

If possible detailed histological types and even subgroups defined by cell biological markers (e.g., in leukemia) should be taken into account when the cancer registration system is being developed to meet the future expectations, both administrative and research oriented.

REFERENCES

1. **Hakulinen, T., Andersen, A., Malker, B., Pukkala, E., Schou, G., and Tulinius, H.,** Trends in cancer incidence in the Nordic countries. A collaborative study of the five Nordic cancer registries, *Acta Pathol. Microbiol. Immunol. Scand. Sect. A,* 94, Suppl. 288, 1986.
2. **Saxén, E. and Teppo, L.,** *Finnish Cancer Registry 1952—1977. Twenty-Five Years of A Nationwide Cancer Registry,* Finnish Cancer Registry, Helsinki, 1978.
3. Finnish Cancer Registry — the Institute of Statistical and Epidemiological Cancer Research, *Cancer Incidence in Finland 1984. Cancer Statistics of the National Board of Health, C*ancer Society of Finland Publication No. 41, Finnish Cancer Registry, Helsinki, 1989.
4. **Parkin, D. M., Stiller, C. A., Draper, G. J., Bieber, C. A., Terracini, B., and Young, J. L., Eds.,** *International Incidence of Childhood Cancer,* International Agency for Research on Cancer Sci. Publ. No. 87, IARC, Lyon, 1988.

5. **Teppo, L.,** Epidemiology of testicular neoplasms, in *Pathology of the Testis. Contemporary Issues in Surgical Pathology,* Talerman, A. and Roth, L. M., Eds., Churchill Livingstone, New York, 1986, 1.

6. **Teppo, L., Pukkala, E., and Saxén, E.,** Multiple cancer - an epidemiological exercise in Finland, *J. Natl. Cancer Inst.,* 75, 207, 1985.

7. **Li, F. P.,** Cancers in children, in *Cancer Epidemiology and Prevention,* Schottenfeld, D. and Fraumeni, J. F., Jr., Eds., W. B. Saunders, Philadelphia, 1982, 1012.

8. **Bithell, J. F. and Stewart, A. M.,** Prenatal irradiation and childhood malignancy. A review of British data from the Oxford survey, *Br. J. Cancer,* 31, 271, 1975.

9. **Salonen, T.,** Risk indicators in childhood malignancies, *Int. J. Cancer,* 15, 941, 1975.

10. **Hakulinen, T., Hovi, L., Karkinen-Jääskeläinen, M., Penttinen, K., and Saxén, L.,** Association between influenza during pregnancy and childhood leukaemia, *Br. Med. J.,* 4, 265, 1973.

11. **Hakulinen, T., Salonen, T., and Teppo, L.,** Cancer in the offspring of fathers in hydrocarbon-related occupations, *Br. J. Prev. Soc. Med.,* 30, 138, 1976.

Chapter 13

TESTICULAR CANCER AND AGE

Guy R. Newell

TABLE OF CONTENTS

Age is the most important determinant of cancer risk.[1] The incidence of most cancers increases progressively and approximately in proportion to a power of age.[2] Different cancers peak at different ages within the life span; some cancers peak at more than one age. Testicular cancer (TC) has three peaks of occurrence: in childhood, young adulthood, and in older adults (Figure 1). The shape of the age curve for TC varies with ethnic group, social class, and over time.[3] TC is rare among children but accounts for 20% of all cancers among 20 to 34-year-old white men in the U.S.[4] As incidence has increased among young white men both in the U.S. and the U.K., it has decreased in the elderly, suggesting dynamic trends related to changing social environments, personal habits, external exposures, or a combination of these.[5]

I. SOURCES OF DATA

In addition to the existing literature, data are derived from the Surveillance, Epidemiology, and End Results (SEER) program of the National Cancer Institute. Procedures for the SEER program have been presented in detail previously.[6] The geographic areas participating in the program are as follows: the states of Connecticut, Iowa, New Mexico, Utah, and Hawaii; the metropolitan areas of San Francisco-Oakland, Atlanta, Detroit, and Seattle; and the Commonwealth of Puerto Rico. Although these areas in the aggregate are not necessarily representative of the population of the U.S. as a whole, they provide complete and accurate cancer ascertainment by site, age, and other variables within defined geographic areas for about 10% of the U.S. population.

Besides reporting on ethnicity, sex, age at diagnosis, residence, and reporting area, the SEER program also routinely collects data on marital status and tumor laterality and documents whether testicular tumors are present in a cryptorchid testis. Histologic codes were defined by ICD-0 for 1976. Only patients with germ cell tumors, including seminoma (9060 to 9064), embryonal carcinoma (9070 to 9073), teratoma (9080 to 9083), and choriocarcinoma (9100 to 9102) were included.

A. CHILDREN

There is an early peak of TC in children under 5 years with a sharp decline between ages 5 and 14. This pattern differs little among the major ethnic groups in this country: whites, blacks, and Hispanics (non-Caucasian whites).

Histologic subclassification of TC is age dependent. Embryonal carcinoma is the most common histologic type in boys under 15 years of age; teratoma in young adults and seminoma increases in frequency with advancing age.[6] Although rates for childhood testicular cancer are based on small numbers, the data suggest equality of rates by ethnic group nationally, although in adulthood ethnic differences are striking. This highlights the potential importance of environmental exposure in pathogenesis.

Of 50 cases of TC in children under age 5, 45 (90%) were embryonal carcinoma (Table 1). This suggests some etiologic influence around the time of conception, factors from the external environment conveyed by one or the other parent, or perhaps an event occurring *in utero*. Li and Fraumeni[7] found that of 70 children with TC in a hospital series, 15 (21%) had inguinal hernia, undescended testis, or other genitourinary defect. Since these developmental defects also accompany children with Wilms' tumors, they suggested a close relationship between oncogenesis and teratogenesis in the developing genitourinary tract.[7]

Seminoma is rare in childhood, but increases progressively with age at diagnosis, accounting for 70% and more of histologic types in adults age 35 and older (Table 2). Teratomas peak during ages 15 to 34 and decrease afterwards. Choriocarcinoma is the least common histologic type.

Incidence among children has not changed significantly between 1973 and 1982. Similarly, among eight reporting SEER areas in the continental U.S. there was little geographic variation in incidence (Table 3). In Puerto Rico, the incidence among children is lower than in the Continental U.S. as are rates among Puerto Rican adults lower than among U.S. adults.

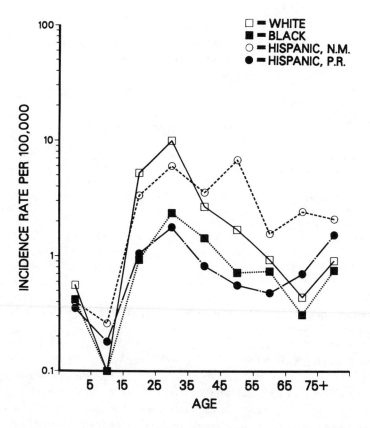

FIGURE 1. Age-specific incidence rates of testicular cancer per 100,000 population in U.S. whites, blacks, and Hispanics, 1973—1982 (NM = New Mexico; PR = Puerto Rico). (Reproduced from *Cancer*, 58, 1785, 1986. With permission.)

TABLE 1
Percent Distribution of Testicular Cancer
by Histologic Type, Ages 0—24

Histologic type	Age at diagnosis				
	0—4 (n = 50)	5—9 (n = 1)	10—14 (n = 9)	15—19 (n = 224)	20—24 (n = 699)
Seminoma	—	—	33.3	8.5	24.3
Embryonal carcinoma	90.0	100.0	11.1	32.5	33.9
Teratoma	10.0	—	44.5	46.9	33.1
Choriocarcinoma	—	—	11.1	12.1	8.7
Total	100.0	100.0	100.0	100.0	100.0

Li and Fraumeni[7] found no evidence of unusual seasonal pattern in birth dates or year-by-year variation between 1960 to 1967. They also found a random geographic distribution of deaths within the U.S.

B. ADULTS

There are distinct ethnic risk differentials in SEER incidence data for TC. White men have significantly higher rates than their black, Puerto Rican, and New Mexican Hispanic counterparts.[3] Higher rates of TC among indigenous U.S. Hispanics relative to their migrant counterparts indicate that environmental factors are important in this disease etiology.[8] However,

TABLE 2
Percent Distribution of Testicular Cancer by
Histologic Type, All Ages[a]

Histologic type	Age at diagnosis			
	<15 (n = 66)	15—34 (n = 2377)	35—54 (n = 1088)	55+ (n = 301)
Seminoma	4.6	38.3	70.0	75.8
Embryonal carcinoma	60.6	28.2	16.6	10.6
Teratoma	12.1	24.5	9.0	2.0
Choriocarcinoma	1.5	7.6	3.2	2.3
NOS[b]	21.2	1.4	1.2	9.3
Total	100.0	100.0	100.0	100.0

[a] Adapted from Spitz et al.[3]
[b] Not otherwise specified.

testicular cancer is rare among all black populations of the world, suggesting a genetic resistance to this tumor among these persons.[9]

C. SOCIAL ENVIRONMENT

Testicular cancer occurs more frequently in men of higher rather than lower social class, even within the same ethnic group.[5] Most studies report a positive relationship between testicular cancer incidence and several indicators of social class. In the lowest social class the curve is bimodal, but assumes a unimodal peak in young adults in the highest social class.[10] Protection is also afforded by large sibship size.[11]

II. POSSIBLE VIRAL ETIOLOGY

In 1970, Newell compared the epidemiologic features of Hodgkin's disease to those of multiple sclerosis and hypothesized that both diseases reflect the rare manifestation of a very prevalent infection of low pathogenicity. Among low socioeconomic groups such infections occur more commonly at an early age, leading to acquired immunity.[12] This behavior is also characteristic of paralytic poliomyelitis infection.

In 1984, we extended the analogy by comparing epidemiologic features of Hodgkin's disease with testicular cancer among young adult men.[13] Although their epidemiologic features had not been compared before, their similarity was remarkable (Table 4). Shared characteristics include an age peak in young adults that, in each malignancy, is probably related to different histologic tumor types. The occurrence of both diseases is increasing in white, urbanized groups. Both occur more frequently in Europe, especially Denmark. They have a north-south gradient within the U.S., and occur very infrequently in blacks and in native Japanese. They are definitely more frequent among higher social classes, according to several measures of social class. They occur more in professionals than in blue-collar workers. All of these features suggest an association with urbanization, westernization, or economic development. Both diseases have a low but definite familial occurrence. The few studies available suggest that the lifetime risk is determined at a young age, and follows the person throughout later life to wherever he may migrate.

III. POSSIBLE ASSOCIATION WITH EPSTEIN-BARR VIRUS (EBV)

EBV antibodies have been reported in Hodgkin's disease both after and before its onset.[14]

TABLE 3
Incidence of Testicular Cancer by Participating
SEER Area and Age at Diagnosis

Age at Diagnosis	San Francisco (n = 155)	Connecticut (n = 152)	Detroit (n = 179)	Hawaii (n = 44)	New Mexico (n = 53)	Seattle (n = 124)	Utah (n = 82)	Atlanta (n = 51)	Puerto Rico (n = 39)
0—4	0.97	0.29	0.58	1.03	0.52	0.37	1.02	0.61	0.31
5—9	—	0.13	0.17	—	—	0.11	—	—	—
10—14	0.07	0.14	0.09	0.33	0.14	0.08	0.07	—	0.15
15—19	2.17	2.88	1.78	1.22	2.11	2.59	1.36	1.73	0.55
20—24	7.65	7.35	7.47	5.25	7.55	7.50	3.48	4.66	1.35

TABLE 4
Epidemiologic Similarities between Testicular Cancer
and Hodgkin's Disease in Young Adult Males[13]

Epidemiologic feature	Similarity between TC and HD
Age	Biomodal in adults with first peak around age 30
Histologic type	Differs in young vs. older adults
Time trend	Increasing in young adults
International variation	High in developed countries except Japan
National variation	North/south gradient in the U.S.
Socioeconomic status	High in upper social class
Familial occurrence	Suggests environmental exposure
Religion	Less frequent in Catholics, more frequent in Jewish patients
Viral etiology	Suggested relationship with EBV

TABLE 5
Percent Positive Viral Titers[15]

Group (no. of cases)	EBV	CMV	Hep A	Hep B
Nonseminoma TC (n = 45)	82	47	14	5
Seminoma TC (n = 11)	73	64	9	27
Physician controls (n = 10)	50	10	10	30

Persons with serologically confirmed infectious mononucleosis have an approximately three-fold increased risk for developing Hodgkin's disease. In a small preliminary serologic survey, we found significantly elevated EBV titers among untreated patients with TC compared with a group of physicians and another group of nonphysicians.[15] Titers to cytomegalovirus (CMV), hepatitis A, and hepatitis B viruses were not elevated in the patients compared with the controls (Table 5). We stress that this represents a preliminary observation requiring further investigation.

IV. TIME TRENDS

One of the most striking features of the epidemiology of testicular cancer is its rapidly increasing occurrence. It has been increasing in young white men in this country and in England and Wales for the last 40 years or more.[5] The largest increases in TC during the 10 years occurred in single men age 20 to 44 years old, followed by those for married men of the same ages. More recently, it may have begun to increase in Hispanic Americans as well.[3] In England and Wales, this increase occurred first among men of higher social class. Davies attributes this to features of modern life which have always affected men in higher social classes and which are becoming more common throughout society.[5] She argues against occupation, exposure *in utero* or in childhood, or cryptorchidism as contributing substantially to this increase.

V. LATERALITY

There is a predominance of right-sided TC at time of diagnosis for all three major ethnic groups for all ages combined (Table 6).[3] Among children, this right-sided excess was more

TABLE 6
Percent Right-Sided Onset by
Age at Diagnosis and Ethnicity[3]

Age at diagnosis	White (n = 3427)	Black (n = 78)	Hispanic (n = 139)
<15	68.2	80.0	55.6
15—34	51.6	60.4	50.6
35—54	54.7	73.3	60.6
55+	47.3	40.0	42.9
All ages	52.4	62.8	52.5

TABLE 7
Incidence of Testicular Cancer
By Ethnicity and Marital Status[16]

Ethnicity	Single	Married	Risk ratio
White	8.4	6.3	1.3
New Mexico Hispanic	3.9	5.3	0.7
Puerto Rico	1.1	1.0	1.1
Black	2.0	1.2	1.7

prominant for whites (68.2%) and blacks (80%). Interestingly, in the oldest age group there was left-sided predominance in each ethnic group. This suggests different etiologic factors might be responsible for laterality among children and older adults than among younger adults.

VI. MARITAL STATUS

An excess of TC among single men with histologic types other than seminoma has been reported.[16] Higher rates of TC were found for white and black, and Puerto Rican single men compared with their married counterparts, despite large differences in actual incidence rates. Excess among single men was not found for Hispanics residing in either New Mexico or Puerto Rico (Table 7). This excess TC among single men was not manifest until age 25 or older and was repeated during three time periods covering 10 years.

The question is whether being single or unmarried and developing TC is a causal association. Alternatively, being married could convey a protective effect. One explanation is that men who are susceptible for the development of TC also are less likely to marry or to marry at older ages. This would account for the increased occurrence of TC in men with cryptorchidism, in those of uncertain sex determination, and in infertile men with atrophic testes.

VII. OCCUPATION

Mortality rates for TC are reported highest among professional, administrative, and clerical workers and lowest among manual workers in England and Wales.[5] In the U.S. high rates have been reported among professionals, white collar, administrative occupations, and lower among manual laborers.[10,17,18] In a hospital-based case-control study of 347 patients with histologically confirmed germ cell TC and 347 randomly selected controls, we found a significant association between TC and work in the agricultural industry (odds ratio = 6.3) and in the crude petroleum and natural gas extraction industry (odds ratio = 2.3).[19] Workers in finance, insurance, real estate, or professional services had slightly, though not significantly, high odds ratios. Although the literature supports an association between agricultural work and TC,[20] it is improbable that this would account for a large number of cases of TC, and the short exposure time (with peak onset of TC in young men ages 25 to 34) mitigates against direct occupational exposure as a major contributor to the etiology of TC. However, following the paralytic polio model of an infectious agent described above, agriculture and farming exposures could be explained in two ways. First, children raised on farms and who later work in farming may have less contact with other children of the same age and thus may escape viral infections while young. This would make them more susceptible to common infections in late childhood or early adolescence, resulting in more severe clinical manifestation of disease, as occurs with mumps infection. Second, farming may produce exposure to zoonotic viruses that could result in testicular damage, although there is no good evidence that zoonotic oncogenic viruses are transmitted to humans. The finding of excess risk among crude petroleum and natural gas extraction workers is not supported by most of the literature.

VIII. CRYPTORCHIDISM

Undescended testicle is the most commonly reported risk factor for the development of TC. There is a predilection of seminoma-type tumors to occur in cryptorchid testes and there is a slightly greater incidence of right-sided cryptorchidism. Given the attributable risk associated with cryptorchidism (about 10% of incident TC cases), this risk factor is not large enough to account for most of the cases of TC.[3]

IX. OTHER RISK FACTORS

An increased risk for TC has been reported associated with a history of hernia surgery independent of a history of undescended testicle.[21] Several cases of TC following mumps orchitis has been reported,[4] but the evidence is not sufficient to implicate this agent in the etiology of TC. We reported an association with hydrocele,[19] but this is not substantiated.

REFERENCES

1. **Newell, G. R., Spitz, M. R., and Sider, J. G.,** Cancer and age, *Semin. Oncol.,* 16, 3, 1989.
2. **Armitage, P. and Doll, R.,** A two-stage theory of carcinogenesis in relation to the age distribution of human cancer, *Br. J. Cancer,* 11, 161, 1957.
3. **Spitz, M. R., Sider, J. G., Pollack, E. S., Lynch, H. K., and Newell, G. R.,** Incidence and descriptive features of testicular cancer among United States whites, blacks, and Hispanics, 1973—1982, *Cancer,* 58, 1785, 1986.
4. **Schottenfeld, D. and Warshauer, M. E.,** Testis, in *Cancer Epidemiology and Prevention,* Schottenfeld, D., Fraumeni, J. F., Jr., Eds., W. B. Saunders, Philadelphia, 1982, 957.
5. **Davies, J. M.,** Testicular cancer in England and Wales: some epidemiologic aspects, *Lancet* 1, 928, 1981.
6. **Young, J. L., Jr., Percy, C., and Asire, A. J., Eds.,** Surveillance, Epidemiology and End Results: incidence and Mortality, 1973—1977, *Natl. Cancer Inst. Monogr.,* 57, 1, 1981.
7. **Li, F. P. and Fraumeni, J. F., Jr.,** Testicular cancers in children: epidemiologic characteristics, *JNCI,* 48, 1575, 1972.
8. **Thomas, D. B.,** Epidemiologic Studies of Cancer in Minority Groups in the Western United States, *Natl. Cancer Inst. Monogr.,* 53, 103, 1979.
9. **Tulinius, H., Day, N., and Muir, C. S.,** Rarity of testis cancer in Negroes, *Lancet,* 1, 35, 1973.
10. **Ross, R. K., McCurtis, J. W., Henderson, B. E., Menck, H. R., Mack, T. M., and Martin, S. P.,** Descriptive epidemiology of testicular and prostate cancer in Los Angeles, *Br. J. Cancer,* 39, 284, 1979.
11. **Henderson, B. E., Benton, B., Jing, J., Yu, M. C., and Pike, M. C.,** Risk factors for cancer of the testis in young men, *Int. J. Cancer,* 23, 598, 1979.

12. **Newell, G. R.,** Etiology of multiple sclerosis and Hodgkin's disease, *Am. J. Epidemiol.,* 2, 119, 1970.
13. **Newell, G. R., Mills, P. K., and Johnson, D. E.,** Epidemiologic comparison of cancer of the testis and Hodgkin's disease among young males, *Cancer,* 54, 1117, 1984.
14. **Evans, A. S. and Comstock, G. W.,** Presence of elevated antibody titers to Epstein-Barr virus before Hodgkin's disease, *Lancet,* 1, 1183, 1981.
15. **Algood, C. B., Newell, G. R., and Johnson, D. E.,** Viral etiology of testicular tumors, *J. Urol.,* 139, 308, 1988.
16. **Newell, G. R., Spitz, M. R., Sider, J. G., and Pollack, E. S.,** Incidence of testicular cancer in the United States related to marital status, histology, and ethnicity, *JNCI,* 78, 881, 1987.
17. **Graham, S., Gibson, R. W., West, D., et al.,** Epidemiology of cancer of the testis in upstate New York, *JNCI,* 58, 1255, 1977.
18. **Mustacchi, P. and Millmore, D.,** Racial and occupational variations in cancer of the testis: San Francisco, 1956—65, *JNCI,* 56, 717, 1976.
19. **Mills, P.K., Newell, G.R., and Johnson, D.E.,** Testicular cancer associated with employment in agriculture and oil and natural gas extraction, *Lancet,* I, 207, 1984.
20. **Mills, P. K. and Newell, G. R.,** Testicular cancer risk in agricultural occupations, *J. Occup. Med.,* 26, 798, 1984.
21. **Morrison, A. S.,** Cryptorchidism, hernia, and cancer of the testis, *JNCI,* 56, 731, 1976.

Chapter 14

HODGKIN'S DISEASE

Bengt Glimelius and Gunilla Enblad

TABLE OF CONTENTS

I. INTRODUCTION

Hodgkin's disease (HD) has, unlike most other neoplastic diseases predominating either in the older age groups, or occasionally in children/adolescents, a bimodal age distribution. A first peak in incidence occurs in early adult life, and a second, sustained increase in incidence occurs from the sixth decade on. In studies where the incidence has been analyzed in patients older than 80 to 85 years, a decreased rate has been noticed among the very old. The characteristic bimodal age distribution which varies between different geographical regions in the world, has suggested that HD is composed of several (at least two) disease entities, one of which occurs in young adults and one, or several, in elderly patients.[1-8]

Although the disease(s) has been recognized for now over 150 years,[9] only recently has the presence of the neoplastic cell(s) been firmly established. The origin of the neoplastic cells, the mononuclear Hodgkin's cell, and the binuclear or multinuclear Reed-Sternberg cell is, however, not yet known.[10] These two cell types display similar, if not identical, markers. The mechanism involving the transformation of Hodgkin's cells to Reed-Sternberg cells is not completely known.[11] Recent evidence suggests that the origin may be heterogenous, further supporting epidemiological and clinical evidence that HD is not one disease. This heterogeneity has been described in histochemical, immunohistochemical, and immunocytochemical studies.[10,12,13] It has also been shown in the eight established HD derived cell lines.[14,15] Whether this heterogeneity is different in different age groups is entirely unknown.

The detection of the Reed-Sternberg cell is mandatory for the diagnosis of HD. In the appropriate pathological environment, these cells, perhaps also including their mononuclear counterpart, are pathognomonic of HD.[16-18] Whereas neoplastic cells of other malignancies are abundantly present in involved tissues, the neoplastic cells in HD usually form only a small minority (less than 1 to 2%) of the cells in the tissues involved with HD.

There is a marked difference in prognosis between younger and older patients. This difference has invariably been ascribed to a number of factors.[19-22] This review first describes the epidemiological evidences for the "two-disease hypothesis", and then focuses on the relation between age and prognosis.

II. DESCRIPTIVE EPIDEMIOLOGY

HD is a relatively rare disease. Although the incidence varies between countries, the overall annual age-specific incidence is in the order of 2 to 3/100,000 with generally higher rates among males.

The bimodal age-specific incidence curve is present in virtually all countries (Figure 1). According to Correa and O'Connor,[2] three distinct epidemiologic patterns related to the economic stratification of different communities can be identified. In well-developed regions, as in most areas in the U.S. and in urban areas of other developed countries, HD is rare in children but has high rates among young adults (type III). This contrasts with the "type I pattern" in developing countries, where no early young adulthood peak is seen but a higher incidence in children. An intermediate form (type II) with moderate rates both in childhood and in young adulthood is seen in the rural areas of developed countries and in central Europe. These patterns have been repeatedly seen in several studies.[1,3,5,6,23-25] In contrast to previous studies, a possible correlation between childhood (5 to 14 years) and young adult HD was, however, seen in a Surveillance, Epidemiology, and End Results (SEER) program of the National Cancer Institute.[7]

There is a clear male predominance in children and in elderly patients, whereas in young adults, females are equally common. Nodular sclerosis (NS) histology is the most common subtype among young adults, whereas mixed cellularity (MC) and lymphocytic depletion (LD) are more common in the other ages.[2,3,6,7,23]

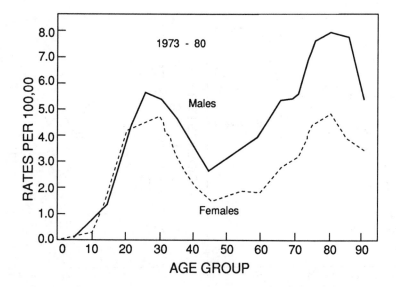

FIGURE 1. Bimodal age distribution of HD. Rates indicate average annual age-specific incidence rates for all SEER regions, by sex, 1973 to 1980.[6] (Reprinted with permission from Dr. Glaser and Pergamon Press.)

III. POSSIBLE ETIOLOGIC FACTORS

In 1966, MacMahon[1] presented a hypothesis to explain the shape of the age-specific incidence curves of HD. According to this theory, HD is composed of three different diseases with different etiology: (1) disease of children, (2) disease of young adulthood, (3) disease of elderly. This idea is mainly supported by the bimodality of the age-specific incidence and mortality curves, by the different sex ratios in different ages, and by differences in the shape of the incidence curves in different countries. Although the different epidemiologic entities do not strictly correspond to the histologic types of the Rye classification,[26] NS represents the young adult disease. MacMahon[1] further proposed that the disease in the first age peak (15 to 34 years) in developed countries is infectious in nature while that seen in the second one (>50 years) results from causes similar to those of other lymphomas.

In contrast, Correa and O'Connor[2] were of the opinion that the different epidemiologic, histologic, and prognostic features of HD were best understood as manifestations of different host responses in different environments. Their idea is mainly supported by the relationship of the prognostically different histologic subtypes to the economic level of the population and the changes of age-specific mortality rates from pattern I to pattern III in the U.S. which may be related to increasing urbanization and economic growth.

The epidemiological patterns have suggested that the pathogenesis of HD involves an infectious agent as has been considered ever since the disease was first described by Thomas Hodgkin in 1832.[9] Several authors have suggested that HD may be an unusual event after a common infection.[8,27,28] An infectious agent has, however, not been identified.

As first suggested by Newell in 1970,[29] the geographic variation among younger persons in relation to socioeconomic conditions is similar to the epidemiology of paralytic polio in the prevaccine era. The epidemiologic features of HD among young adults have also been reminiscent of that of infectious mononucleosis.[30] The association between HD and EBV has been extensively studied.[8] In several studies, there is a consistent finding of an increased diagnosis of HD among persons who have been diagnosed with mononucleosis. Several studies have also shown elevated titers of antibodies against major determinants of the EBV.

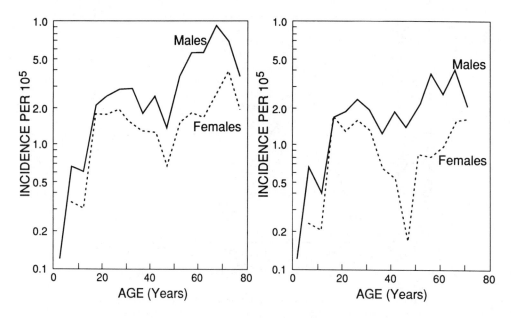

FIGURE 2.   Annual age-specific incidence rates of HD in Finland, 1961 to 1964 before (left) and after re-examination of the histological slides.[3] Note the decrease particularly among elderly patients. (Reprinted with permission from Dr. Franssila and Lippincott/Harper & Row.)

Altered EBV antibodies have been noted in all age groups.[31] In contrast, other risk factors such as small family size, early birth order, high maternal education, and tonsillectomy noted in different studies have only been noticed in young adulthood or in middle-aged persons.[5] None of the many correlations between different exposures or social class and HD in younger persons have yet solved the etiology of HD. All findings do, however, suggest that the pathogenesis of HD among elderly is independent of that among younger persons.

IV. PROPORTION OF ELDERLY PATIENTS

A large proportion of patients with HD belongs to the "elderly" age group. It varies, however, considerably between different hospital based series and between different more or less population-based series. This proportion, however, also varies depending upon whether the histopathological diagnosis is made by experienced hematopathologists only or made by routine. The latter is usually the case in register-based studies.

The proportion of erroneous histologic diagnosis in HD is higher than in almost any other malignant disease, varying from 15 up to 60% in different series.[3,23,25,32,33] The overdiagnosis of HD is mainly due to inclusion of non-Hodgkin's lymphomas (NHL). Since NHL is more common in the elderly, the proportion of erroneous cases is higher in the elderly. Thus, the proportion of elderly patients is lower after histopathological reclassification than before (Figure 2).

Data from reclassified register-based series indicate that between 35 to 50% of the patients are 50 years or older and between 15 to 25% are older than 60 years.[2,3,7,23] The median age in these series varies between 35 to 50 years. These figures contrast to the usually much lower ones in hospital-based series or series from many cooperative groups. In this aspect, the Stanford series of totally 1169 patients constitutes an extreme with only 10% of the patients over 50 years and 4% over 60 years of age, with a median age of 26 years (Figure 3).[34] In most American and European clinical series, the proportion of patients over 50 ranges between 10 to 25%, and over 60 between 5 to 10%, with median ages of about 30 years.[35-38] An exceptional series is the Danish

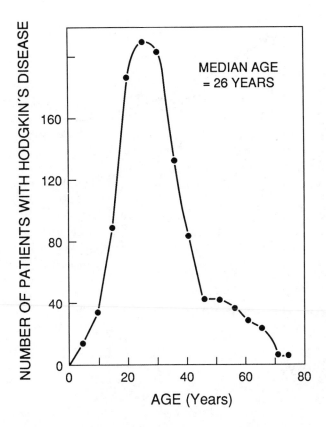

FIGURE 3. Histogram of age at presentation of patients with HD at Stanford University.[34] Note the difference in age distribution in this hospital-based series compared to the population-based series shown in Figure 1. (Reproduced with permission from Dr. Rosenburg and *Ann. Intern. Med.*)

LYGRA-project. In their 10 year material of 809 patients, 35% were over 50 and 22% over 60 years of age.[4] Two Swedish hospital-based, reclassified series also have high numbers of elderly patients (43 and 50%, respectively, over 50 years of age).[19,33]

The differences in the proportion of elderly patients must reflect referral bias to specialized centers. In several clinical trials, an upper age limit is present. Even if no upper age limit is defined, elderly patients are not always referred. Fears of excessive toxicity have often led to reluctance of physicians to recommend intensive staging and treatment. Also, the possible outcome in relation to toxicity of treatment has not been considered justified.[39] Due to the organization of the medical systems, the referral bias is probably lower in Scandinavian countries than (particularly) in the U.S. This referral bias, with an often strong selection of the patients, also complicates the judgment of the outcome of treatment in elderly patients.

V. AGE IS AN IMPORTANT PROGNOSTIC FACTOR

Most studies in HD have identified age as an important prognostic factor.[4,19-21,37,38,40]

In large cooperative series, the decline in prognosis usually starts at about the age of 40 or slightly above. In the Danish LYGRA-project, probably being one of the least selected, but large series, survival was reduced already in the age group between 40 to 49 years compared to survival in younger patients.[4] In the large survey of 6314 patients with HD reported to the Cancer Commission of the American College of Surgeons, the projected 10 year survival rate for ages

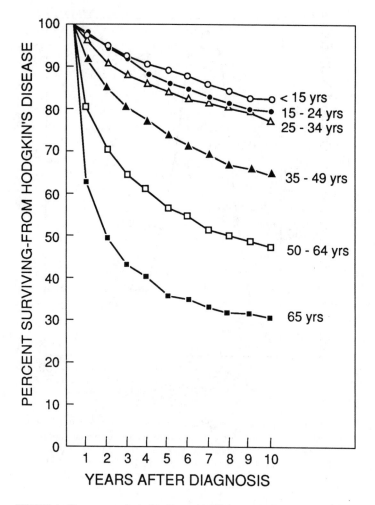

FIGURE 4.   Ten-year survival of patients with HD by age at diagnosis, specific to HD.[41] (Reprinted with permission from Dr. Kennedy and Lippincott/Harper & Row.)

up to 34 years was between 80 to 85% compared to below 70% for those between 35 to 49 years (Figure 4).[40] Survival for the older age groups became progressively worse. Similar findings were also noted in the British National Lymphoma Investigation (BNLI) study.[37] In that study encompassing 1500 patients, the decline in prognosis was, however, not detectable until after 50 years of age.

In all studies with sufficient numbers of patients, age has been (one of) the most important prognostic factor(s) as noticed in univariate and multivariate analyses.[19-21,37,38] An age of 40 or 50 years has often been used as a cut-off point when age was dichotomized. This importance of age has been present whether all stages have been included in the analysis, or only subsets of stages. In the BNLI study, age maintained its prognostic importance in both sexes, all histologies, all stages, A and B symptoms, and in all treatment response categories. When developing a prognostic index to be used in treatment selection of patients with early stages, age was included together with mediastinal involvement and pathological grade.[20]

VI. TREATMENT OUTCOME IN ELDERLY PATIENTS

Very few studies have analyzed treatment outcome in elderly patients with HD. Most studies were small, retrospective, and not specifically designed to address the problems of the elderly.

Lokich et al.[42] reviewed the case records of 47 patients with HD representing essentially all elderly patients seen at two institutions in Boston between 1960 to 1972. Radical radiotherapy and combination chemotherapy were used in less than one third (15/47) of the patients. Actuarial survival in all stages together was below 20% at 42 months. This figure was low compared to a matched group of young patients.

In two phase III trials of the Cancer and Leukemia Group B (CALG B), 385 patients with advanced stage received different combination chemotherapy regimens.[40] There was no upper age limited. Standardized dose adjustments were prescribed for myelosuppression, irrespective of age. The 73 (19%) patients over 60 years of age had significantly lower complete remission rate, shorter median time to progression, and duration of survival than younger patients. The median survival time in the patients over 60 yers of age was 18 months. The poor outcome in elderly patients was true even if the analysis was restricted to those 11 patients who received >90% of the projected amount of nitrosurea or mechlorethamine during the first three treatment cycles. An unstated number of patients failed to complete three treatment cycles.

Eghbali et al.[43] reviewed the total experience of 30 patients over 70 years of age with HD seen in Bordeaux Cancer Center over a 20 year period (1962 to 1981). The material formed 7% of all primary HD cases. Treatment varied considerably. Overall survival was below 20% at 5 years and below 10% at 10 years. Although most patients died from HD, a considerable proportion died of other causes. The disease-free survival curve plateaued after 2 years, indicating that one third of the patients could be considered cured.

The experience of 52 patients aged 60 to 75 years representing 4% of totally 1169 patients seen at Stanford University between 1968 and 1980 was reviewed by Austin-Seymour et al.[34] These patients, having a median age of 64 years, were in the majority of cases intensively, and adequately staged and treated according to the same intensive program as younger patients. The survival for this group of patients was unfavorable (25% alive after 10 years) compared to younger ages at the same institution (17 to 49 years, 75%; 50 to 59 years, about 40%), but favorable compared to virtually all other series of elderly patients. Adequately staged and treated elderly patients had a 86% 5 year survival rate compared to only 35% for the remaining patients.

Comparably favorable results were recently reported by an Italian group.[44] In a group of 61 patients aged over 60 years (mean age 68 years) constituting 16% of 387 patients seen between 1969 and 1986, the 5 year survival rate was 55%. In younger patients, it was 76%. Staging was considered inadequate in only three patients. Almost every other patient had clinical stage II. Virtually all patients received chemotherapy, mostly intensive combination therapy.

In a series of 182 patients diagnosed between 1973 and 1978 and seen at two hospitals in Stockholm, the mean age was 47 years and 78 (43%) patients were 50 years of age or older.[19] Although these figures indicate that the extent of patient selection is less than in the series described above, it is still substantial in that during the same time period 18 (19%) elderly patients with HD (in the original publication, 57 patients, but the majority of those did not have HD after reexamination of the pathological slides)[60] reported to the Regional Cancer Registry were not referred. The 5 year survival for patients over 50 years was only 28% compared to 74% in the remainder. This difference was still considerable after correction for background mortality. The prognosis in the elderly age group was unrelated to factors like stage and systemic symptoms, being of prognostic importance in the young. Staging in the Stockholm series was not as intense as, e.g., in the Stanford series. However, differences in patient selection, rather than differences in staging intensity, as concluded by Austin-Seymour et al.,[34] may explain the marked difference in 5 year survival rates.

VII. WHY DO ELDERLY PATIENTS HAVE POOR SURVIVAL?

The poor survival in elderly patients has been invariably attributed to an association of high age with advanced stage and aggressive histologic subtypes, i.e., another disease;[40,42] to differences in therapy or therapeutic response in the elderly;[37,40,42] to difficulties to tolerate the intensive treatment due to high age as such or to the frequency of other diseases in the elderly;[34,40] to a decreased capacity of (immunological?) host response;[19] or to a failure of investigators to correct their data for intercurrent deaths.[17] The last reason is not a major explanation, since several authors have convincingly shown that the survival difference is still substantial after correction for intercurrent deaths or background mortality.[19,37]

A. ANOTHER DISEASE

Besides the epidemiological evidences that HD in the elderly is (an)other disease(s) than the one(s) in younger individuals, as discussed above, there are a number of clinico-pathological differences. Several authors have shown that stage is more advanced in the elderly, that B-symptoms, primary abdominal presentation, and MC- and LD-histologies are more common among the elderly.[19,37,42,45] All these factors are associated with poor prognosis. A couple of findings indicate, however, that the accumulation of "adverse prognostic factors" is not the (main) reason for the poor prognosis. First, Wedelin et al.[19] could not detect any prognostic importance of these parameters in the elderly patients, only in the young ones. Second, in the large BNLI study,[20,37] the difference in prognosis was present in all stages, all histologies, and whether the patients had A- or B-symptoms.

B. DECREASED TOLERANCE TO THERAPY

There are several physiological and pharmacological reasons for decreased tolerance to both intensive radiotherapy and chemotherapy in elderly patients, as recently discussed.[46-48]

The tolerance to extended-field radiotherapy like mantle therapy is diminished in elderly. Age is claimed to be a risk factor for anthracycline cardiotoxicity,[50] for bleomycin-induced pulmonary fibrosis,[51] and for neurotoxicity by vinca alkaloids.[40] Probably more important is the increased cytostatic drug-induced myelotoxicity. In the CALG B study described above,[40] hematological toxicity increased in frequency and severity with age. It was described to be severe or life threatening in 33% of those over 60 years of age compared to only 14% for those less than 40 years of age and 24% for those between 40 and 59 years. The increased hematological toxicity was also reflected in the extent of dose reductions of myelotoxic agents being significantly higher in patients over 60 years of age.

C. IMMUNOLOGIC DEFECT IN HD

The existence of an immunologic defect in patients with HD has been shown by both clinical and laboratory findings. In HD, the impaired immune function is inherent and not a complication of advanced disease, as in many other advanced tumors.[17,52-54] Evidence indicates that the immune deficiency in HD is a preexisting phenomenon. Some of the immune alterations may persist in long-term survivors with HD and some have also been noted in relatives of HD patients.[17,55] Elderly patients usually have a more pronounced immune defect than younger persons. Aging as such is, however, also associated with a progressive T-cell defect which in turn is connected with a short survival.[56,57] Much of the immune deficiency in HD can be associated with defects in T-cell responses, although altered functions are also numerous in the B-cell system and in monocytic cells.[53] The complexity of the immune system with numerous interactions between different immunologic cells makes such a distinction inappropriate.

The extent of the immune deficiency is closely connected to survival in most HD series.[57,58] Whether the poorer survival in elderly HD patients can, at least in part, be ascribed to the usually more marked immunologic defects in these age groups is not known. They may, e.g., result in an increased susceptibility to bacterial, viral, and disseminated fungal infections which may be more serious in an elderly patient under treatment than in a young one. The increased risk of second malignancies in long-term survivors of treated patients may also be ascribed to immune alterations. It has been noted that the risk of developing a secondary acute nonlymphocytic leukemia is higher in middle-aged patients than in younger ones.[59]

VIII. CONCLUSIONS

1. The bimodal age-distribution in HD indicates that HD is composed of at least two separate disorders. Descriptive and analytical epidemiological data further indicate that the pathogenesis of elderly patients is different from the one in younger patients. The limited understanding of the etiology in older persons has made it difficult to identify relevant exposures.

2. A considerable number of patients with HD belongs to the older age group. This proportion is higher than what can be read in most clinical patient materials due to referral bias but lower than seen in cancer registries due to a number of erroneous diagnoses. With increasing age of the population, the proportion will further increase.

3. Age is probably the most important prognostic factor in HD. Because of patient selection due to a more or less hidden referral bias in virtually all patient series, it is difficult to draw any general conclusions of treatment outcome in elderly patients. In those series being "least selected", overall survival for elderly patients is still very poor. Data from certain series do, however, suggest that there is a group (how large?) of elderly patients with HD (in good general physical and mental health?) who are able to accept and tolerate the same intensive staging and treatment as young patients and who has a favorable outcome.

4. The reasons for the poor outcome in elderly patients are probably many, such as another disease(s), accumulation of poor prognostic factors, lower tolerance to treatment, and depressed immunologic response. Large unselected, homogenously staged, and treated patient series must be analyzed before the importance of each of these and other parameters can be better understood. Not until then will specially devised treatment protocols have the chance of truly improving prognosis among elderly patients.

REFERENCES

1. **MacMahon, B.,** Epidemiology of Hodgkin's disease, *Cancer Res.,* 26, 1189, 1966.
2. **Correra, P. and O'Connor, G. T.,** Epidemiologic patterns of Hodgkin's disease, *Int. J. Cancer,* 8, 192, 1971.
3. **Franssila, K. O., Heiskala, M. K., and Heiskala, H. J.,** Epidemiology and histopathology of Hodgkin's disease in Finland, *Cancer,* 39, 1280, 1977.
4. **Nordentoft, A. M., Pedersen-Bjergaard, J., Brincker, H., Andersen, E., Pedersen, M., Boye Nielsen, J., Björn Jensen, K., Nissen, N. I., Skov Jensen, T., Vidbaek, Aa., Krogh Jensen, M., and Walbom-Jörgensen, S.,** Hodgkins disease in Denmark. A national clinical study by the Danish Hodgkin study group, LYGRA, *Scand. J. Haematol.,* 24, 321, 1980.
5. **Guthenson, N. M.,** Social class and age at the diagnosis of Hodgkin's disease: new epidemiologic evidence for the "two-disease-hypothesis", *Cancer Treat. Rep.,* 66, 689, 1982.
6. **Glaser, S. L.,** Recent incidence and secular trends in Hodgkin's disease and its histologic subtypes, *J. Chron. Dis.,* 39, 789, 1986.
7. **Glaser, S. L.,** Regional variation in Hodgkin's disease incidence by histologic subtype in the US, *Cancer,* 60, 2841, 1987.
8. **Mueller, N.,** Epidemiologic studies assessing the role of the Epstein-Barr virus in Hodgkin's disease, *Yale J. Biol. Med.,* 60, 321, 1987.
9. **Hodgkin, T.,** On some morbid appearances of the absorbent glands and spleen, *Med. Chir. Trans.,* 17, 68, 1832.
10. **Poppema, S., Brinker, M. G. L., and Visser, L.,** Evidence of a B-cell origin of the proliferating cells, in *Hodgkin's Disease in Children,* Kamps, W. A., Humphrey, G. B., and Poppema, S., Eds., Kluwer Academic Publishers, Boston, 1989, 5.
11. **Hsu, S.-M., Chakraborty, Y.-F. L., Wang-Peng, J., Lok, M. S., and Fukuhara, S.,** Reed-Sternberg cells in Hodgkin's cell lines HDLM, L-428, and KM-H2 are not actively replicating: lack of bromodeoxyuridine uptake by multinuclear cells in culture, *Blood,* 71, 1382, 1988.

12. **Stein, H.,** Useful markers for the definition of Hodgkin and Sternberg-Reed cells in Hodgkin's disease, in *Tumour Markers in Clinical Practice: Concepts and Applications,* Paar, A. S., Ed., Blackwell Scientific, Oxford, U.K., 1987, 228.

13. **Raghavachar, A., Binder, T., and Bartram, C. R.,** Immunoglobulin and T-cell receptor rearrangements in Hodgkin's disease, *Cancer Res.,* 48, 3591, 1988.

14. **Drexler, H. G., Amlot, P. L., and Miniwada, J.,** Hodgkin's disease-derived cell lines- Conflicting clues for the origin of Hodgkin's disease?, *Leukemia,* 1, 629, 1987.

15. **Burrichter, H., Schaadt, M., and Diehl, V.,** Conclusions from Hodgkin-derived cell lines, in *Hodgkin's Disease in Children,* Kamps, W. A., Humphrey, G. B., and Poppema, S., Eds., Kluwer Academic Publishers, Boston, 1989, 29.

16. **Carbone, P. P., Kaplan, H. S., Musshof, K., Smithers, D. W., and Tubiana, M.,** Report on the committee on Hodgkin's disease staging classification, *Cancer Res.,* 31, 1860, 1971.

17. **Kaplan, H. S.,** Hodgkin's disease: unfolding concepts concerning its nature, management and prognosis, *Cancer,* 45, 2439, 1980.

18. **Dorfman, R. F. and Colby, T. V.,** The pathologist's role in management of patients with Hodgkin's disease, *Cancer Treat. Rep.,* 66, 675, 1982.

19. **Wedelin, C., Björkholm, M., Biberfeld, P., Holm, G., Johansson, B., and Mellstedt, H.,** Prognostic factors in Hodgkin's disease with special reference to age, *Cancer,* 53, 1202, 1984.

20. **Haybittle, J. L., Easterling, M. J., Bennet, M. H., Vaughan Hudson, B., Hayhoe, F. G., Jelliffe, A. M., Vaughan Hudson, G., and MacLean, K. A.,** Review of British national lymphoma investigation studies of Hodgkin's disease and development of prognostic index, *Lancet,* 967, 1985.

21. **Tubiana, M., Henry-Amar, M., van der Werf-Messing, B., Henry, J., Abbatucci, J., Burgers, M., Hayat, M., Somers, R., Laugier, A., and Carde, P.,** A multivariate analysis of prognostic factors in early stage Hodgkin's disease, *Int. J. Radiat. Oncol. Biol. Phys.,* 11, 23, 1985.

22. **Loeffler, M., Pfreundschuh, M., Hasenclever, D., Hiller, E., Gerhartz, H., Wilmanns, W., Rohloff, R., Rühl, U., Kühn, G., Fuchs, R., Kirchner, H., Teichmann, J., Schoppe, W., Petsch, S., Wilhelmy, W., Worst, P., Pflüger, K. H., Hecht, T., Bartels, H., Gassman, W., Krüger, G., Schmitz, G., Oertel, W., and Diehl, V.,** Prognostic risk factors in advanced Hodgkin's lymphoma, *Blut,* 56, 273, 1988.

23. **Silverman, D. T., Correra, P., O'Connor, G., Myers, M. H., Axtell, L. M., and Bragg, K. U.,** A comparison of Hodgkin's disease in Alameda county, California, and Connecticut, *Cancer,* 39, 1758, 1977.

24. **Gimbrere, K., Mc Kay, F. W., and Li, F. P.,** Geographic patterns of Hodgkin's disease in the United States, *JAMA,* 254, 1033, 1985.

25. **Agnarsson, B. A., Olafsdottir, K., and Benediktsson, H.,** Tumours in Iceland, *Acta Pathol. Microbiol. Immunol. Scand.,* Sect. A 95, 23, 1987.

26. **Lukes, R. J., Craver, L. F., Hall, T. C., Rappaport, H., and Rubin, P.,** Report of the nomenclature committee, *Cancer Res.,* 26, 1311, 1966.

27. **Evans, A. S.,** The spectrum of infections with Epstein-Barr virus: a hypothesis, *J. Infect. Dis.,* 124, 330, 1971.

28. **Guthenson, N. and Cole, P.,** Epidemiology of Hodgkin's disease in the young, *Int. J. Cancer,* 19, 595, 1977.

29. **Newell, G., Cole, S., Miettinen, O., and MacMahon, B.,** Age differences in the histology of Hodgkin's disease. *J. Natl. Cancer Inst.,* 45, 311, 1970.

30. **Hallee, T. J., Evans, A. S., Niederman, J. C., Brooks, C. M., and Voegtly, J. H.,** Infectious mononucleosis at the United States military academy. A prospective study of a single class over four years, *Yale J. Biol. Med.,* 47, 182, 1974.

31. **Evans, A. S. and Guthensson, N. M.,** A population-based control study of EBV and other viral antibodies among persons with Hodgkin's disease and their siblings, *Int. J. Cancer,* 34, 149, 1984.

32. **Symmers, W. S.,** Survey of the eventual diagnosis in 600 cases referred for a second histological opinion after an initial biopsy diagnosis of Hodgkin's disease, *J. Clin. Pathol.,* 21, 650, 1968.

33. **Norberg, B., Dige, U., Johansson, H., Roos, G., and Lenner, P.,** Hodgkin's disease in northern Sweden 1971—1981 - a retrospective study with morphological review, Meeting Abstract ECCO, 3, 1985, 189.

34. **Austin-Seymor, M. M., Hoppe, R. T., Cox, R. S., Rosenberg, S. A., and Kaplan, H. S.,** Hodgkin's disease in patients over sixty years old, *Ann. Intern. Med.,* 100, 13, 1984.

35. **Bonadonna, G.,** Chemotherapy strategies to improve the control of Hodgkin's disease. The Richard and Hinda Rosenthal foundation award lecture, *Cancer Res.,* 42, 4309, 1982.

36. **Young, C. W., Straus, D. J., Myers, J., Passe, S., Nisce, L. Z., Lee, B. J., Koziner, B., Arlin, Z., Kempin, S., Gee, T., and Clarkson, B. D.,** Multidisciplinary treatment of advanced Hodgkin's disease by an alternating chemotherapeutic regimen of MOPP/ABVD and low-dose radiation therapy restricted to originally bulky disease, *Cancer Treat. Rep.,* 66, 907, 1982.

37. **Vaughan Hudson, B., Mac Lennan, K. A., Easterling, M. J., Jelliffe, A. M., Haybittle, J. L., and Vaughan Hudson, G.,** The prognostic significance of age in Hodgkin's disease. Examination of 1500 patients (BNLI Report No. 23), *Clin. Rad.,* 34, 503, 1983.

38. **Horwich, A., Easton, D., Nogueira-Costa, R., Liew, K. H., Colman, M., and Peckham, M. J.,** An analysis of prognostic factors in early stage Hodgkin's disease, *Rad. Oncol.,* 7, 95, 1986.

39. **Carbone, P. P., Begg, C., and Moorman, J.,** Cancer in the elderly: clinical and biological considerations, in *Inter-Relationships Among Aging, Cancer and Differentiation,* Pullman, B., et al., Eds., Dordrecht, Reidel, 1985, 313.

40. **Peterson, B. A., Pajak, T. F., Cooper, M. R., Nissen, N. I., Glidewell, O. J., Holland, J. F., Bloomfield, C. D., and Gottlieb, A. J.,** Effect of age on therapeutic response and survival in advanced Hodgkin's disease, *Cancer Treat. Rep.,* 66, 889, 1982.

41. **Kennedy, B. J., Loeb, V., Peterson, V. M., Donegan, W. L., Natarajan, N., and Mettlin, C.,** National survey of patterns of care for Hodgkin's disease, *Cancer,* 56, 2547, 1985.

42. **Lokich, J. J., Pinkus, G. S., and Moloney, W. C.,** Hodgkin's disease in the elderly, *Oncology,* 29, 484, 1974.

43. **Eghbali, H., Hoerni-Simon, G., deMascarel, I., Durand, M., Chauvergne, J., and Hoerni, B.,** Hodgkin's disease in the elderly, *Cancer,* 53, 2191, 1984.

44. **Ferrini, P. R., Bosi, A., Casini, C., Messori, A., and Bellesi, G.,** Hodgkin's disease in the elderly: a retrospective clinicopathologic study of 61 patients aged over 60 years, *Acta Haemat.,* 78(Suppl. 1), 163, 1986.

45. **Frederick, P., Lokich, J., Costanza, M., Moloney, W. C., and Hellman, S.,** Hodgkin's disease in the elderly, *Lancet,* 774, 1973.

46. **Dodion, P.,** Chemotherapy in the elderly, *Eur. J. Cancer Clin. Oncol.,* 23, 1833, 1987.

47. **Kennedy, B. J.,** Aging and cancer, *J. Clin. Oncol.,* 6, 1903, 1988.

48. **Joseph, R. R.,** Aggressive management of cancer in the elderly, *Clin. Geriatr. Med.,* 4, 749, 1988.

49. **Gunn, W. G.,** Radiation therapy for the aging patient, *Cancer,* 30, 337, 1980.

50. **Bristow, M. R., Mason, J. W., Billingham, M. E., and Daniels, J. R.,** Doxorubicin cardiomyopathy: evaluation by phonocardiography, endomyocardial biopsy and cardiac catheterisation, *Ann. Intern. Med.,* 88, 168, 1978.

51. **Blum, R. H., Carter, S. K., and Agre, K.,** A clinical review of bleomycin — a new antineoplastic agent, *Cancer,* 31, 903, 1973.

52. **Matchett, K. M., Huang, A. T., and Kremer, W. B.,** Impaired lymphocyte transformation in Hodgkin's disease. Evidence for depletion of circulating T-lymphocytes, *J. Clin. Invest.,* 52, 1908, 1973.

53. **Björkholm, M., Wedelin, C., Holm, G., and Essy-Ehsing, B.,** Familial longevity and prognosis in Hodgkin's disease, *Cancer,* 54, 1088, 1984.

54. **Romagnini, S., Maggi, E., and Parronichi, P.,** The immune derangement and strategies for immunotherapy, in *Hodgkins Disease in Children,* Kamps, W. A., Humphrey, G. B., and Poppema, S., Eds., Kluwer Academic Publishers, Boston, 1989, 53.

55. **Björkholm, M., Holm, G., and Mellstedt, H.,** Immunological family studies in Hodgkin's disease: is the deficiency horizontally transmitted?, *Scand. J. Haematol.,* 20, 297, 1978.

56. **Greenberg, L. J.,** Aging and immune functions in man: influence of sex and genetic background, *Aging and Immunity,* Singhal, S. K., Sinclair, N. R., Stiller, C. R., Eds., Elsevier/North-Holland, New York, 1979, 43.

57. **Wedelin, C., Björkholm, M., Holm, G., Ogenstad, S., Johansson, B., and Mellstedt, H.,** Lymphocyte function in untreated Hodgkin's disease: an important predictor of prognosis, *Br. J. Cancer,* 45, 70, 1982.

58. **van Rijswijk, R. E. N., deMeijer, A. J., Sybesma, B., and Kater, L.,** Five-year survival in Hodgkin's disease, *Cancer,* 57, 1489, 1986.

59. **Coleman, C. N.,** Secondary malignancy after treatment of Hodgkin's disease: an evolving picture, *J. Clin. Oncol.,* 4, 821, 1986.

60. **Björkholm, M.,** personal communication.

Chapter 15

RELATIONSHIP OF AGE TO CANCER OF THE CERVIX

John A. Carmichael

TABLE OF CONTENTS

The association of age and aging to carcinoma of the cervix has commanded considerable attention in the gynecological literature over the past 1 to 2 decades. The sexual revolution of the mid-1960s and our understanding of the epidemiology of carcinoma of the cervix have resulted in numerous reports claiming to identify a relative increase of cervical cancer in the younger age group, and that this particular age group is demonstrating a cervical cancer more aggressive in its natural history, less responsive to traditional treatment methods, and less susceptible to preventive cervical screening programs than the traditional cervical cancer seen in the older patient.[1-4]

This chapter reviews the impact of age on cervical cancer as it relates to etiology and epidemiology, screening susceptibility, tumor virulence, treatment response, and survival rates.

I. ETIOLOGY

Of the many etiological variables studied, only two, age of onset of coitus[5,6] and multiple partners, are consistently related to squamous carcinoma of the cervix.[7] Evidence has been offered to suggest the importance of one variable over the other, however, it is generally accepted that both have an important etiological role. This observation implies a greater vulnerability in the young to whatever is the ultimate cause of carcinoma of the cervix.

A possible explanation for this early vulnerability is the observaion made by Colposen et al. of the natural history of squamous metaplasia of the cervix. He describes three "dynamic phases" when the metaplastic activity is most active:[8]

1.   During fetal life
2.   Early adolescence
3.   The middle trimester of the first pregnancy

During these periods there is rapid replacement of columnar epithelium by immature squamous epithelium within the transformation zone. It is suggested that some or all of the immature metaplastic cells develop a "neoplastic potential" or suspectibility to the many carcinogenic agents currently being suspected in the etiology of cancer of the cervix. This observation may be offered to explain the first independent variable, i.e., early onset of sexual activity.

The second independent variable, multiple partners, obviously increases the likelihood of exposure of the cervix to whatever is necessary to induce a malignant change.

A number of studies have attempted to identify a "high risk" male[9] whose sperm may have an enhanced carcinogenic effect. These males have more than one sexual partner who develops carcinoma of the cervix.

Many infectious agents have been identified as the possible agent(s), syphilis, Chlamydia, trichomonas, Herpes Simplex Virus I and II,[1,10,11] and more recent human papillomavirus (HPV).[12]

Regardless of the cofactor(s), sperm DNA or infection, cancer of the cervix can be labeled, in the broadest sense of the term, a venereal disease. The more partners, the more likelihood of exposure to that particular etiological agent or cofactor. These agents or cofactors are most effective in the younger age group.

HPV infection appears to be almost indigenous to the female genital tract in some societies. Some have placed the incidence as high as 30%.[13] Clinically apparent HPV infection is most common, but not exclusive, to the younger coitally active female, suggesting a possible spontaneous cure over time.[14] Recent evidence suggests that HPV is "necessary but not sufficient" for the development of lower genital tract cancer.[15] There are apparent determinants as to who in this large population will develop preinvasive and invasive cancer of the cervix: (1) age at time of infection, (2) viral virulence (subtype), and possibly (3) duration of exposure to the viral infection.

Whatever the ultimate etiologic sequence or sequences prove to be, and all current concepts fit satisfactorily into the etiological observation, early onset of sexual activity, multiple partners, the implication is very clear that the cervix of the younger woman is more susceptible to the development of squamous carcinoma than that of the older woman.

II. SCREENING

There have been a number of poorly documented observations given to suggest that precancerous changes in the younger age group may be less susceptible to the cervical screening program, that there is some difference in the cell character premalignant and malignant. The cytological review of a small number of patients developing invasive cancer under 35 years of age as compared to the older sisters fails to support this observation. This study showed the same number of false positives in both age groups, and the same histologic patterns.[16]

The fact that a woman develops an invasive cancer of the cervix at an early age implies a reasonably rapid progression through the dysplasias, carcinoma *in situ* (CIS) to invasive cancer. Preinvasive disease does not appear to be more rapidly progressive in younger women[17] and therefore should not imply a different disease pattern but simply a biological variance to be experienced at any age.

If we understand correctly the changing sexual patterns of the early sixties which resulted in more frequent onset of early coitus and higher incidence of multiple partners, and if our etiological understanding is correct, then it could be assumed that we should see an endemic of carcinoma of the cervix in subsequent decades. In Canada this has not happened. While the universal decrease in the incidence of invasive cancer in all provinces has tended to level off and in two of the western provinces there was a transient but slight increase in incidence of carcinoma of the cervix in the under 35 age group, there has been little change in the incidence of carcinoma of the cervix in the past 20 years.[1,16] Recent figures from the Province of Ontario confirm the slight but persistent decrease in incidence of carcinoma of the cervix in all ages.[18] Although accurate incidence figures for preinvasive cancer are difficult to obtain and must be held somewhat suspect, there has been an apparent dramatic increase in the incidence of CIS since the mid-1960s.[1]

In Canada, by the early 1960s there were well-established screening programs in most provinces.[19] The fact that this endemic of preinvasive change was identified and effectively treated is offered to explain the level rate of invasive squamous cancer of the cervix in the past 2 decades.[1] It also strengthens the argument that preinvasive cancer of the cervix in the younger age group can be effectively identified by cervical screening programs.

III. CLINICAL PATTERNS OF DISEASE

A. STAGING

One of the recognized effects of a cervical screening program is a decrease in the mortality rate from cervical cancer, the result of the increased diagnosis of invasive disease in its earlier stages.[20] Voluntary screening programs are more regularly attended by younger women.[16,20,21] The decreased staging therefore in the younger aged population must be considered a factor of increased screening rather than any particular biological pattern of disease in the younger age group. This observation must also be taken into consideration when comparing treatment results and survival of the younger vs. the older patient.

B. CELL TYPE

Cell type and degree of differentiation are considered by some to be related to prognosis. Poorly differentiated, small cell, and possibly adenocarcinoma having a less favorable outcome.[22] In a small number of series addressing this question, there was no difference in the distribution of cell type or degree of differentiation between young and old.[16,23,24]

C. SIZE OF LESION AND POSITIVE LYMPH NODES

Size of primary tumor affects both the incidence of positive nodes and survival.[25,26] It has been stated[27] that younger patients have a higher incidence of positive nodes, stage for stage. A study of 10,002 cases of invasive cervical cancer from 1957 to 1981 failed to show an increase in either large lesions or positive nodes in the young age group during the period of review.[24] This discourages the concept that a more virulent and more rapidly progressive tumor type has developed in the younger age group.

IV. TREATMENT RESPONSE

The literature is divided regarding treatment response and the prognosis for young patients with carcinoma of the cervix.[3,4,28-30] Stuart[30] concluded from his review of the literature that young age implied a poorer prognosis and poorer response to treatment, surgery, radiation, or both. Stanhope et al.,[31] in a review of a large series reported a significant decrease in survival in the under thirty five year-old group, particularly Stage IIB. LeVecchia[27] went as far as to say that a young woman with recurrent carcinoma of the cervix could not be salvaged. Meanwell,[24] in a more contemporary and larger statistical study, concluded that age by itself had no impact on survival and should not influence treatment policies. Others, including our own experience,[16] have failed to show a difference in time to, or site of recurrences, or survival. Lybeert et al.[32] have claimed the failure to identify a difference in survival is the size of the reported series, and the lack of very young patients. In their experience a significant difference was demonstrated when the 28 year old and younger age group were compared.

Most series reviewing treatment of younger patients indicate a preference for primary surgery (radical hysterectomy and pelvic node dissection) with or without postoperative pelvic irradiation. There are no reported prospective trials comparing treatment modalities. However, what comparisons have been made, and the numbers are small, have failed to show any difference between primary radiotherapy and primary surgery.[14,30]

V. CONCLUSION

The relation of age or aging to carcinoma of the cervix is much debated. However, the only impact of age appears to be based on the epidemiologic observation which suggests an increase of vulnerability of the younger patient to the etiological factor(s) that cause carcinoma of the cervix. There is no apparent influence of age on method of presentation, distribution of cell type, degree of differentiation, preinvasive cytological picture, or rate of spread. The literature is mixed regarding the influence of age on treatment response and prognosis although treatment methods do not appear to be influenced by age.

REFERENCES

1. Canadian Task Force on Cervical Cancer Screening Programs — Cervical Cancer Screening Programs 1982, Department of Health and Welfare, Ottawa, Ontario, Canada, 1982.
2. **Fedorkow, D. M., Rob ertson, D. I., Duggan, M. A., Nation, J. G., McGregor, S. E., and Stuart, G. C. E.,** Invasive squamous cell carcinoma of the cervix in women less than 35 years old: recurrent versus nonrecurrent disease, *Am. J. Obstet. Gynecol.,* 158, 307, 1988.
3. **Lindell, A.,** Carcinoma of the uterine cervix; incidence and influence of age; statistical study, *Acta Radiol.,* 1(Suppl. 92), 102, 1952.
4. **Prempree, T., Patanaphan, V., Sewchand, W., and Scott, R. M.,** The influence of patients' age and tumour grade on prognosis of carcinoma of the cervix, *Cancer,* 51, 1764, 1983.

5. **Lombard, H. L. and Potter, E. A.,** Epidemiological aspects of cancer of the cervix; hereditary and environmental factors, *Cancer,* 3, 960, 1950.

6. **Martin, C. E.,** Epidemiology of cancer of the cervix, II. Marital and coital factors in cervical cancer, *Am. J. Public Health,* 57, 830, 1967.

7. **Rotkin, I. D.,** A comparison review of key epidemiological studies in cervical cancer related to current searches for transmissible agents, *Cancer Res.,* 33, 1353, 1974.

8. **Coppleson, M., Pixley, E., and Reid, B.,** *A Scientific and Practical Approach to the Cervix and Vagina in Health and Disease,* 2nd ed., *Colposcopy,* American Lecture Series, Charles C Thomas, Springfield, IL, 76.

9. **Kessler, I. I.,** Human cervical cancer as a veneral disease, *Cancer Res.,* 36, 783, 1976.

10. **Schachter, J., Hill, E. C., King, E. B., et al.,** Chlamydia trachomatis and cervical neoplasia, *JAMA,* 248, 2134, 1982.

11. **Fenoglio, C. M. and Ferenezy, A.,** Etiologic factors of cervical neoplasia, *Semin. Oncol.,* 3, 349, 1982.

12. **ZurHausen, H., DeVilliers, E. M., and Gissmann, L.,** Papilloma virus infections and human genital cancer, *Gynecol. Oncol.,* 12, S124, 1981.

13. **Schneider, A., Hotz, M., and Gissmann, L.,** Increased prevalence of human papillomaviruses in the lower genital tract of pregnant women, *Int. J. Cancer,* 40, 198, 1987.

14. **Kaminski, P. F., Sorosky, J. I., Wheelock, J. B., and Stevens, C. W., Jr.,** The significance of atypical cervical cytology in an older population, *Obstet. Gynecol.,* 73, 13, 1989.

15. **Richart, R. H.,** Causes and management of cervical intraepithelial neoplasia, *Cancer,* 60, 1951, 1987.

16. **Carmichael, J. A., Clarke, D. H., Moher, D., Ohlke, I. D., and Karchmar, E. J.,** Cervical carcinoma in women aged 34 and younger, *Am. J. Obstet. Gynecol.,* 154, 264, 1986.

17. **Robertson, J. H., Woodend, B. E., et al.,** Risk of cervical cancer associated with mild dyskariosis, *Br. Med. J.,* 297, 18, 1988.

18. Ontario Cancer Treatment and Research Foundation, Cancer registry, 1989, chap. 20.

19. Cervical Cancer Screening Programs — The Walton Report, *Can. Med. Assoc. J.,* 114, 11, 1976.

20. **Carmichael, J. A., Jeffrey, J., Steele, H. D., and Ohlke, D.,** The cytologic history of 245 patients developing invasive cervical carcinoma, *Am. J. Obstet. Gynecol.,* 148, 685, 1984.

21. **Rodney, A. H., Shapiro, M. F., Freeman, H. E., and Corey, C. R.,** Who gets screened for cervical and breast cancer? Results from a new national survey, *Arch. Intern. Med.,* 148, 1177, 1988.

22. **Ferenczy, A. and Winkler, B.,** Carcinoma and metastatic tumours of the cervix, *Blaustein's Pathology of the Female Genital Tract-Third Edition,* Kurman, R., Ed., Springer-Verlag, New York,, 281.

23. **VanNagell, J. R., Donaldson, E. S., Parker, J. C., VanDyke, A. H., and Wood, E. G.,** The prognostic significance of cell type and lesions size in patients with cervical cancer treated by radical surgery, *Gynecol. Oncol.,* 5, 142, 1977.

24. **Meanwell, C. A., Kelly, K. A., Wilson, S., et al.,** Young age as a prognostic factor in cervical cancer: analysis of population based data from 10,022 cases, *Br. Med. J.,* 296, 386, 1988.

25. **Piver, M. S. and Chung, W. S.,** Prognostic significance of cervical lesion size and pelvic node metastases in cervical carcinoma, *Obstet. Gynecol.,* 46, 507, 1975.

26. **O'Brien, D. M. and Carmichael, J. A.,** Presurgical prognostic factors in carcinoma of the cervix, Stages IB and IIA, *Am. J. Obstet. Gynecol.,* 158, 250, 1988.

27. **LeVecchia, C., Franceschi, S., Decarli, A., Gallus, G., Parazzini, F., and Merlo, E.,** Invasive cervical cancer in young women, *Br. J. Obstet. Gynecol.,* 91, 1149, 1984.

28. **Kjorstad, K. E.,** Carcinoma of the cervix in the young patient, *Obstet. Gynecol.* 50, 28, 1977.

29. **Berkowitz, R. S., Ehrmann, R. L., Lavizzo-Mourey, R., and Knapp, R. C.,** Invasive cervical carcinoma in young women, *Gynecol. Oncol.,* 8, 311, 1979.

30. **Stuart, G. C. E., Robertson, D. I., Fedorkow, D. M., Duggan, M. A., and Nation, J. G.,** Recurrent and persistent squamous cell cervical carcinoma in women under age 35, *Gynecol. Oncol.,* 30, 163, 1988.

31. **Stanhope, C. R., Smith, J. P., Wharton, J. T., Rutledge, F. N., Fletcher, G. H., and Gallager, H. S.,** Carcinoma of the cervix: the effect of age on survival, *Gynecol. Oncol.,* 10, 188, 1980.

32. **Lybeert, M. L. M., Meerwaldt, J. H., and van Putten, W. L. J.,** Age as a prognostic factor in carcinoma of the cervix, *Chem. Oncol.,* 9, 147, 1987.

Chapter 16

AGE AT BREAST CANCER DIAGNOSIS AS A PREDICTOR OF SUBSEQUENT SURVIVAL

Janet Mohle-Boetani

TABLE OF CONTENTS

I. INTRODUCTION

Prognosis in breast cancer is correlated with clinical stage of presentation, the number o positive axillary lymph nodes found at operation, and the hormone receptor status of the tumor Some researchers consider age at diagnosis a prognostic indicator, while others conclude tha age is unrelated to survival and thus differ in their assessment of whether those diagnosed at ₑ young, middle, or old age have the best relative survival. This chapter reviews the literature on the relation between age at diagnosis and survival and attempts to clarify this issue.

In 1934, in his treatise on neoplastic diseases, Ewing stated that "Before 30 years of age mammary cancer is extremely fatal..." and that "In aged women, on the other hand, the disease runs a prolonged course...."[1] The literature from 1940 through 1988 contains many reports of age at diagnosis of breast cancer and survival, most of which are based on small sample sizes. The studies from 1970 through 1988 that used small sample sizes in their analyses are listed in Table 1.[2-24] In general these studies compare survival in patients using broad age groups. Results of these studies are summarized in Table 2. No clear pattern of age-specific prognosis emerges from these studies.

In contrast to the studies listed in Table 1 which use small numbers of patients, several large studies in different countries and spanning different time periods reveal a consistent finding. Diagnosis at 45 to 49 years of age confers a significant survival advantage over diagnosis at all other ages.

In 1955 McKenzie reported on the survival of 10,025 patients in the Cancer Registration Scheme of England and Wales in whom diagnosis was made between 1945 and 1947.[25] The highest 5-year survival percentage overall and within each stage at diagnosis was found in the age group 45 to 49 years at diagnosis (Figure 1). In a second large study Hakama analyzed 12,125 breast cancer patients who were diagnosed between 1953 and 1968 in Finland.[26] In this study broad age groups were used and the best survival was found in those less than 50 years of age when compared with those between 50 to 64 years of age and those greater than 64 years of age.

In 1983 Ries et al.[27] reported the survival of 46,959 breast cancer patients in the U.S. in whom diagnosis was made between 1973 and 1979. The best 5-year relative survival rate was in patients diagnosed between ages 45 and 49 years. A subset of this study of 12,994 patients in the San Francisco Bay area diagnosed between 1973 and 1982, was analyzed by both stage and by 5-year age groups.[28] In this study those diagnosed at age 45 to 49 had the best overall survival and the best survival in each stage of disease at diagnosis (Figure 2).

In a fourth large study Adami et al.[29] examined the survival of 57,068 Swedish patients diagnosed between 1960 and 1978. The best relative 5-year survival was among patients aged 45 through 49 years at diagnosis (Figure 3). Rutquist[8] analyzed a subset of this study, 1730 patients in Stockholm County diagnosed between 1961 and 1963, using the following age groups: less than 50 years, 50 through 69 years, and greater than 69 years. When analyzed with these broad age groups and the smaller sample size there was no difference in the survival between the three groups of patients.

A final large study included 31,594 patients who were diagnosed between 1955 and 1980 in Norway.[30] The relative 5-year survival rate was again found to be best in the age group 45 through 49 years at time of diagnosis (Figure 4).

These data suggest that women diagnosed in the middle years of life, specifically between ages 45 and 49 years, enjoy a longer relative survival than women who are diagnosed either at younger or at older ages. The most convincing evidence comes from the large studies in the Scandinavian countries, the U.K., and the U.S. Survival data from other countries either have not been reported by age groups or have been reported only as small samples of the population. Therefore, the correlation between the age at diagnosis and survival may not be applicable to breast cancer in southern Europe, the East, or other regions. For example, the age-specific incidence in Japan decreases after age 50 in contrast to the incidence in the U.S. and northern

TABLE 1
Breast Cancer Survival Studies with Small Sample Sizes

Study author and year of report		Place/country	Time of data collection	No. of patients	Grouping of ages at diagnosis (years)
King et al.[2]	1985	Minnesota, U.S.	1950—80	63	22—44
Nugent et al.[3]	1985	Los Angeles, U.S.	1970—80	176	<40
				1224	≥40
Aareleid et al.[4]	1985	Estonia, U.S.S.R.	1968—81	4090	<35
					35—64
					>64
Rosen et al.[5]	1985	New York, U.S.	1964—70	101	<35
			1976—79	65	<35
				262	All ages
Tabbane et al.[6]	1985	Tunis, Tunisia	1973—80	48	<35
				94	45—49 and premeno
Hibberd et al.[7]	1983	New Zealand	1950—54	2019	35—44
					45—54
					55—64
					>64
Rutquist et al.[8]	1983	Stockholm Co., Sweden	1961—63	1730	<50
					50—69
					>69
Noyes et al.[9]	1982	Texas, U.S.	1945—77	310	<30
				3380	≥30
Palmer et al.[10]	1982	Manchester, U.K.	1970—75	1022	
Ribiero et al.[11]	1981	Manchester, U.K.	1955—70	803	≤30
					31—35
					36—39
Nikkanen et al.[12]	1981	Turku, Finland	1961—70	644	<50
					50—64
					>64
Langlands et al.[13]	1979	Edinburgh, U.K.	1954—64	102	<40
				102	40—44
				151	>44
Redding et al.[14]	1979	London, U.K.	1977	214	21—49
				382	50—69
				211	70—93
Mueller et al.[15]	1978	New York, U.S.	1955—74	3558	21—50
					51—70
					71—100
Valagussa et al.[16]	1978	Milan, Italy	1964—68	737	Premeno
					Postmeno
Wallgren et al.[17]	1977	Gothenburg, Sweden	1958—68	91	<30
			1968—71	263	All ages
Schwartz et al.[18]	1976	Pennsylvania, U.S.	1951—64	111	<30
				9003	All ages
Gogas and Skalkeas[19]	1975	Athens, Greece	1950—69	138	<41
				690	>40
Birks et al.[20]	1973	Vancouver, Canada	1941—66	58	<30
				4980	>29
Crosby et al.[21]	1971	Saskatchewan, Canada	1932—65	2612	<35
					≥35
Devitt et al.[22]	1970	Ontario, Canada	1946—62	1530	<35
					35—44
					45—54

TABLE 1 (continued)
Breast Cancer Survival Studies with Small Sample Sizes

Study author and year of report		Place/country	Time of data collection	No. of patients	Grouping of ages at diagnosis (years)
					55—64
					65—74
					75—84
Norris et al.[23]	1970	Washington, D.C.		135	<30
Brightmore et al.[24]	1970	London, U.K.	1947—66	101	<35

TABLE 2
Results of Breast Cancer Survival Studies with Small Sample Sizes

Author, year of report		Results
King et al.[2]	1985	5-year survival of pregnant patients aged 22—44 years was 59%.
Nugent et al.[3]	1985	5-year survival of patients <40 years was 55%, and of those >40 years was 75%. 11% of cases that were <40 years were pregnant, 71% of pregnant patients were estrogen receptor negative.
Aareleid[4]	1985	5-year relative survival of patients <35 years was 69%, 35—64 years was 59%, and >65 years was 46%.
Rosen et al.[5]	1985	10 year survival of patients <35 years was 60% and in patients of all ages was 60%.
Tabbane et al.[6]	1985	Poorer histological grade and poorer survival in the younger group.
Hibberd et al.[7]	1983	5-year relative survival: 20—34 years - 49% 35—44 years - 55% 45—54 years - 51% 55—64 years - 44% >64 years - 43%
Rutquist et al[8]	1983	No difference in survival overall or when divided by node involvement at diagnosis in the age groups <50, 50—69, >69 years.
Noyes et al.[9]	1982	5-year survival of patients <30 years old was 43%, and was 59% for those >30 years of age.
Palmer et al.[10]	1982	Patients aged 40—49 years at diagnosis had the best survival at 5 and 10 years.
Ribiero et al.[11]	1981	5-year survival of those <30 years was 34%, of those 31—35 years was 51%, and of those 36—39 years was 57%.
Nikkanen et al.[12]	1981	Patients aged <50 years had the best 10 year survival in each of three stages, patients aged >64 years had the worst survival.
Langlands et al.[13]	1979	Patients aged 40—44 years had the best survival, those less than 35 years had the worst survival, those diagnosed within 5 years of menopause had a poorer survival in stages I and III than other menopausal groups.
Redding et al.[14]	1979	No difference in survival between age groups.
Mueller et al.[15]	1978	The longest time to 50% mortality was in the age group 21—50 years.
Valagussa et al.[16]	1978	No difference in survival between pre- and postmenopausal patients.
Wallgren et al.[17]	1977	5-year survival for those <30 years was 63% and for all ages was 71%. When comparing those <30 years with all ages there was no significant survival difference when separated by nodal status.

TABLE 2 (continued)
Results of Breast Cancer Survival Studies with Small Sample Sizes

Author, year of report		Results
Schwartz et al.[18]	1976	10-year survival of patients, 30 years of age was similar to that of older patients in the group without axillary node involvement or stage A. Patients <30 years old with axillary node involvement had poorer survival than older patients with similar involvement.
Gogas and Skalkeas[19]	1975	There was no significant difference in the survival rates between those less than 41 years and those 41 years or older.
Birks et al.[20]	1973	No difference in survival between those <30 years and older patients.
Crosby et al.[21]	1971	5-year survival for patients <35 years old was 58%, for all ages was 62%, and for pregnant or lactating patients was 38%.
Devitt et al.[22]	1970	Crude 5-year survival rates for patients with stage I or stage II breast cancer in ten year age groups were <35 years - 76%, 35—44 years - 69%, 45—54 years - 72%, 55—64 years - 65%, 65—74 years - 72%, 75—84 years - 64%.
Norris et al.[23]	1970	5-year survival of patients <30 years old was 56%. Patients with 1 to 2 axillary nodes survived shorter than expected.
Brightmore et al.[24]	1970	Patients <35 years had a 5-year survival of 35% which was compared by the author to other large series that reported a 5-year survival of 50% for all ages.

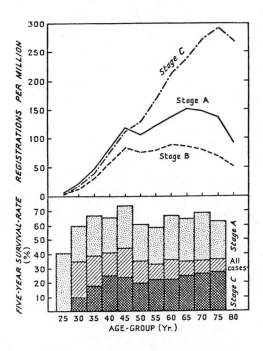

FIGURE 1. Registration rates and five-year survival rates of cancer of the female breast at different clinical stages by 5-year age groups in England, 1955. (From *Lancet*, 1130, November 26, 1955, Figure 2.)

Europe, which increases after age 50.[31] The genetic or environmental factors that result in the difference in the age-specific incidence pattern may also influence survival. Therefore, the age at diagnosis that correlates with the best survival may also be different.

The improved survival among women in the perimenopausal years has led to theorizing

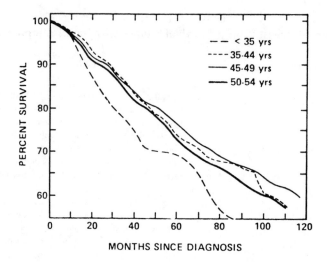

FIGURE 2.   Survival after diagnosis of breast cancer by age at diagnosis in the U.S. in 1986. (From Mohle-Boetani, J., *N. Engl. J. Med.*, 315, 9, 587, Figure 1.)

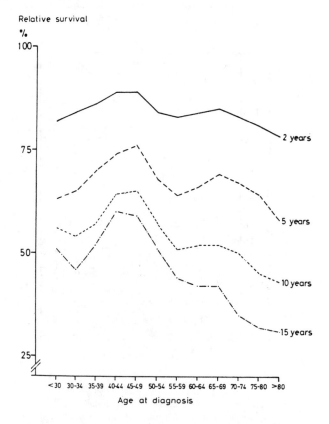

FIGURE 3.   Cumulative relative survival for consecutive 5-year age groups in Sweden, 1986. (From Adami, H. O., *N. Engl. J. Med.*, 315, 9, 561, Figure 1.)

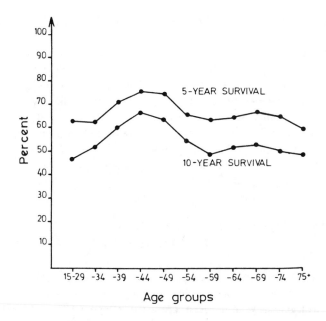

FIGURE 4. Relative 5- and 10-year survival rates by age in Norway, 1986. (From H. Host and *Cancer*, 57, 2218, Figure 2.)

concerning possible biological explanations. Speculations concerning both the disadvantage of young or old ages at diagnosis and the advantages of a middle age at diagnosis have been proposed.

II. THE DISADVANTAGE OF YOUNG AGE AT DIAGNOSIS

Several reports emphasize apparent differences in tumor biology of young patients compared with that seen in older patients. Tabbane et al.[6] noted a higher percentage of tumor necrosis and a lower percentage of histologic grade I at diagnosis in Tunisian patients aged less than 30 years of age compared with premenopausal patients aged 45 to 49 at diagnosis. Brightmore reported that patients less than 35 years of age had a smaller proportion of grade I malignancy compared with the proportion seen in all age groups combined.[24] Norris, however, reported a high percentage of noninvasive tumors in women less than 30 years of age at diagnosis.[23] Several studies note a high percentage of bilateral breast cancer and of axillary node involvement at presentation in young women when compared with older women.[24,32-34] Two studies reported that young patients with positive axillary lymph nodes had a decreased survival compared with that of older age groups with positive axillary nodes.[19,23] Kurtz et al. reported a high local recurrence rate among patients who were less than 40 years of age but no overall survival disadvantage compared with that of patients without recurrences.[34]

A possible explanation for the disadvantage of young age at diagnosis is that 5 to 10 % of young women are pregnant at the time of diagnosis and that pregnant breast cancer patients as a group have diminished survival time. Deemarsky emphasized the poor prognosis among patients who were lactating at diagnosis(30% survival at 5 years).[35] This group is characterized by a high percentage of advanced tumors and metastatic disease. Some investigators have concluded that pregnancy is less important prognostically than age, estrogen receptor status, and the stage at presentation. Pregnant patients present at young ages, with a high percentage of estrogen receptor negative tumors,[3] with a high percentage of axillary lymph node involvement[36,23] and at more advanced stages.[2] The prognosis of pregnant patients is equivalent to that of others of the same age and stage.[3,23]

III. THE DISADVANTAGE OF OLD AGE AT DIAGNOSIS

The reason for the poorer survival experienced by older patients when compared with perimenopausal patients has been incompletely explored. Mueller's[15] study in 1978 reported that 25% of the elderly are not staged at diagnosis. Thus, an accurate comparison between these patients and younger patients by extent of disease is impossible. A high prevalence of comorbidity in elderly women may decrease their survival. Mor's[37] study of 1986 reported the presence of cardiac disease in 29% of women diagnosed with breast cancer at age 80 or older. Finally, age is inversely related to receipt of chemotherapy independent of stage at diagnosis and cardiac comorbidity.[37] Thus, older patients may experience poorer survival because of less aggressive treatment. Further study is clearly necessary to determine the reasons for the relatively poor survival of elderly breast cancer patients.

IV. THE ADVANTAGE OF PERIMENOPAUSAL AGE AT DIAGNOSIS

The survival advantage of breast cancer patients who are diagnosed between ages 45 and 49 may be due to a lack of the poor prognostic conditions observed in the younger or older age groups. Women in the middle years of life in contrast to younger women are less likely to present with advanced breast cancer. When compared with older women they are less likely to have comorbid disease at presentation.

The average age of menopause is 51,[38] in close proximity to the 45 to 49-year-old age group. This association has led authors to speculate that the growth of breast tumors may be curtailed when estrogen stimulation decreases with menopause.[28,30,39] Adami et al.[29] argued against this theory because they did not observe an increase in the survival rates when younger age groups survived to a menopausal age. Although there has been theorizing, there have been no large studies with direct analysis of this issue. For example, a study of survival among those who become menopausal soon after diagnosis compared to those who enter menopause many years after diagnosis would be of interest.

The survival advantage could also be due to a less malignant tumor or to a physiological or hormonal milieu in middle-aged women that is less conducive to tumor progression. The tumor biology issue has been addressed by evaluation of the proportion of estrogen or progesterone receptor positive tumors within age groups. In general, hormone receptors suggest differentiation and tumors with these receptors are less malignant than tumors that are receptor negative. Estrogen receptor positivity is correlated with increased survival in patients with clinical stage I and II cancer.[40] Progesterone receptor positivity is correlated with increased survival amoung patients with stage II breast cancer.[40] The Danish Cancer Cooperative Group reported that the progesterone receptor predominates in women less than 50 years of age at diagnosis and in premenopausal women.[41] The estrogen receptor predominates in postmenopausal women and is positively correlated with age.[41] There is a presumed high false negative estrogen receptor rate amoung premenopausal women because endogenously produced estrogens are likely to block estrogen receptors.[42] The tumors in older premenopausal patients are more likely to be progesterone positive than the tumors in younger premenopausal patients.[41,43] Therefore, women aged 45 to 49 are more likely than younger women to have progesterone positive tumors and consequently a better prognosis.

V. SUMMARY

Large studies from Northern Europe and the U.S. show a survival advantage among women diagnosed with breast cancer between ages 45 and 49 years. Further analysis is necessary to determine whether this finding is generalizable to breast cancer diagnosed in other geographic regions where the age-specific incidence pattern differs substantially from that noted in northern Europe.

At the present time there is no satisfactory explanation for the improved survival of the 45 to 49-year-old women. Since the epidemiologic data are strong and consistent, laboratory and clinical investigation directed at the mechanism of the survival advantage of women diagnosed at 45 to 49 years of age is now warranted.

REFERENCES

1. **Ewing, J.,** *Neoplastic diseases; a Treatise on Tumors,* 4th ed., W. B. Saunders, Philadelphia, 1940.
2. **King, R. M., Welch, J. S., Martin, J. K., and Coulam, C. B.,** Carcinoma of the breast associated with pregnancy, *Surg. Gynecol. Obstet.,* 160, 228, 1985.
3. **Nugent P., O'Connell, T. X.,** Breast cancer and pregnancy, *Arch. Surg.,* 120, 1221, 1985.
4. **Aareleid, T.,** Survival patterns of female breast cancer patients in the Estonian SSR in 1968-1981, *Neoplasma,* 32, 257, 1985.
5. **Rosen, P. P., Lesser, M. L., Kinne, D. W., and Beattie, E. J.,** Breast carcinoma in women 35 years of age or younger, *Ann. Surg.,* 199, 133, 1984.
6. **Tabbane, F., May, A. E., Hachiche, M., Bahi, J., Jaziri, M., Cammoun, M., and Mourali, N.,** Breast cancer in women under 30 years of age, *Breast Cancer Res. Treat.,* 6, 137, 1985.
7. **Hibberd, A. D., Horwood, L. J., and Wells, J. E.,** Long term prognosis of women with breast cancer in New Zealand: Study of survival to 30 years, *Br. Med. J.,* 286, 1777, 1983.
8. **Rutquist, L. E. and Wallgren, A.,** Influence of age on outcome in breast carcinoma, *Acta Rad. Oncol.,* 22, 289, 1983.
9. **Noyes, R. D., Spanos, W. J., and Montague, E. D.,** Breast cancer in women aged 30 and under, *Cancer,* 49, 1302, 1982.
10. **Palmer, M. K., Lythgoe, J. P., and Smith, A.,** Prognostic factors in breast cancer, *Br. J. Surg.,* 69, 697, 1982.
11. **Ribieiro, G. G. and Swindell, R.,** The prognosis of breast carcinoma in women aged less than 40 years, *Clin. Rad.,* 32, 231, 1981.
12. **Nikkanen, V., Linna, M., and Toikkanen, S.,** Treatment results in mammary carcinoma stages I-IV, *Acta Rad. Oncol.,* 20, 9, 1981.
13. **Langlands, A. O. and Kerr, G. R.,** Prognosis in breast cancer: the effect of age and menstrual status, *Clin. Oncol.,* 5, 123, 1979.
14. **Redding, W. H., Thomas, J. M., Powles, T. J., Ford, H. T., and Gazet, J. C.,** Age and prognosis in breast cancer, *Br. Med. J.,* 1465, 1979.
15. **Mueller, C. B., Ames, F., and Anderson, G. D.,** Breast cancer in 3,558 women: age as a significant determinant in the rate of dying and causes of death, *Surgery,* 83, 123, 1978.
16. **Valagussa, P., Bonadonna, G., and Veronesi, U.,** Patterns of relapse and survival following radical mastectomy, *Cancer,* 41, 1170, 1978.
17. **Wallgren, A., Silfversward, C., and Hultborn, A.,** Carcinoma of the breast in women under 30 years of age, *Cancer,* 40, 916, 1977.
18. **Schwartz, G. F. and Zeok, J. V.,** Carcinoma of the breast in young women, *Am. J. Surg.,* 131, 570, 1976.
19. **Gogas, J. and Skalkeas, G.,** Prognosis of mammary cancer in young women, *Surgery,* 78, 339, 1975.
20. **Birks, D. M., Crawford, G. M., Ellison, L. G., and Johnstone, F. R. C.,** Carcinoma of the breast in women 30 years of age or less, *Surg. Gynecol. Obstet.,* 137, 21, 1973.
21. **Crosby, C. H. and Barclay, T. H. D.,** Carcinoma of the breast: surgical management of patients with special conditions, *Surg. Breast Cancer,* 28, 1628, 1971.
22. **Devitt, J. E.,** The influence of age on the behavior of carcinoma of the breast, *Can. Med. Assoc. J.,* 103, 923, 1970.
23. **Norris, H. J. and Taylor, H. B.,** Carcinoma of the breast in women less than thirty years old, *Cancer,* 26, 953, 1970.
24. **Brightmore, T. G. J., Greening, W. P., and Hamlin, I.,** An analysis of clinical and histopathological features in 101 cases of carcinoma of breast in women under 35 years of age, *Br. J. Cancer,* 644, 1970.
25. **McKenzie, A.,** Cancer of the female breast, mortality and the menopause, *Lancet,* 1129, 1955.
26. **Hakama, M. and Riihimaki, H.,** End results of breast cancer patients in Finland 1953-1968, *Ann. Clin. Res.,* 6, 115, 1974.

27. **Ries, L. G., Pollack, E. S., and Young, J. L.,** Cancer patient survival: surveillance, epidemiology and end results program, 1973-79, *JNCI*, 70, 693, 1983.

28. **Mohle-Boetani, J., Grosser, S., Malec, M., and Whittemore, A. S.,** Survival advantage among patients with breast cancer diagnosed at 45 to 49 years of age (letter), *N. Engl. J. Med.,* 315, 587, 1986.

29. **Adami, H. O., Malker, B., Holmberg, L., Persson, I., and Stae, B.,** The relation between survival and age at diagnosis in breast cancer, *N. Engl. J. Med.,* 315, 559, 1986.

30. **Host, H. and Lund, E.,** Age as a prognostic factor in breast cancer, *Cancer,* 57, 2217, 1986.

31. **Seidman, H.,** *Cancer of the Breast: Statistical and Epidemiological Data,* American Cancer Society, New York, 1972.

32. **Kleinfeld, G., Haagensen, C. D., and Cooley, E.,** Age and menstrual status as prognostic factors in carcinoma of the breast, *Ann. Surg.,* 157, 600, 1962.

33. **Cutler, S. J., Asire, A. J., and Taylor, S. G.,** An evaluation of ovarian status as a prognostic factor in disseminated cancer of the breast, 26, 938, 1970.

34. **Kurtz, J. M., Spitalier, J. M., Amalric, R., Brandone, H., Ayme, Y, Bressac, C., and Hans, D.,** Mammary recurrences in women younger than forty, *Int. J. Rad. Oncol. Biol. Phys.,* 15, 271, 1988.

35. **Deemarsky, L. J. and Neishtadt, E. L.,** Breast cancer and pregnancy, *Dis. Breast,* 7, 17, 1981.

36. **Ribieiro, G. G. and Palmer M. K.,** Breast carcinoma associated with pregnancy : a clinician's dilemma, *Br. Med. J.,* 2, 1524, 1977

37. **Mor, V., Masterson-Allen, S., Goldberg, R. J., Cummings, F. J., Glicksman, A. S., and Fretwell, M. D.,** Relationship between age at diagnosis and treatments received by cancer patients, *J. Am. Geriatr. Soc.,* 33, 585, 1985.

38. **Cecil, R. L.,** *Textbook of Medicine,* Vol. 18, W.B. Saunders, Philadelphia, 1988, 1444.

39. **Stoll, B. A.,** Does the malignancy of breast cancer vary with age?, *Clin. Oncol.,* 2, 73, 1976.

40. **McGuire, W. L.,** Prognostic factors in primary breast cancer, *Cancer Surv.,* 5, 527, 1986.

41. **Thorpe, S. M., Rose, C., Pederson, B. V., and Rasmussen, B. B.,** Estrogen and progesterone receptor profile patterns in primary breast cancer, *Breast Cancer Res. Treat.,* 3, 103, 1983.

42. **Barbi, G. P., Marroni, P., Bruzzi, P., Nicolo, G., Paganuzzi, M., and Perrara, G. B.,** Correlation between steroid hormone receptors and prognostic factors in human breast cancer, *Oncology,* 44, 265, 1987.

43. **Beex, L. V. A. M., Mackenzie, M. A., Raemaekers, J. M. M., Smals, A. G. H., Benraad, P. Th. J., and Kloppenborg, P. W. C.,** Adjuvant chemotherapy in premenopausal patients with primary breast cancer; relation to drug induced amenorrhoea, age and the progesterone receptor status, *Eur. J.Cancer Clin. Oncol.,* 24, 719, 1988.

Chapter 17

RELATIONSHIP BETWEEN AGE AND THE INCIDENCE OF LIVER METASTASES

Stanislav Pejchl

TABLE OF CONTENTS

I. INTRODUCTION

The liver is a frequent site for the location of metastases from a majority of malignant tumors. The presence of liver metastases in patients with a malignant tumor is regarded as a prognostically unfavorable sign. Little is known yet of the mechanisms initiating metastatic processes of malignant tumors in general and namely of a secondary involvement of the liver. They appear to be influenceed by a number of factors,[1-8] of which one might be age. Since the rate of liver metastases in relation to age has not been examined both from a theoretical and a clinical point of view, the present study is intended to contribute to a better understanding of this problem.

II. MATERIALS AND METHODS

The material available for study consisted both of clinical and autopsy records of patients who died between the years 1957 and 1976 in the Department of Internal Medicine, and the Department of Surgery, Medical School Hospital, Pod Petřínem, Prague.

We selected autopsy records containing a reliable histological confirmation of primary malignant tumors in any organ except the liver. If there were two or more tumors in a patient, each was evaluated separately. Only histologically confirmed secondary involvements of the liver were considered as metastases. A direct infiltration of the liver by a malignant tumor or tumorous implantation on the liver capsule was excluded.

Our cases of malignant tumors obtained from a total of 2,203 autopsies, were divided into 10 groups according to the organs where the tumors were present:

1. Colon, rectum
2. Stomach
3. Gallgladder, bile ducts
4. Pancreas
5. Bronchus
6. Breast
7. Ovary, uterus
8. Prostate
9. Kidney
10. Other organs

All cases were divided into two main groups:

1. Malignant tumors in the area of the portal circulation (colon, rectum, stomach, gallbladder, bile ducts, pancreas)
2. Malignant tumors in the area of the systemic circulation (bronchus, breast, ovary, uterus, prostate, kidney, others)

Out of a total of 2270 malignant tumors, 1166 were from male and 1104 from female patients; mortality occurred at an average age of 67.8 years. Carcinomas were identified in 94% of patients. The primary site, sex, and age of the patients and the frequency of liver metastases are given in Table 1.

In order to evaluate the incidence of liver metastases in relation to age, the cases were divided both into six age groups (16 to 40, 41 to 50, 51 to 60, 61 to 70, 71 to 80, above 80 years) and into two age groups (16 to 60 and more than 70 years), ruling out age group 61 to 70.

Autopsies and histological examinations were performed at the 2nd Pathologico-Anatomical Institute, School of General Medicine, Charles University, Prague and at the Pathologico-Anatomical Institute, Faculty of Paediatrics, Charles University, Prague. The chi-square test was used for statistical evaluation.

TABLE 1
Number of Malignant Tumors Arranged by Organs, Sex, Liver Metastases, and Average Age at Death

Primary site	Malignant tumors				Liver metastases		
	Male	Female	Total	Age	Male	Female	Total
Colon, rectum	228	209	437	68.1	77[a]	69[a]	146
Stomach	240	213	453	68.4	76[a]	68[a]	144
Gallbladder, bile ducts	57	151	208	70.5	30[a]	77[a]	107
Pancreas	57	85	142	68.9	36[a]	48[a]	84
Bronchus	266	46	312	66.7	105[a]	18[a]	123
Breast	2	140	142	66.0	1[a]	54[a]	55
Ovary, uterus	—	118	118	66.3	—	26	26
Prostate	102	—	102	72.0	11	—	11
Kidney	67	40	107	67.4	14[a]	11[a]	25
Others	147	102	249	64.8	39[a]	25[a]	64
Total	1166	1104	2270	67.8	389[a]	396[a]	785

[a] Difference in frequency of liver metastases not significant (chi-square test, $p > 0.05$).

III. RESULTS

As can be seen in Table 1, male and female patients did not differ significantly in the incidence of liver metastases from malignant tumors of the different organs ($p > 0.05$). The results were also not significant ($p > 0.05$) when using a division into six age groups. Therefore, we tested all our groups without separating the sexes.

Table 2 illustrates our division of malignant tumors into six age groups. Apart from malignant tumors of the stomach, the incidence of liver metastases was lower in the older patients, particularly in those older than 70 years. However, when using the chi-square test, the differences between age groups in the incidence of liver metastases were statistically significant only in the case of malignant tumors of the prostate ($p < 0.01$).

A division of malignant tumors into two age groups is shown in Table 3. Apart from malignant tumors of the stomach, liver metastases from all other organs were less frequent in the older patients. Although this relationship was not significant for any malignant tumor located in the area of the portal circulation (always $p > 0.05$), it was statistically significant for malignant tumors located in the area of the systemic circulation, with the exception of the tumors of the kidney and those of the inhomogeneous group "others". The values were $p < 0.01$ for bronchus and prostate and $p < 0.05$ for breast, ovary, and uterus.

The results of Tables 4 and 5 show that differences in the incidence of liver metastases among the six age groups were significant both for the total of tumors ($p < 0.05$) and for all tumors from the systemic circulation ($p < 0.01$), but were not significant for all tumors from the portal circulation ($p > 0.05$). With a division into two age groups, the relationship between age and the incidence of liver metastases was significant both for the total of tumors and for all tumors from the systemic circulation ($p < 0.01$), but was not significant for all tumors from the portal circulation ($p > 0.05$).

IV. DISCUSSION

The relationship between age and the incidence of liver metastases can be approached by intra vitam and postmortem studies.

The probability of a clinical diagnosis of a malignant tumor depends *inter alia* upon the site of its primary location, the age of the patient, and concomitant diseases. A relatively large

TABLE 2
Relationship between Age and the Incidence of Liver Metastases in Males and Females when the Cases were Divided into Six Age Groups

Primary site	Age	(a) No. of malignant tumors (b) No. of liver metastases (in %) 16—40	41—50	51—60	61—70	71—80	> 80	Total
Colon, rectum	(a)	8	27	71	139	144	48	437
	(b)	50.0	33.3	36.6	33.8	31.9	29.2	33.4
Stomach	(a)	6	30	73	144	143	57	453
	(b)	33.3	26.7	28.8	32.6	32.2	35.1	31.8
Gallbladder,	(a)	0	5	28	72	77	26	208
bile ducts	(b)	0.0	60.0	67.9	48.6	50.6	42.3	51.4
Pancreas	(a)	3	4	25	41	53	16	142
	(b)	66.7	50.0	68.0	58.5	54.7	62.5	59.2
Bronchus	(a)	5	12	69	105	101	20	312
	(b)	60.0	41.7	50.7	39.0	32.7	30.0	39.4
Breast	(a)	2	22	22	49	28	19	142
	(b)	50.0	54.5	40.9	44.9	25.0	21.1	38.7
Ovary, uterus	(a)	2	7	27	41	28	13	118
	(b)	50.0	42.9	29.6	24.4	10.7	7.7	22.0
Prostate[a]	(a)	0	1	9	34	44	14	102
	(b)	0.0	0.0	44.4	8.8	9.1	0.0	10.8
Kidney	(a)	0	7	18	44	30	8	107
	(b)	0.0	42.9	22.2	27.3	13.3	25.0	23.4
Others	(a)	18	14	44	83	66	24	249
	(b)	33.3	28.6	27.3	26.5	24.2	16.7	25.7

[a] Chi-square test, $p < 0.01$.

TABLE 3
Relationship between Age and the Incidence of Liver Metastases in Males and Females when the Cases were Divided into Two Age Groups

Primary site	Age	(a) No. of malignant tumors (b) No. of liver metastases (in %) 16—60	>70	Statistical significance
Colon, rectum	(a)	106	192	
	(b)	36.8	31.3	NS
Stomach	(a)	109	200	
	(b)	28.4	33.0	NS
Gallbladder,	(a)	33	103	
bile ducts	(b)	66.7	48.5	NS
Pancreas	(a)	32	69	
	(b)	65.6	56.5	NS
Bronchus	(a)	86	121	
	(b)	50.0	32.2	S, $p < 0.01$
Breast	(a)	46	47	
	(b)	47.8	23.4	S, $p < 0.05$
Ovary, uterus	(a)	36	41	
	(b)	33.3	9.8	S, $p < 0.05$
Prostate	(a)	10	58	
	(b)	40.0	6.9	S, $p < 0.01$
Kidney	(a)	25	38	
	(b)	28.0	15.8	NS
Others	(a)	76	90	
	(b)	28.9	22.2	NS

Note: Chi-square test, NS = not significant, $p > 0.05$; S = significant.

TABLE 4
Relationship between Age and the Incidence of Liver Metastases for Tumors of the Portal and Systemic Circulations Divided into Six Age Groups

Primary site		16—40	41—50	51—60	61—70	71—80	>80	Total
	(a) No. of malignant tumors							
	(b) No. of liver metastases (in %)							
	Age							
Portal	(a)	17	66	197	396	417	147	1240
circulation	(b)	47.1	33.3	42.1	38.6	38.4	37.4	38.8
Systemic	(a)	27	63	189	356	297	98	1030
circulation[a]	(b)	40.7	42.9	38.1	30.9	22.6	17.3	29.5
Total[b]	(a)	44	129	386	752	714	245	2270
	(b)	43.2	38.0	40.2	35.0	31.8	29.4	34.6

[a] Chi-square test: $p < 0.01$.
[b] Chi-square test: $p < 0.05$.

TABLE 5
Relationship between Age and the Incidence of Liver Metastases for Tumors of the Portal and Systemic Circulations Divided into Two Age Groups

Primary site	Age	16—60	>70	Statistical significance
	(a) No. of malignant tumors			
	(b) No. of liver metastases (in %)			
Portal	(a)	280	564	
circulation	(b)	40.4	38.1	NS
Systemic	(a)	279	395	
circulation	(b)	39.4	21.3	S, $p < 0.01$
Total	(a)	559	959	
	(b)	39.9	31.2	S, $p < 0.01$

Note: Chi-square test, NS = not significant, p >0.05; S = significant.

proportion of malignant tumors are diagnosed only at autopsy. Thus, Berndt and Berndt[9] identified more than 10% of malignant tumors that had not been diagnosed clinically. In patients older than 70 years, more than 30% of malignant tumors had not been diagnosed clinically, whereas more than 50% had not been identified if located in certain organs (male: rectum and kidney; female: colon, bronchus, and gallbladder).[10] Older age is frequently associated with an incidence of other diseases.[10-12] This explains the observation that more than 30% of patients with a malignant tumor, who were older than 70 years, died of a cause not directly related to the tumor.[10]

Autopsy studies comprise not only tumors identified at autopsy, but also cases supported by clinical and histological evidence. However, several other facts ought to be considered in an evaluation of this type of data. On the one hand, there is a limitation in the selection of patients available for autopsy; on the other hand, the various sites of location of a malignant tumor (e.g., colon) might influence the incidence of liver metastases.[13] Furthermore, different histological types of a malignant tumor (e.g., bronchus) establish liver metastases at a diferent rate, and their distribution changes with age.[14]

Treatment policies, including a targeted local treatment of liver metastases, might influence the final incidence of metastases in general and that of liver metastases in particular. In general, treatment of malignant tumors becomes less aggressive in the older patients because of the presence of other serious diseases. Noltenius and Tetzner[10] observed in patients older than 70 years that untreated malignant tumors established fewer metastases than treated tumors.

Our observations were collected from patients from one district who died in the Clinic of

Internal Medicine and in the Surgical Department. In Czechoslovakia, patients with malignant tumors originally treated in specialized clinics (e.g., gynecological tumors, tumors of the larynx, prostate, etc.) are hospitalized in the final stages in departments of internal medicine, mainly if there is an incidence of other complicating diseases. This explains the composition of our cases.

Our records date back to a time at which targeted, local treatment of liver metastases was not a common procedure and, if performed, was usually liver resection, irradiation, or targeted chemotherapy of the liver by way of the vena portae.[15]

Inaccurracies may well have occurred when dividing the cases into two groups (portal circulation, systemic circulation), because some tumors of the rectum are drained both by the vena portae (portal circulation) and the vena cava, inferior (systemic circulation). In our opinion, this division of malignant tumors must not necessarily have influenced our results.

Barz and Barz observed in their study on a total of 5708 carcinomas, confirmed by histological sections, that the number both of hematogenous and lymphogenous metastases declined significantly after the age of 67.5 years. There was also a significant decrease in the number of organs involved in the metastatic process.[16] Most of the carcinomas from 14 primary locations established fewer metastases in older patients than in the younger age groups. Similar results were obtained by Langsch and Uhlig who examined histological sections of carcinomas of the bronchus, stomach, colon, and rectum, and by Zschoch and Kober, who did the same type of studies on carcinomas of the bronchus.[17,18] Other observations of carcinomas of the stomach, colon, and rectum (identified by histological sections) suggested that age did not substantially influence the frequency of incidence of liver metastases.[13,17,19,20]

According to our results, liver metastases from malignant tumors located in the area of the portal circulation occurred with an equal frequency in the younger and older age groups. In contrast, malignant tumors from the area of the systemic circulation (bronchus, breast, ovary and uterus, prostate, but not those of the kidney and the unhomogeneous group "others'") established fewer liver metastases in the older age group. At present, we have no satisfactory explanation for these findings.

The liver is an organ interposed between the portal and systemic circulations. Both its position in the body, its structure, and vascular supply provide favorable conditions for the attachment and growth of tumor cells. A metastatic involvement of the liver might be due to the transport of tumor cells either along hematogenous (vena portae, hepatic artery) or lymphogenous routes, the former route being more common.[2] A question is whether the difference observed between tumors of the portal and systemic circulations might be due to the fact that the time of transport of the tumor cells along the vena portae to the liver is too short to allow the action of putative factors prevalent in older patients, that counteract the metastasizing power.

V. SUMMARY

The relationship between age and the incidence of metastases from malignant tumors (carcinomas in 94%) in the liver was evaluated from a total of 2270 malignant tumors identified histologically. For statistical evaluation, the cases were divided both into six and two age groups: 16 to 40, 41 to 50, 51 to 60, 61 to 70, 71 to 80, above 80; 16 to 60, above 70 years of age, ruling out age group 61 to 70. Five additional points need to be made:

1. The relationship between age and the incidence of liver metastases was not significant for any malignant tumor from the area of the portal circulation (colon and rectum, stomach, gallbladder and bile ducts, pancreas) — always $p > 0.05$.
2. The incidence of liver metastases from several malignant tumors from the area of the systemic circulation decreased as the patients grew older, and the difference was more marked in the older patients. When using six age groups to test the relationship, the results were statistically not significant except for malignant tumors of the prostate ($p < 0.01$). On the other hand, when these cases were divided into two groups, the results were significant

for malignant tumors of the following organs: bronchus, prostate ($p < 0.01$), breast, ovary, and uterus ($p < 0.05$). They were not significant for malignant tumors of the kidney and those of the unhomogeneous group "others" located in the area of the systemic circulation ($p > 0.05$).

3. The differences between the six age groups were also significant for all tumors combined ($p < 0.05$) and for all tumors from the systemic circulation ($p < 0.01$). They were not significant for all tumors from the portal circulation ($p > 0.05$). When the cases were divided into two age groups, the relationship between age and the incidence of liver metastases was significant both for all tumors combined and for all tumors from the area of the systemic circulation ($p < 0.01$), but was not significant for all tumors from the area of the portal circulation ($p > 0.05$).

4. Higher age was not a risk factor for the development of metastases in the liver.

5. Too little is yet understood of the relationship between age and the incidence of liver metastases to justify a convincing, theoretical explanation.

REFERENCES

1. **Walther, H. E.,** *Krebsmetastasen,* Benno Schwabe, Basel, 1948, 55.
2. **Pack, G. T. and Islami, A. H.,** Metastatic cancer to and from the liver, in *Tumors of the Liver, Recent Results in Cancer Research 26,* Pack, G. T. and Islami, A. H., Eds., Springer-Verlag, Berlin, 1970, 72.
3. **Kellner, B.,** *Die Ausbreitung des Krebses,* Akadémiai Kiadó, Budapest, 1977, 140.
4. **Viadana, E., Bross, I. D. J., and Pickren, J. W.,** The metastatic spread of cancers of the digestive system in man, *Oncology,* 35, 114, 1978.
5. **Clark, R. L.,** Systemic cancer and the metastatic process, *Cancer,* 43, 790, 1979.
6. **Pejchl, S., Pejchlová, J., and Chaloupka, F.,** Relationship of age and sex to the incidence of liver metastases in malignant tumors (in Czech), *Vnitr. Lek.,* 27, 1073, 1981.
7. **Pejchl, S., Chaloupka, F., and Krivohlavy, A.,** A contribution to the problem of metastases from malignant tumors into cirrhotic liver (in Czech), *Vnitr. Lek.,* 24, 338, 1978.
8. **Pejchl, S. and Chaloupka, F.,** The relationship between the blood-groups ABO and Rh factor and the frequency of malignant liver metastases (in Czech), *Cesk. Gastroenterol. Vyz.,* 35, 105, 1981.
9. **Berndt, R. and Berndt, H.,** Inzidenz und Mortalität an bösartigen Neubildungen in der DDR, *Dtsch. Gesundheitswes.,* 34, 268, 1979.
10. **Noltenius, H. and Tetzner, C.,** Vorkommen, Metastasen und natürlicher Verlauf von behandelten und unbehandelten malignen Tumoren bei über 70 Jahre alten Patienten, *Onkologie,* 7, 100, 1984.
11. **Howel, T. H. and Piggot, A. P.,** Morbid anatomy of old age, *Geriatrics,* 6, 85, 1951.
12. **Lake, B.,** Morbid conditions at death in old men, *J. Chron. Dis.,* 21, 761, 1969.
13. **Bengmark, S. and Hafström, L.,** The natural history of primary and secondary malignant tumors of the liver. I. Prognosis for patients with hepatic metastases from colonic and rectal carcinoma by laparotomy, *Cancer,* 23, 198, 1969.
14. **Auerbach, C., Garfinkel, L., and Parks, V. R.,** Histologic type of lung cancer in relation to smoking habits, year of diagnosis and sites of metastases, *Chest,* 67, 382, 1975.
15. **Kalny, J., Pejchl, S., Cholt, M., Zárubová, V., and Zuntová, A.,** Transumbilical administration of cytostatics into the portal circulation in liver tumors (in Czech), *Cesk. Gastroenterol. Vyz.,* 33, 200, 1979.
16. **Barz, H. and Barz, D.,** Altersabhängigkeit der Metastasierung. Eine Untersuchung an über 5000 Karzinomtodesfällen, *Arch. Geschwulstforsch.,* 54, 77, 1984.
17. **Langsch, H. G. and Uhlig, M.,** Carcinommetastasierung in verschiedenem Lebensalter, *Z. Krebsforsch.,* 63, 575, 1960.
18. **Zschoch, H. and Kober, B.,** Sektionsstatistische Untersuchungen zur Metastasierung des Bronchialkarzinoms, *Arch. Geschwulstforsch.,* 30, 126, 1967.
19. **Bengmark, S. and Hafström, L.,** The natural history of primary and secondary malignant tumors of the liver. II. The prognosis for patients with hepatic metastases from gastric carcinoma verified by laparotomy and post-mortem examination, *Digestion,* 2, 179, 1969.
20. **Sakamoto, M.,** Differential metastatic mode of gastric cancer by age and histological type (in Japanese), *Nippon Geka Gakkai Zasshi,* 88, 440, 1987.

Chapter 18

THE EFFECT OF AGING ON THE DEVELOPMENT AND PROGRESSION OF CANCER: FROM THE LABORATORY ANIMAL TO THE CLINIC

Paul R. Kaesberg and William B. Ershler

TABLE OF CONTENTS

As a result of the aging trend in industrialized populations and the increased incidence of cancer with advancing age, the problem of cancer in the elderly will become increasingly more apparent. Nevertheless, many clinicians have misunderstandings regarding the development and progression of cancer in the elderly and these may result in incorrect or inadequate clinical management. This chapter aims to examine the biology of cancer in aging, beginning with sentinel observations in the laboratory animal and then examining how these observations relate to clinical findings of cancer in the elderly.

For cancer as a whole, and for many specific cancers, advanced age is the single greatest risk factor.[1] The concept that the immune system eliminates "early" cancers (immune surveillance theory), combined with the currently well-defined age-associated decline in cellular immune competence of humans and all other mammalian species, implies that an increased incidence of cancer is, at least in part, due to immune senescence. Extending this idea, one might predict that once cancers become clinically evident, they might be more aggressive in hosts of advanced age. However, it has been our experience that in many instances, the opposite is true; that is, the presence of a competent immune system often confers a distinct disadvantage to the tumor bearing animal. These observations, combined with several others, have raised doubt regarding the immune surveillance theory. Alternate theories have been developed explaining the increased incidence of cancer in the elderly, and these are explored briefly below.

Of considerable interest are the observations made in laboratory animals of the unexpected beneficial effects to the host of immune senescence on the progression of certain transplanted tumors. The elucidation of the underlying mechanisms for the restrained growth of tumors in old animals may ultimately lead to improvement in the clinician's ability to control cancer in both young and old patients.

I. THE USEFULNESS OF ANIMAL MODELS IN THE STUDY OF TUMOR BIOLOGY

The use of animal models has clearly expanded our knowledge of tumor biology by allowing experimentation that would not be possible in humans. Nevertheless, it has brought with it its own set of problems, not the least of which is the degree of relevance a tumor model may have to an analogous human tumor. It should be realized that a given tumor model may be relevant to human tumors only in very limited aspects. It is therefore necessary to choose a tumor model carefully, based on a specific question to which an answer is sought.

The development of identical syngeneic rodents, by continued inbreeding, has been a major advance in the study of tumor biology. As compared to human studies or to studies on noninbred animals, it allows the use of sufficiently large numbers of animals in a given experiment to give statistically significant results, while eliminating confounding variables that occur from genetic variability within an experimental subgroup, and allows the transplantation of tumors from animal to animal (or culture dish to animal) without immunologic rejection due to allogeneic antigens. Rejection may still occur via nonallogeneic mechanisms.

While other mammalian species are similar to humans in many ways, especially with regard to the senescence of the cellular immune system, the differences must be considered when comparing experimental animal results to humans. The human life span is an order of magnitude greater than that of the typical rodent. How this may relate to the biology of aging is not fully appreciated. Inbreeding seems to have minimal deleterious effects on these animals, however, subtle effects may alter tumor biology in ways not yet determined. Other concerns regarding transplanted tumors also need to be considered. For example, when a tumor is implanted into an otherwise healthy animal, that animal has not been exposed to the original carcinogen that induced the tumor. Because a human tumor bearing host would have had that exposure, there may be differences in tumor biology.

Better methods of culturing tumors *in vitro* have led to the ability to implant tumor lines that are genetically identical into animals with much greater ease than if tumors had to be transplanted directly from animal to animal. It also allows the dissemination of identical, well-characterized tumor lines among laboratories for further study. There are again problems that can occur with the study of the biology of cultured tumor lines after injection into animals. Most experimental tumors in animals are induced by irradiation or carcinogens, while most human tumors appear to be spontaneous or induced by carcinogens at a much lower level of exposure. Thus, while the cell type may be similar, human and animal tumors may differ in antigenicity, hormonal receptors, growth characteristics, site of origin, and oncogene activation.

Cell lines grown in culture are, by their very nature, selected to grow well in culture, while human tumor cells in the body are selected to grow well *in vivo*. Cells grown in culture may pick up allogeneic antigens on their surface from the combination of synthetic tissue culture medium and serum in which the cells are grown. This, in turn, may affect the immunologic characteristics of the cells. Because of the ease in working with cultured cell lines, they are used almost to the exclusion of directly transplanted tumors, but the limitations listed above must be considered. The use of human tumor xenografts transplanted into athymic nude mice has overcome some of these limitations, but of course, this system does not allow the investigation of the competent immune system on tumor progression. Most epithelial tumor lines can be grown only by transplantation from animal to animal. This has been a major drawback to their study, and is especially problematic because most human tumors are of epithelial origin.

II. CELLULAR IMMUNITY DECLINES WITH AGE

Cellular immune senescence can be defined as a progressive mild to moderate decline in several cellular immune functions that occurs in all mammalian species coincident with the onset of sexual maturation. It is unrelated to underlying illness, but predisposes to various infectious diseases, such as tuberculosis, influenza, and reactivation of Varicella-Zoster, and has been thought to predispose to neoplastic diseases such as endemic Kaposi's sarcoma. Whether immune senescence predisposes to other tumors whose incidence increases with age is subject to debate.

The progression of cellular immune senescence appears to relate to the involution of the thymus gland that, in humans, begins at puberty and is complete by age 45 to 50. The thymus gland retains only about 10% of its prepubertal weight beyond the age of 50.[2] What thymic epithelium remains may lose the ability to cause T-cell differentiation.[3-5] Levels of thymic hormones are undetectable by age 60.[6] Several changes in the immune system with age have been reasonably well documented. These include reduction or loss of delayed cutaneous hypersensitivity,[7] decreased proliferative response of T-cells to mitogens[8-12] or antigens such as Varicella-Zoster Virus antigen,[13] decreased proliferative response to IL-2,[14] possibly secondary to inability of these cells to express high affinity IL-2 receptor,[15] reduction in IL-2 production by T-cells, and decrease in cytotoxic T-cell[16-17] and natural killer cell number and function.

Caloric restriction appears to delay or slow the progression of immune senescence in rodent models.[18] These studies need to be done in primates or humans to better evaluate their relevance. Thymic hormone administration may enhance immune function, one study showing enhancement of sheep red blood cell rosette formation, lymphocyte number and immunoglobulins, as well as decreased infections[6] and another showing enhancement of antibody response to influenza vaccine.[18]

III. IMMUNE SENESCENCE IS NOT THE MAJOR CAUSE OF THE INCREASED INCIDENCE OF CANCER WITH AGING

The immune surveillance theory, as advanced by Thomas[19] and Good[20] states that the immune system eliminates malignant cells soon after their development. It has been proposed that perhaps more than 1 million cells become "malignant" over a person's lifetime, but the development of clinical cancer occurs only rarely, and represents a breakdown in the ability of the immune system to control the cancer. While one might suppose that several aspects of the immune system might be involved, it is the cellular immune system that has been thought to play the most important role.

Natural killer (NK) cells are able to destroy certain tumor cells independently of the major histocompatability (MHC) antigens on the cell surface.[21-24] The MHC antigens are involved in antigen presentation, therefore, it is assumed that NK cells can kill susceptible targets independently of antigenic stimulation, possibly via an "NK receptor" on tumor cells.[25,26] NK cells are known to kill cells without prior sensitization to them or their antigens. NK cells may act primarily on blood-borne cells and can act to inhibit experimental metastasis.[27-30] This was particularly well illustrated in an experiment where Fisher F344 rats were treated with rabbit anti-asialo GM_1 antiserum which specifically inhibits NK activity, preserving cytotoxic T-cell activity.[31] These rats developed greater than tenfold more metastases than rats treated with normal rabbit serum, after i.v. injection with a syngeneic mammary adenocarcinoma MADB106. This tumor was induced by dimethylbenzanthracene, and would therefore be expected to be immunogenic (see Section V). When radiolabeled tumor cells were used, there was a 6- to 7-fold increase in radioactivity retention in the lungs at 2 h in rats treated with anti-asialo GM_1 at doses that enhanced metastasis, but also a 4-fold enhancement in lung retention of radioactivity in rats treated with doses of anti-asialo GM_1 that did not enhance metastasis. Enhancement of metastasis in anti-asialo GM_1 treated rats could be reversed by treatment with large granular lymphocytes (a lymphocyte fraction high in NK activity) but not by treatment with T-cells. In a separate experiment, depletion of NK-cells in C57B1/6 mice by monoclonal antibody NK-1.1 increased the metastatic potential of B16 melanoma and CT38 colon carcinoma.[32]

Cytotoxic T-lymphocytes are involved in killing cells which express foreign antigens on their surface and also have identical MHC antigens.[33] They are therefore able to kill only cells with analogous MHC class II antigens as themselves (so-called "MHC-restricted killing"). They require prior sensitization. Their main function is probably in the killing of virus-infected cells that express viral antigens on their surfaces, but many examples of antitumor effects of cytotoxic T-lymphocytes exist, some of which will be described in Section VI. Many human tumors exhibit greatly reduced cell surface MHC class I antigens.[34]

Lymphokine-activated killer (LAK) cells and tumor-infiltrating lymphocytes (TILs) are recently discovered cells with potent tumor killing activity. Their significance *in vivo* is yet undetermined. LAK cells can kill both fresh and cultured tumor cells that are resistant to NK cell killing.[35,36] TILs may be cytotoxic T-cells that are specific for the tumor they are infiltrating.[37,38]

Thus, it can be demonstrated that active antitumor cell-mediated immunity does exist in humans. It has also been noted above that cellular immunity declines with age. Why then do we believe that immune senescence is not the major cause of increased incidence of cancer in the elderly?

Certain types of tumors develop in persons who are immunosuppressed. This immunosuppression must be severe, such as in patients treated with the potent immunosuppressive agent, cyclosporine,[39] which inhibits T-cell activation at several levels, but especially at early stages of activation, and in persons infected with the human immunodeficiency virus (HIV) which infects and destroys T-helper cell function.[40] The range of tumors that occur with greater frequency include aggressive B-cell lymphomas, many of which are related to infection with Epstein-Barr virus, a transforming herpesvirus, and Kaposi's sarcoma, a rare disease prior to the HIV epidemic.[41-44] While Kaposi's sarcoma is more common in elderly persons, the disease is different in this population. In the elderly, it is slow growing and relatively benign, whereas in HIV-infected persons it is aggressive and widely metastatic. EBV-related lymphomas are uncommon to rare in elderly populations. The spectrum of increased tumors in elderly persons is quite different, and includes colon, lung, prostate, and breast cancer.[1] This difference in tumor spectrum is one major argument against immune senescence as a cause of cancer.

Experimental animal models for cancer reveal that for highly antigenic tumors, immune suppression is a disadvantage, but for poorly antigenic tumors, which most closely resemble the majority of human tumors, immune suppression is not necessarily disadvantageous and is, in fact, probably advantageous. These experiments are discussed in detail later. The fact that most human tumors are only weakly immunogenic or not immunogenic at all is a second piece of evidence to argue against immune senescence as a cause of cancer.

Penn, in a review of immunodeficiency and the development of cancer,[45] summarizes animal data to say that transplantation of malignant cells is easier (more is said on this later), and metastatic growth is accelerated, in immunodeficient animals. Viral oncogenesis is often enhanced. Effects on chemical oncogenesis are unclear and spontaneous tumors do not occur more frequently in immune-deficient animals.

It is unlikely that the immune system would be very effective on small tumor burdens (such as a small clone of a newly developed tumor) if it is ineffective against larger tumor burdens. Small antigenic loads initiate small immune responses and will even condition the immune system to tolerate that antigen.[46] Small inocula of highly immunogenic tumors can occasionally escape immune destruction by the induction of tolerance whereas larger inocula may not.[47] Therefore, the argument that the immune system may be functional against early tumors even if it is not evident in established tumors may not be valid (but see examples in Section VI).

IV. IF NOT IMMUNE SENESCENCE, THEN WHAT CAUSES THE INCREASED INCIDENCE OF CANCER WITH AGING?

There are multiple potential causes for increased tumor incidence with aging, all of which probably play some role. Carcinogens appear to have different effects on old and young animals. Hormonal milieus may alter with age. Long latency periods or slow growth of some tumors may only allow them to present clinically at an advanced age even when induction of the tumors has occurred at a young age.

The most likely of these possibilities, in many cases, is the effect of carcinogens in advanced age. Obviously, as people or animals age, there is prolonged exposure to multiple potential environmental carcinogens, nitrosamines, aflatoxins, or other food-born carcinogens, UV and other types of irradiation, chemicals or mutagens found in the home or workplace, cigarettes or tobacco in other forms, and viral carcinogens. While this could manifest in cancer on a random basis as a single effective "hit" on a cell, prolonged or multiple exposure may be required for some tumors.[48,49] The initiator/promoter theory of carcinogenesis states that an initial event "initiates" carcinogenesis, but that multiple, subsequent qualitatively different events "promote" the already initiated cell to form a tumor.[50,51] These promoter effects may be due to multiple exposures to carcinogenic agents. It has been clearly shown that multiple events are needed in cellular transformation by carcinogens and even by some highly oncogenic retroviruses.[52] These multiple steps could include activation of multiple oncogenes, sequential changes that enhance expression of a single oncogene, sequential inactivation of both copies of an anti-oncogene, or other mechanisms. Therefore, multiple random mutations by carcinogens may be absolutely essential for cancer formation.

There may also be enhanced effects of carcinogens on animals with advanced age. Metabolic inactivation of carcinogens via cytochrome P-450 and NADP-cytochrome P-reductase may be impaired with advancing age, as demonstrated by levels of these enzymes in aged vs. young rat livers.[53] While these systems may detoxify active carcinogens, they may also activate carcinogens, muddying the water substantially.

DNA repair appears to be impaired with aging. It was thought that accumulation of DNA damage might acually be a (or perhaps, the) cause of aging,[54] and suppor was seen in data on DNA repair in fibroblasts of species with different life spans. Longer-living species had better DNA repair capacity of *in vitro* cells post-UV irradiation, and this observation was made in a wide range of species,[55] including primates.[56] Data showing lack of correlation also exist.[57-58]

One problem with these studies is when to test the cells. Should all test animals be the same age, or relative age with regard to their life span, or somewhere inbetween?

Many reports show that DNA repair capacity declines in cells taken from aging animals or humans, including human peripheral blood lymphocytes after UV irradiation[59,60] and aging rat hepatocytes after UV irradiation.[61,62] Again, conflicting data exist.[63,64]

The data on the influence of aging on development of tumors after carcinogen exposure are so scattered as to be almost uninterpretable (see Reference 65 for review), but some specifics can be determined. It appears that there may be an increased susceptibility of skin to carcinogens (for example, to DMBA[66,67]), while breast tissue may show a decrease. Other tissues are somewhat more variable. Possible reasons for such scatter are different carcinogens having different actions, different metabolic pathways of activation or inactivation, different dosing schedules (amount, or acute vs. chronic administration), difference in animal species, or by chance hitting a particularly sensitive or insensitive portion of the animal life cycle.

Certain drugs or other manipulations thought to affect the aging process may affect tumor incidence. Antioxidants are thought to work directly to inhibit the effects of carcinogens.[67] Studies have been mixed as to whether they can reduce tumor occurrence.[68-71] Caloric restriction or treatment with thymic factors, which appear to have wide ranging metabolic effects on aging animals, including partial restoration of cellular immune defects, can cause a decrease in tumor incidence in experimental animals.[72-76]

Alterations in hormonal milieu with aging may play some role in increased tumor incidence, however, this has not been documented. Some possibilities might include tumors of cells responsive to follicle stimulating hormone (FSH) or lutenizing hormone (LH), hormones which increase dramatically in women after menopause, and in men more gradually with advancing age. Also, decreases in testosterone levels or estrogen/progesterone levels may promote some tumors, but this seems less unlikely. Other "physiologic" hormonal changes with age such as diminished insulin response to glucose load or diminished thyroid responsiveness would seem unlikely to be related to cancer incidence. One argument against this proposal is the age-related increased incidence of tumors responsive to hormones that decline with age, such as prostate carcinoma and estrogen receptor positive breast carcinoma.

The possible effect of long latency periods or slowly growing tumors on increased incidence in the elderly is illustrated in Figure 1. Note how a slowly growing tumor or a tumor with a long latency period would present later in life even if the carcinogenic event occurred early in life. Note also that this is one possible explanation for the slower growth of tumors in older animals or humans.

V. IMMUNE SENESCENCE IS IMPORTANT: TUMORS GROW MORE SLOWLY IN OLD ANIMALS

The B16 murine melanoma tumor injected subcutaneously or intravenously into the C57B1/6 mouse is one of the most studied tumor models. This tumor has the advantages of having occurred spontaneously and of being very weakly immunogenic, features typical of human malignancies. The C57B1/6 mouse, the source of B16 melanoma, is an excellent experimental animal of aging studies. It is a highly inbred strain in which growth and longevity characteristics are well known. The life expectancy of these animals is nearly rectangular with most mice dying in a 3-month period surrounding their 26th month of life. For these reasons, our laboratory chose B16 melanoma and the C57B1/6 strain as the model for our early investigations of the effect of host age on tumor growth and spread. Where this model was not used, comparisons and contrasts to this model will be indicated.

There is a correlation between spontaneous occurrence of a tumor and lack of immunogenicity, and between virus or chemical carcinogen-induced tumors and strong immunogenicity. Prehn and Main[77] showed in 1957 that mice immunized against spontaneous tumors showed

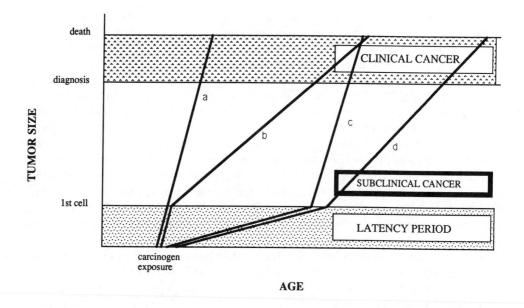

FIGURE 1. Four clinical situations: (a) Fast growing tumor, short latency. Presents at early age as aggressive tumor. (b) Slow growing tumor, short latency. Presents at mid-life as relatively benign tumor. (c) Fast growing tumor, long latency. Presents at mid-life as aggressive tumor. (d) Slow growing tumor, long latency period. Presents late in life as relatively benign tumor.

weak or absent response to a challenge inoculum of the tumor (i.e, growth is identical in immunized and nonimmunized mice), while animals immunized against 3-methylcholanthrene (MCA) induced tumors are often highly resistant to growth of the same tumor. This immunity is tumor specific (i.e., not cross reactive between tumors).

In an early experiment, B16 melanoma F10 cells, a subline developed by Fidler,[78] were injected subcutaneously into young (2 months) or old (24 months) mice, 10^5 cells per animal.[79] The tumor grew more slowly (at 26 d, vol. 3.5 cm^3 for young and 1.0-3.5 cm^3 for old) in old mice. Survival was slightly longer in older mice but all mice died near 30 to 35 d. Tumor volume at death in old mice was about 40% of what it was in young mice. After i.v. injection of 10^5 B16 F1 cells (also from Fidler[78]) into C57B1/6 mice, old mice developed fewer pulmonary colonies (mean = 6) than young mice (mean = 29) at 14 d. Survival was also substantially longer in old mice. Ninety percent of young mice were dead by 45 d, at which time all the old mice were alive. Three of the ten old mice survived the tumor challenge. Median survivals were 32 d for young and 63 d for old animals.

Lewis lung carcinoma, injected into the flank of C57B1/6 mice gives similar results. Tumor growth is approximately 50% as fast in old compared to young mice and final tumor volume in old mice was about 33% that of young mice.[80] The number of tumors that develop after injection of Lewis lung carcinoma was found to be different, with 100% of 24-month-old, 90% of 10-month-old, and 70% of 2-month-old mice developing tumors.[81] No report on the growth rate of tumors was given. Lewis lung carcinoma differs from B16 melanoma in its difficulty in being maintained in culture, and by being an epithelial tumor instead of a mesenchymal tumor. It also arose spontaneously in C57B1/6 mice.[82]

Two other experimental tumors have been shown to have decreased growth rate with advanced age: teratocarcinoma OTT60-50 in 129/Sv mice,[83] and line 1 alveolar carcinoma in BALB/c mice.[84] The last study is especially important because of the correlative studies (actually the main point of the paper) that were performed on immunosuppression and growth of the tumor.

Teratocarcinoma OTT60-50 arose after embryo transplantation into the testis of an F1 hybrid mouse.[85] Compared to B16, it is a transplantable tumor, but cannot be grown in culture. It can be passaged by intraperitoneal injection where it develops a form similar to a 5-d embryo. Because of its sensitivity to host environments, it is considered a good model to study host-tumor relationships.[83] Tumor doubling time in mice was 2.1 d for juvenile (2- to 3-week-old) mice and 3.0 d for adult (10- to 30-week-old) mice. Adult and old (50- to 70-week-old) mice did not differ. When eliminating mice that died of old age, survival time after tumors reached 100 mm³ increased linearly with age.

Line 1 alveolar cell carcinoma is a tumor that arose spontaneously in a BALB/c female mouse.[84] It was studied for tumor growth rate in old animals and immunosuppressed animals. The growth rate of the tumor decreased linearly with age in BALB/c mice from 8 to 28 months of age. Growth rate at 4 months was similar to that at 20 months and greater than that at 28 months. Immunosuppression of 3-month-old BALB/c mice by 500 rad γ-irradiation or by injection of hydrocortisone also suppressed tumor growth rate without changing the tumor take.[84]

There are notable exceptions to decreased tumor growth rate with advanced age. Tumor 1591, induced by repeated exposure of a mouse to UV light, is more likely to form a progressively growing tumor in 10-month-old C3H/HeN mice than 6-month-old mice. Two-month-old mice do not form tumors after inoculation of this tumor.[86] CMCA V is a tumor derived from a male CBA mouse treated with MCA. Growth rates for this tumor in CBA mice are lowest in 3- or 6-month-old mice and higher in 1- or 10-month-old mice. The highest growth rate was seen in 15- and 22-month-old mice or very young mice. UV light- and MCA-induced tumors share the property of having specific highly immunogenic tumor antigens on their surfaces, and therefore differ from B16 melanoma. EMT6 is a mouse mammary tumor virus-induced mammary carcinoma syngeneic to BALB/c KaRw mice.[87] Similar to the MCA-induced tumors, the tumor grew slowest in young adult mice, with faster growth in old and weanling mice. Again, virus-induced tumors often display surface tumor-associated antigens, differing from B16 melanoma. P815 mastocytoma caused a higher mortality in old BALB/c (H2-d) mice than in young mice.[88] This tumor was derived from a different strain of mouse that had H2-d at its MHC locus. It is unknown how immunogenic this tumor is in BALB/c mice.

MC-26 murine colon adenocarcinoma was injected into the flank of weanling, 3- to 4-week-old or 20- to 22-month-old BALB/c, at 10⁴ cells per mouse.[89] In this experiment, the 3- to 4-week-old mice had the greatest resistance to tumor development. Median time to development of a tumor was 37 d, while the 20- to 22-month-old mice had a median of 25 d and the weanling mice, 9 d. Of 3- to 4- week-old mice, 73% developed tumors, while 92% of old mice and 100% of weanling mice developed tumors. Once tumors developed, survival was the same for all age groups. When a higher inoculum of tumor cells was used, these differences disappeared. The differences demonstrated in this model are curious because mice of 3 to 4 weeks are not fully immunocompetent,[90] and in fact may be less competent than 20- to 22- month-old BALB/c mice, which is an age that is several months younger than the median survival for that strain.

How can these results be summarized? Some models show a slower growth of tumors in older animals, whereas some others show a faster, more malignant growth. While data remains somewhat conflicting, it appears that the strongly immunogenic tumors have a growth advantage in older animals, while more poorly antigenic tumors may have a growth advantage in younger animals (Figure 2). The underlying mechanism for this is most probably related to senescence of the immune system. Before exploring immune senescence, some alternatives will be considered.

Hormonal factors influence the growth of B16 melanoma.[91-93] The proposal that decreased testosterone levels may be the cause of decreased B16 growth in old mice was excluded by results showing that B16 had an increased growth rate in castrated young mice.[91] This does, however, reveal the importance of considering hormonal influences in tumor models other than ones traditionally thought to be hormonally responsive tumors.

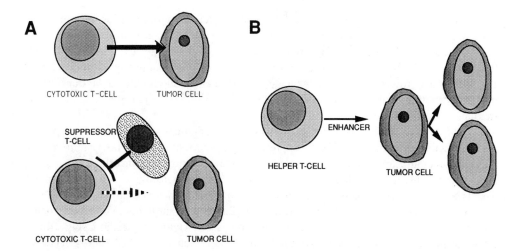

FIGURE 2. Two possible mechanisms of immunologic enhancement of tumor growth: (A) Suppressor T-cell inhibition of anti-tumor immunity. (B) Helper T-cell production of tumor mitogenic or enhancer molecules.

Nutritional factors may be important, as aging in mice brings about dietary changes such as decreased total food consumption while gaining weight.[94] Dietary changes, especially calorie restriction, may have profound effects on the aging immune system. In mice, a 30% reduction in calories leads to a delay in immune senescence[95] and prolonged survival.[96] The effects of this on tumor growth and spread are as yet incompletely determined. We have previously reported that B16 melanoma grows more slowly in calorie restricted mice,[97] and it is possible that the beneficial effects of undernutrition, which might occur spontaneously in old mice, might actually account for some of the observed "age-advantage" in certain of these models.

The ability of the body to heal wounds is decreased with age.[98] Wound healing shares many characteristics of tumor growth and spread: cell localization with specific receptors, mitogenesis, tissue invasion, angiogenesis, and extracellular matrix deposition. Changes in these factors with age may result in changes in tumor growth. Collagens are known to change with age, mainly demonstrating increased crosslinking[99] without primary sequence alteration.[100] Fibrosis surrounding B16 melanoma implants is enhanced in old mice.[79] All of these "alternative" mechanisms deserve further study. What we are considering below, however, is how the immune system may act to enhance as well as inhibit the growth of tumors.

VI. THE IMMUNE SYSTEM CAN STIMULATE TUMOR GROWTH

While under some circumstances the immune system can function as an inhibitor of tumor growth, there are certainly cases in which the immune system is not effective. The varied response perhaps reflects the degree of tumor antigenicity, but this does not mean that the immune system has no effect on poorly immunogenic tumors.

Prehn initially hypothesized that a weak immunologic reaction to a tumor may stimulate its growth. He showed that tumor cells injected into immunosuppressed mice grew better if injected along with specifically immune spleen cells, compared to when injected alone, or with normal or nonspecifically immune spleen cells.[102] Thymus-derived (theta positive) cells were found to be the cells that stimulated Lewis lung carcinoma growth in irradiated, thymectomized, or intact C57B1/6 mice. [103] These T-cells had been sensitized to syngeneic fibroblasts. Similar findings were seen when spleen cells from C3H mice were sensitized with syngeneic fibrosarcoma cells. The autosensitized spleen cells increased fibrosarcoma growth. They did not increase Lewis lung carcinoma (a tumor that is not syngeneic to C3H mice, therefore not having similar antigens to the fibroblasts to which the T-cells were sensitized) growth in C3H mice, suggesting that growth stimulation was by sensitization of the lymphocytes to determinants on the tumor rather than by causing a nonspecific action on the host to increase tumor growth.

B16 melanoma also grows more slowly in mice previously subjected to thymectomy.[104] Prior thymectomy and subsequent treatment with anti-theta (anti-T-cell) antiserum further decreased B16 melanoma growth. The "age-advantage" in B16 melanoma growth can be transferred to young mice either by the transfer of old spleen cells[104] or old bone marrow cells[80] to lethally irradiated, thymectomized young recipients.

The most studied mechanism that seems to be active in immune-competent hosts to promote tumor growth is the tumor-specific T-suppressor cell. When splenic lymphocytes from MCA-induced sarcoma-bearing mice are injected into mice immunized against these tumors, they again become susceptible to lethal tumor growth.[105,106] The responsible cells were shown to be T-cells bearing surface markers of a suppressor phenotype as shown by elimination of the tumor promoting effects of these cells by treatment of mice either with antithymocyte serum[107] or anti-I-J alloantiserum, specific for an antigen on suppressor T-lymphocytes.[108] Using a highly immunogenic methylcholanthrene-induced fibrosarcoma (Meth A) in BALB/c mice, it has been shown that T-cells from immunized mice are not able to mediate rejection when injected into tumor-bearing, immunologically intact mice, but were able to mediate tumor rejection when injected into mice rendered immune deficient by irradiation and thymectomy.[109] When the immune-deficient mice were pretreated with T-cells from tumor-bearing mice, the immune T-cells were unable to mediate tumor rejection. These results suggest that T-cells from tumor-bearing mice suppress anti-tumor activity.

Our laboratory has explored this phenomenon with B16 melanoma, finding that the tumor grew faster in mice injected with spleen cells from tumor-bearing mice than mice injected with normal mouse spleen cells.[110] Cell depletion studies showed that tumor enhancement occurred even when T-helper or T-suppressor cells were depleted.

Splenic cells from tumor-bearing mice enhanced the development of methylcholanthrene- or benzpyrene-induced fibrosarcomas or Lewis lung carcinoma after injection.[111] When fractionated by sedimentation, large cells mediated tumor growth enhancement, while smaller cells mediated tumor growth inhibition. Mixtures of fractions showed only the effect of tumor growth-enhancing cells. These cells may be immature thymocytes, for thymus-derived cells that cause enhancement of Lewis lung carcinoma growth can be matured with thymic humoral factor, which causes T-cell maturation, after which they lose their enhancing activity.[112]

In the Lewis lung carcinoma model, initial T-cell response to the tumor was found to be protective (in seeming contrast to the proposal of Stillstrom,[46] described in Section III) but later was stimulatory.[113] It was found that the T-cells from Lewis lung carcinoma-bearing mice also produced a soluble factor that enhance the growth of this and other tumors.[114] This factor (or factors) is a small (less than 70,000 mol. wt.) molecule and its activity is destroyed by proteolytic enzymes. It appears not to be an immunoglobulin. Antigenically, it is similar to a portion of the MHC complex of the mouse.[115]

Suppressor cells also form in DBA/2 mice bearing syngeneic mastocytoma. These suppressor cells direct their activity against the formation of cytotoxic T-cells. They can be eliminated by anti-T-cell (anti-theta) antiserum and can be separated from NK cell activity-bearing cells by density gradient sedimentation.[116,117]

There is also evidence of suppressor cell activity in humans with cancer. For example, in a patient with melanoma, peripheral blood lymphocytes, and lymphocytes from a tumor-infiltrated lymph node were examined for *in vitro* effects on autologous tumor cells.[118,119] A cytotoxic response against the melanoma cell line could be established from autologous peripheral blood lymphocytes if they were co-cultured with the melanoma cell line, but not from lymphocytes from the tumor-bearing lymph node. Addition of mixed lymphocytes, or CD4 or CD8 enriched lymph node lymphocytes to peripheral blood lymphocytes, blocked the induction of a cytotoxic response to the melanoma cell line. This suppression was specific, at least to the extent that it did not inhibit reaction to allogeneic antigens. Further studies showed that lymphocytes from an uninvolved lymph node also inhibited the cytotoxic response. To achieve full suppressor activity, cells needed antigen presentation *in vitro* followed by expansion with interleukin-2. This suppressor activity was also found in cells from a tumor-bearing lymph node form a patient with a paraganglioma.[120] The suppressor activity was not effective in suppressing reactivity to an allogeneic tumor line. The suppressor cells carried a CD8 phenotype.

Cytotoxic and suppressor T-cells can be differentially activated in a manner that is consistent with above results.[121] Cytotoxic T-cell activity is induced by mitomycin C treated live cells that do not proliferate. Suppressor cells can be generated with soluble tumor extracts. The suppressor cells generated in this manner were specific to individual tumors and had surface determinants controlled by the I-J subregion of the mouse MHC complex. Live tumor cells inhibited cytotoxic T-cell activity, but not suppressor activity, *in vitro*.

Suppressor cells that inhibit cytotoxic T-cell responses appear to be generated as a response to tumor cells in spontaneously occurring tumors, as seen in the examples described above. In carcinogen-induced tumor, suppressor T-cell responses may be generated by the carcinogen. Repeated exposure of mice to UV light induces suppressor cells that are effective *in vivo* against the general class of UV light-induced tumors.[122] These suppressor cells act to inhibit immunity against UV light-induced tumor. This inhibition appears to result from the blocking of the generation of T-helper cells. This effect is not seen *in vitro*.

Macrophages may also act as suppressor cells in MCA-induced fibrosarcoma-bearing BALB/c mice.[123] Macrophage induced suppression of tumor immunity required a much greater number of cells than anti-theta sensitive suppressor activity.

These examples show that the regulatory functions of the immune system are capable of suppressing antitumor immunity and, in this way, may promote tumor growth. Tumor-bearing animals are especially likely to have suppressor cells that inhibit immunity directed at that particular tumor, which overwhelms previously developed antitumor immunity. Often it appears that the antigens that cytotoxic and suppressor cells are reacting to are different, with cytotoxic cells reacting to cell surface antigens, and suppressor cells reacting to soluble shed antigens. If this proposal were to have validity in models of poorly antigenic tumors, then despite the relative lack of antigenicity, antitumor immunity must exist. Indeed, there is evidence that such immunity does exist, even to the poorly immunogenic B16 melanoma,[110] and that tumor growth does indeed occur via escape from this immunity via tumor-antigen induced suppressor activity during its normal growth pattern in the C57B1/6 mouse.[124]

A second mechanism by which the immune system may enhance the growth of tumors is via the production of tumor stimulating factors by immune competent T-cells. This mechanism would not necessarily require that the tumor be antigenic, however, a slightly antigenic tumor may recruit T-cells that enhance its growth without inducing a lytic reaction by the T-cells. One of the mechanisms may be via lymphocyte-induced angiogenesis (LIA). As tumors grow, they require the formation of new blood vessels for nourishment. It has been proposed that tumors produce an angiogenic factor themselves,[125] and this is almost certainly true of at least some tumors. Tumors may also be able to trick the immune system into inducing new vessels for it. LIA was first described in 1975 as an allogeneically mediated induction of new blood vessel formation by Lyt 1 + 2,3-T-lymphocytes injected subcutaneously into mice.[126,127] This reaction, as first described, was mainly active when injected cells differed at the H2 locus of the MHC of the mouse but some non-H2 differences also were involved. Because of this, it was described as a manifestation of the graft vs. host response. The authors proposed, however, that this may be an explanation for restricted tumor growth that was seen in nude mice, whose lymphocytes do not induce this phenomenon. It was later shown that *in vitro* activated lymphocytes could be reinjected into a syngeneic animal and induce angiogenesis,[128,129] showing that GVH is not necessary for LIA. Probably several molecules are involved in this activity and likely they will turn out to be growth factors such as basic fibroblast growth factor.[130] LIA activity has been

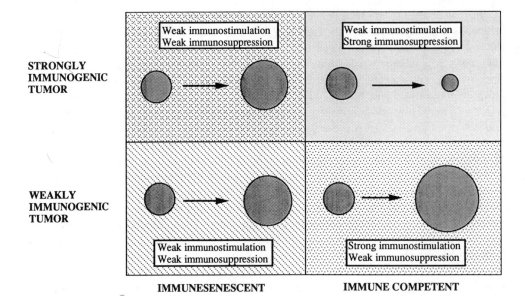

FIGURE 3. Effects of the senescence of the immune system on tumor growth: in immune senescent hosts, strongly immunogenic tumors and weakly immunogenic tumors have identical growth characteristics, because of the absence of immune suppressing or immune stimulating factors. In immune competent hosts, strongly immunogenic tumors are rejected by immune suppressing factors, while weakly immunogenic tumors are enhanced by immune stimulating factors.

shown to decline with age.[131] Figure 3 illustrates our interpretation of how intact and senescent immune systems affect the growth of strongly and weakly immunogenic tumors.

VII. CORRELATIONS WITH CLINICAL FINDINGS OF CANCER IN AGING HUMANS

Studying the human system is generally more difficult than studying a well-controlled animal system. All patients with a given disease are not necessarily comparable. Cancers of the same histologic appearance may have diverse etiologies and different clinical expressions. Is this due to the cancer or to the host reaction to the cancer? Defense systems may be altered by physical illnesses or their treatments, or by environmental exposures that differ from person to person, or, of course, by age.

Two large studies have been performed examining the stage of tumors at presentation in relationship to age.[132,133] Both found that breast, cervical, endometrial, ovarian, and bladder carcinoma presented at more advanced stages in the elderly while lung cancer presented at an earlier stage. Goodwin's study[133] also found that pancreatic, rectal, and gastric cancer presented at earlier stages in the elderly. What is the explanation for these results? Are some tumors more aggressive in the elderly, and therefore present at a more advanced stage, or are these tumors less aggressive and therefore do not cause symptoms until they are at a later stage? Perhaps older people are more or less likely to get symptoms from a given tumor at a given stage because of decreased reserve of an infected organ, decreased inflammatory response, or other factors. Is the willingness of an older person to seek medical care for a given symptom different from a younger person? Perhaps the older person is more likely to think of a symptom as simply a manifestation of aging. Are physicians less or more likely to screen for a given tumor type in an elderly asymptomatic person? These questions for the most part remain unanswered, and the data are therefore intriguing, but difficult to interpret.

Autopsy and clinical studies show that tumor metastasis is less likely in the elderly.[134-136]

Tumors are more likely to be discovered only at autopsy in older people,[134] a finding that might correlate with experimental observation of less aggressive tumors in aged animals. This may well be due to immune senescence, but this has not been determined.

The difficulties in interpreting the literature in clinical cancer in the elderly is well illustrated by reviewing some studies that have been done in breast cancer in the elderly. Breast carcinomas present with a less malignant histologic grade in the elderly.[137,138] Again, is this the tumor, or the body's reaction to the tumor? Also, the percentage of estrogen receptor positive tumors increase with age, independent of menopausal status.[139] Despite this, two large studies [140,141] conclude that survival is poorer in older women; the overall death rate was higher, and death occurred more rapidly, in older women. Neither of these studies relates age to tumor burden at the time of death, which might be important. Reports to the contrary exist, indicating that older women have improved survival from breast cancer.[142,143] It is difficult to explain these results based on the biology of the tumor, since estrogen receptor positive tumors are usually less aggressive,[144,145] and these occur more frequently in the elderly. One problem with interpreting these results is that adequate local and systemic therapy are often withheld from the elderly, which can skew the results.

VIII. SUMMARY AND CONCLUSION

Studies have been presented that support the following: a progressive decline in many functions of the cellular immune system with age, relating to the involution of the thymus gland; a lack of correlation of this immune senescence with the increased development of cancer with age; that the growth of weakly immunogenic tumors is enhanced by the immune response, while the growth of strongly immunogenic tumors is suppressed by the immune response; that this is the likely cause of the decreased growth rate of poorly immunogenic tumors in old animals; and that suppressor cells may inhibit the antitumor cytotoxic response or that T-cells may release tumor growth promoting substances as a mechanism for immune enhancement of tumor growth.

As yet, there are no clear studies to correlate animal data to human data with regard to the effects of immune scenescence on tumor growth. The phenomenologic studies exist, but are often contradictory, and the mechanistic studies have not been done, nor will they be easy to do. The contradictory data suggests a delicate balance between tumor growth control and enhancement in the elderly, a balance that can easily be tipped by underlying secondary illnessses.

As it becomes more clear which cells or molecules mediate antitumor immunity and which mediate tumor enhancement, and as we become better at isolating those cells and propagating them *in vitro,* or eliminating them *in vivo,* we will obtain a better picture of how the aging immune system regulates growth of cancer in humans. This eventually will be important not only for the treatment of elderly but also young cancer patients, as treatment strategies are developed that enlist immune cell functions in the therapeutic effort.

ACKNOWLEDGMENTS

Supported by Public Health Service Award AG007831 and VA Merit Award to W. B. E. and Public Health Service Award T32CA09614-01 to P. R. K.

REFERENCES

1. **Young, J. L., Jr., Percy, C. L., and Asire, A. J., Eds.,** Surveillance, epidemiology, and end results, incidence and mortality data, 1973—1977, National Cancer Institute Monogr. 1981, 1.
2. **Boyd, E.,** The weight of the thymus gland in health and disease, *Am. J. Dis. Child,* 43, 1162, 1935.

3. **Moody, C. E., Innes, J. B., Staiano-Colico, L., Incefy, G. S., Thaler, J. T., and Weksler, M. E.,** Lymphocyte transformation induced by autologous cells: XI. The effect of age on the autologous mixed lymphocyte reaction, *Immunology,* 44, 431, 1981.

4. **Pahwa, S. E., Pahwa, R. N., and Good, R. A.,** Decreased *in vitro* humoral immune responses in aged humans, *J. Clin. Invest.,* 67, 1094, 1981.

5. **Singh, J. and Singh, A. K.,** Age related changes in the thymus, *Clin. Exp. Immunol.,* 37, 507, 1979.

6. **Lewis, V. M., Twomey, J. J., Bealmar, P., Goldstein, G., and Good, R. A.,** Age, thymic involution and circulating thymic hormone activity, *J. Clin. Endocrinol. Metab.,* 47, 145, 1978.

7. **Waldorf, D. S., Wilken, R. F., and Decker, J. L.,** Impaired delayed hypersensitivity in an aging population: association with anti-nuclear reactivity and rheumatoid factor, *JAMA,* 203, 831, 1968.

8. **Pisciotta, A. V., Westring, D. W., Deprey, C., and Walsh, B.,** Mitogenic effects of phytohemagglutinin at different ages, *Nature,* 215, 193, 1967.

9. **Goodwin, J. S., Searles, R. P., and Tung, K. S. K.,** Immunological responses of a healthy elderly population, *Clin. Exp. Immunol.,* 48, 403, 1982.

10. **Inkeles, B., Innes, J. B., Kuntz, M. M., Kadish, A. S., and Weksler, M. E.,** Immunological studies of aging. III. Cytokinetic basis for the impaired response of lymphocytes from aged humans to plant lectins, *J. Exp. Med.,* 145, 1176, 1977.

11. **Weksler, M. E. and Hutteroth, T. H.,** Impaired lymphocyte function in aged humans, *J. Clin. Invest.,* 53, 99, 1974.

12. **Fernandez, L. A., MacSween, J. M., and Langley, G. R.,** Lymphocyte responses to phytohemagglutinin, age related effects, *Immunology,* 31, 583, 1976.

13. **Berger, R., Florenti, G., and Just, M.,** Decrease of the lymphoproliferative response to Varicella-Zoster Virus antigen in the aged, *Infect. Immun.,* 32, 24, 1981.

14. **Gillis, S., Kozak, R., Durante, M., and Weksler, M. E.,** Immunological studies of aging: decreased production of and response to T-cell growth factor by lymphocytes from aged humans, *J. Clin. Invest.,* 67, 937, 1981.

15. **Schwab, R., Walters, C. A., and Weksler, M. E.,** Host defense mechanisms and aging, *Semin. Oncol.,* 16, 20, 1989.

16. **Bach, M.,** Influence of aging on T-cell subpopulations involved in the *in vitro* generation of allogeneic cytotoxicity, *Clin. Immunol. Immunopathol.,* 13, 220, 1979.

17. **Gottesman, S. R., Kristie, J. A., and Walford, R. L.,** Proliferative and cytotoxic immune functions in aging mice. I. Sequence of decline of reactivities measured under optimal and suboptimal sensitization conditions, *Immunology,* 44, 607, 1981.

18. **Gravenstein, S., Duthie, E. H., Miller, B. A., Roecker, E., Drinka, P., Prathipati, K., and Ershler, W. B.,** Augmentation of anti-influenza antibody response in elderly men by Thymosin Alpha One, *J. Am. Geriatr. Soc.,* 36, 1, 1989.

19. **Thomas, L.,** Reactions to homologous tissue antigens in relation to hypersensitiviy, in *Cellular and Humoral Aspects of the Hypersensitivity Status,* Lawrence, H. S., Ed., Hoeber-Harper, New York, 1959.

20. **Good, R. A.,** Disorders of the immune system, in *Immunobiology,* Good, R. A. and Fisher, D. W., Eds., Sinauer, Sunderland, MA, 1971.

21. **Kiessling, R., Klein, E., and Wigzell, H.,** "Natural" killer cells in the mouse. I. Cytotoxic cells with specificity for mouse Moloney Leukemia cells. Specificity and distribution according to genotype, *Eur. J. Immunol.,* 5, 112, 1975.

22. **Kiessling, R., Petranyi, G., Klein, G., and Wigzell, H.,** Non-T-cell resistance against a mouse Moloney lymphoma, *Int. J. Cancer,* 17, 275, 1976.

23. **Haller, O., Kiessling, R., Orn, A., Karre, K., Nilsson, K., and Wigzell, H.,** Natural cytotoxicity to human leukemia mediated by mouse non-T cells, *Int. J. Cancer,* 20, 93, 1977.

24. **Herberman, R. B. and Ortaldo, J. R.,** Natural killer cells: their role in defenses against disease, *Science,* 214, 24, 1981.

25. **Kay, H. D., Bonnard, G. D., West, W. H., and Herberman, R. B.,** A functional comparison of human Fc-receptor bearing lymphocytes active in natural cytotoxicity and antibody-dependent cellular cytotoxicity, *J. Immunol.,* 118, 2058, 1977.

26. **Shih, H. S., Johnson, R. J., Pasternack, G. R., and Economou, J. S.,** Mechanisms of tumor immunity: the role of antibody and non-immune effectors, *Prog. Allergy,* 25, 163, 1978.

27. **Hanna, N. and Burton, R.,** Definitive evidence that natural killer (NK) cells inhibit experimental metastasis *in vivo, J. Immunol.,* 121, 1754, 1981.

28. **Gorelik, E., Wiltrout, R. H., Okumumura, K., Habu, S., and Herberman, R. B.,** Role of NK cells in the control of metastatic spread and growth of tumor cells in mice, *Int. J. Cancer,* 30, 107, 1982.

29. **Talmadge, J., Meyers, K., Prieur, D., and Starkey, J.,** Role of NK cells in tumor growth and metastasis in beige mice, *Nature,* 284, 622, 1980.

30. **Hanna, N.,** Role of natural killer cells in control of cancer metastasis, *Cancer Metast. Rev.,* 1, 45, 1982.

31. **Barlozzari, T., Leonhardt, J., Wiltrout, R. H., Herberman, R. B., and Reynolds, C. W.,** Direct evidence for the role of LGL in the inhibition of experimental tumor metastasis, *J. Immunol.,* 134, 2783, 1985.

32. **Seaman, W. E., Sleisenger, M., Eriksson, E., and Koo, C.,** Depletion of natural killer cells in mice by monoclonal antibody to NK-1.1. Reduction in host defence against malignancy without loss of cellular or humoral immunity, *J. Immunol.,* 138, 4539, 1987.

33. **Zinkernagel, R. M. and Doherty, P. C.,** MHC-restricted cytotoxic T-cells: studies on the biological role of polymorphic major transplantation antigens determining T-cell restriction-specificity, function, and responsiveness, *Adv. Immunol.,* 27, 51, 1979.

34. **Tanaka, K., Yoshioka, T., Bieberich, C., and Jay, G.,** Role of the major histocompatability complex class I antigens in tumor growth and metastasis, *Ann. Rev. Immunol.,* 6, 359, 1988.

35. **Yron, I., Wood, T. A., Spiess, P., and Rosenberg, S. A.,** *In vitro* growth of murine T-cells. V. The isolation and growth of lymphoid cells infiltrating syngeneic solid tumors, *J. Immunol.,* 125, 238, 1980.

36. **Lotze, M. T., Grimm, E., Mazumder, A., Strausser, J. L., and Rosenberg, S. A.,** Lysis of fresh and cultured autologous tumor by human lymphocytes cultured in T-cell growth factor, *Cancer Res.,* 41, 4420, 1981.

37. **Speiss, P. J., Yang, J. C., and Rosenberg, S. A.,** *In vivo* antitumor activity of tumor infiltrating lymphocytes expanded in recombinant interleukin 2, *JNCI,* 79, 1067, 1987.

38. **Rosenberg, S. A., Spiess, P., and Lafreniere, R.,** A new approach to the adoptive immunotherapy of cancer with tumor-infiltrating lymphocytes, *Science,* 223, 1318, 1986.

39. **Kay, J. E. and Benzie, C. R.,** Effects of cyclosporine A on metabolism of unstimulated and mitogen-activated lymphocytes, *Immunology,* 49, 153, 1983.

40. **Fauci, A. S., Macher, A. M., Longo, D. L., Lane, C., Rook, A. H., Masur, H., and Gelman, E. P.,** Acquired immunodeficiency syndrome: epidemiologic, clinical, immunologic and therapeutic considerations, *Ann. Intern. Med.,* 101, 92, 1984.

41. **Friedman-Kien, A. E., Laubenstein, L. J., Rubenstein, P., Buimovici-Klein, E., Marmor, M., Stahl, R., Spigland, I., Kim, K. S., and Zolla-Pazner, S.,** Disseminated Kaposi's sarcoma in homosexual men, *Ann. Intern. Med.,* 96, 693, 1982.

42. **Ziegler, J. L., Drew, W. L., and Miner, R. C.,** Outbreak of Burkitt's-like lymphoma in homosexual men, *Lancet,* 2, 631, 1982.

43. **Penn, I.,** Kaposi's sarcoma in organ transplant recipients: report of 20 cases, *Transplantation,* 27, 8, 1979.

44. **Cleary, M. L., Warnke, R., and Sklar, J.,** Monoclonality of lymphoproliferative lesions in cardiac transplant recipients, *N. Engl. J. Med.,* 310, 477, 1984.

45. **Penn, I.,** Depressed immunity and the development of cancer, *Clin. Exp. Immunol.,* 46, 459, 1981.

46. **Stillstrom, J.,** The importance of dose and proliferation of SV-40-transformed cells with different oncogenic potential to the level of tumor immunity, *Int. J. Cancer,* 13, 273, 1974.

47. **Bonnassar, A., Menconi, E., Goldwin, A., and Cudkowicz, G.,** Escape of small numbers of allogeneic lymphoma cells from immune surveillance, *J. Natl. Cancer Inst.,* 53, 475, 1974.

48. **Doll, R. and Peto, R.,** The causes of cancer, *JNCI,* 66, 1193, 1981.

49. **Peto, R.,** Influence of dose and duration of smoking on lung cancer rates, in *Tobacco: A Major Health Hazard,* Zaridze, D. and Peto, R. Eds., IARC Sci. Publ. No. 74, International Agency for Research on Cancer, Lyon, 1986, 23.

50. **Day, N. E.,** Time as a determinant of risk in cancer epidemiology: the role of the multistage model, *Cancer Surv.,* 2, 577, 1983.

51. **Montesano, R. and Slaga, T. J.,** Initiation and promotion in carcinogenesis: an appraisal, *Cancer Surv.,* 2, 613, 1983.

52. **Boutwell, R. K.,** Some biological aspects of skin carcinogenesis, *Prog. Exp. Tumor Res.,* 4, 207, 1964.

53. **McMartin, D. N., O'Conner, J. A., Fasco, M. J., and Kaminsky, L. S.,** Influence of aging and induction of rate liver and kidney mixed function oxidase systems, *Toxicol. Appl. Pharmacol.,* 54, 411, 1980.

54. **Szillard, L.,** On the nature of the aging process, *Proc. Natl. Acad. Sci. U.S.A.,* 45, 30, 1959.

55. **Hart, R. W. and Setlow, R. B.,** DNA repair in late passage human cells, *Mech. Ageing Dev.,* 5, 67, 1976.

56. **Hall, J. D., Almy, R. E., and Sherer, K. L.,** DNA repair in cultured human fibroblasts does not decline with donor age, *Exp. Cell Res.,* 139, 351, 1982.

57. **Kato, H. M., Harada, K., Tsuchija, K. and Moriwaki, K.,** *Jpn. J. Genet.,* 55, 99, 1980.

58. **Collier, I. E., Popp, D. M., Lee, W. H., and Regan, J. D.,** DNA repair in congeneic pair of mice with different longevities, *Mech. Ageing Dev.,* 19, 141, 1982.

59. **Lambert, B., Ringborg, U., and Skoog, L.,** Age-related decrease of ultraviolet light-induced DNA repair synthesis in human leukocytes, *Cancer Res.,* 39, 2792, 1986.

60. **Hartwig, M. and Korner, I. J.,** *Mech. Ageing Dev.,* 38, 73, 1987.

61. **Plesko, M. M. and Richardson, A.,** Age-related changes in unscheduled DNA synthesis by rat hepatocytes, *Biochem. Biophys. Res. Commun.,* 118, 730, 1983.

62. **Weraarchakul, N., Strong, R., Wood, W. G., and Richardson, A.,** The effect of aging and dietary restriction on DNA repair, *Exp. Cell Res.,* 181, 197, 1989.

63. **Ebbson, P.,** Aging increases the susceptibility of mouse skin to DMBA carcinogenesis independent of general immune status, *Science,* 183, 217, 1974.

64. **Anisimov, V.,** Carcinogenesis and aging, *Adv. Cancer Res.,* 40, 365, 1981.

65. **Anisimov, V.,** Age-related mechanisms of susceptibility to carcinogenesis, *Semin. Oncol.,* 16, 10, 1989.

66. **Stenback, F., Peto, R., and Shubik, P.,** Initiation and promotion at different age and doses in 2200 mice. III. Linear extrapolation from high doses may underestimate low dose tumor risk, *Br. J. Cancer,* 44, 24, 1981.

67. **Wattenberg, L. W.,** Chemoprevention of cancer, *Cancer Res.,* 45, 1, 1985.

68. **Heidrick, M. L., Hendricks, L. C., and Cook, D. E.,** Effect of dietary 2-mercaptoethanol on lifespan, immune system, tumor incidence and lipid peroxidation damage in spleen lymphocytes of aging BC3F$_1$ mice, *Mech. Ageing Dev.,* 27, 341, 1984.

69. **Emmanuel, N. M. and Obukhova, L. K.,** Types of experimental delay in aging patterns, *Exp. Gerontol.,* 13, 25, 1978.

70. **Harman, D.,** Free radical theory of aging: dietary implications, *Am. J. Clin. Nutr.,* 25, 839, 1972.

71. **Aslan, A., Vrabikescu, A., Domilescu, C., Campeanu, L., Costiniu, M., and Stanescu, S.,** Long term treatment with procaine (gerovital H$_3$) in albino rats, *J. Geronotol.,* 20, 1, 1965.

72. **Tannenbaum, A. and Silverstone, H.,** Nutrition in relation to cancer, *Adv. Cancer Res.,* 1, 451, 1953.

73. **Anisimov, V. N., Khavinson, V. K., and Morozov, V. G.,** Carcinogenesis and aging. IV. Effect of low-molecular factors of thymus, pineal gland and anterior hypothalamus on immunity, tumor incidence and lifespan of C3H/Sn mice, *Mech. Ageing Dev.,* 19, 245, 1982.

74. **Anisimov, V. N., Morozov, V. G., and Khavinson, V. K.,** Effect of polypeptide factors of thymus, bone marrow, pineal gland and vessels on life span and spontaneous tumor development in mice, *Dokl. Akad. Nauk. SSSR,* 293, 1000, 1987.

75. **Ross, M. H. and Bras, G.,** Tumor incidence patterns and nutrition in the rat, *J. Nutr.,* 87, 245, 1965.

76. **Ross, M. H. and Bras, G.,** Lasting influence of early caloric restriction on prevalence of neoplasms in the rat, *J. Natl. Cancer Inst.,* 47, 1095, 1971.

77. **Prehn, R. T. and Main, J. M.,** Immunity to methylcholanthrene-induced tumors, *J. Natl. Cancer Inst.,* 19, 1053, 1957.

78. **Fidler, I. J.,** Selection of successive tumor lines for metastasis, *Nature,* 242, 148, 1973.

79. **Ershler, W. B., Stewart, J. A., Hacker, M. P., Moore, A. L., and Tindle, B. H.,** B16 murine melanoma and aging: slower growth and longer survival in old mice, *JNCI,* 72, 161, 1984.

80. **Ershler, W. B., Moore, A. L., Shore, H., and Gamelli, R. L.,** Transfer of age-associated restrained tumor growth in mice by old-to-young bone marrow transplantation, *Cancer Res.,* 44, 5677, 1984.

81. **Gozes, Y. and Trainin, N.,** Enhancement of Lewis lung carcinoma in a syngeneic host by spleen cells of C57B1/6 mice, *Eur. J. Immunol.,* 7, 159, 1977.

82. **Sigiura, K. and Stock, C. C.,** Studies in a tumor spectrum. III. The effect of phosphoramides on the growth of a variety of mouse and rat tumors, *Cancer Res.,* 15, 38, 1955.

83. **Kubota, K., Kubota, R., Takeda, S., and Matsuzawa, T.,** Effects of age and sex of host mice on growth and differentiation of teratocarcinoma OTT60-50, *Exp. Gerontol.,* 16, 371, 1984.

84. **Yuhas, J. M., Pazimo, N. H., Procter, J. O., and Toya, R. E.,** A direct relationship between immune competence and subcutaneous growth rate in a malignant lung tumor, *Cancer Res.,* 34, 722, 1974.

85. **Stevens, L. C.,** The development of transplantable teratocarcinomas from intratesticular grafts of pre- and post-implantation mouse embryos, *Dev. Biol.,* 21, 364, 1970.

86. **Flood, P. M., Urban, J. L., Kripke, M. L., and Schreiber, H.,** Loss of tumor specific and idiotype specific immunity with age, *J. Exp. Med.,* 154, 275, 1980.

87. **Rockwell, S. C., Kallman, R. F., and Fajardo, L. F.,** Characteristics of a serially transplanted mouse mammary tumor and its tissue-culture-adapted derivative, *J. Natl. Cancer Inst.,* 49, 735, 1972.

88. **Perkins, E. H. and Cacheiro, L. H.,** A multiple parameter comparison of immunocompetence and tumor resistance in aged Balb/c mice, *Mech. Ageing Dev.,* 6, 15, 1977.

89. **Walker, J. P., Townsend, C. M., Singh, P., James, E., and Thompson, J. C.,** The effect of aging on the growth of colon cancer, *Mech. Ageing Dev.,* 37, 241, 1987.

90. **Rabinowitz, S. G.,** Comparative mitogenic and antigenic responses of T-cells and B-cells in spleens of mice of varying ages, *Fed. Proc.,* 35, 1032, 1975.

91. **Simon, C. R. and Ershler, W. B.,** Hormonal influences on growth of B16 murine melanoma, *JNCI,* 74, 1085, 1985.

92. **Proctor, J. W., Auclair, B. G., and Stokowski, L.,** Endocrine factors and the growth and spread of B16 melanoma, *J. Natl. Cancer Inst.,* 57, 1197, 1976.

93. **Proctor, J. W., Yammamura, Y., Gaydos, D., and Matromatteo, W.,** Further studies on endocrine factors and growth and spread of B16 melanoma, *Oncology,* 38, 102, 1981.

94. **Greene, E. L.,** *Handbook on Genetically Standardized Mice,* 2nd ed., Bar Harbor Time Publishing, Bar Harbor, ME, 1977.

95. **Weindruch, R. H., Kristie, J. A., Cheney, K. E., and Walford, R. L.,** Influence of controlled dietary restriction on immunologic functioning and aging, *Fed. Proc.,* 38, 2007, 1979.

96. **Weindruch, R. and Walford, R. L.,** Dietary restriction in mice beginning at one year of age: effect on life span and spontaneous cancer incidence, *Science,* 215, 1415, 1982.

97. **Ershler, W. B., Berman, E., and Moore, A. L.,** B16 melanoma growth is slower, but pulmonary colonization is greater in calorie restricted mice, *JNCI,* 76, 81, 1986.

98. **Cohen, B. J., Danon, D., and Roth, G. S.,** Wound repair in mice is influenced by age and antimacrophage serum, *J. Gerontol.,* 42, 295, 1987.

99. **Miyahara, T., Murai, A., Tanaka, T., Shiozawa, S., and Kameyama, M.,** Age-related differences in human skin collagen: solubility in solvent, susceptibility to pepsin digestion, and the spectrum of solubilized polymeric collagen molecules, *J. Gerontol.,* 37, 651, 1982.

100. **Miyahara, T., Shiozawa, S., and Murai, A.,** The effect of age on amino acid composition of human skin collagen, *J. Gerontol.,* 33, 498, 1978.

101. **Ershler, W. B., Gamelli, R. L., Moore, A. L., Hacker, M. P., and Blow, A. J.,** Experimental tumors and aging: local factors that may account for the observed age advantage in the B16 murine melanoma model, *Exp. Gerontol.,* 19, 367, 1984.

102. **Prehn, R. T.,** The immune reaction as a stimulator of tumor growth, *Science,* 176, 170, 1972.

103. **Carnaud, C., Ilfeld, D., Levo, Y., and Trainin, N.,** Enhancement of 3LL tumor growth by autosensitized T-lymphocytes independent of the host lymphatic system, *Int. J. Cancer,* 14, 168, 1974.

104. **Tsuda, T., Kim, Y. T., Siskind, G. W., DeBlasio, A., Schwab, R., Ershler, W., and Weksler, M. E.,** Role of the thymus and T-cells in slow growth of B16 in old mice, *Cancer Res.,* 47, 3097, 1987.

105. **Fujimoto, S., Greene, M. I., and Sehon, A. H.,** Regulation of the immune response to tumor antigens. I. Immunosuppressor cells in tumor-bearing hosts, *J. Immunol.,* 116, 791, 1976.

106. **Fujimoto, S., Greene, M. I., and Sehon, A. H.,** Regulation of the immune response to tumor antigens. II. The nature of the immunosuppressor cells in tumor-bearing hosts, *J. Immunol.,* 116, 800, 1976.

107. **Greenberg, A. and Greene, M. I.,** Non-adaptive rejection of small tumor inocula as a model of immune surveillance, *Nature,* 264, 356, 1976.

108. **Greene, M. I., Dorf, M. E., Pierres, M., and Benacerraf, B.,** Reduction of syngeneic tumor growth by an anti-I-J- alloantiserum, *Proc. Natl. Acad. Sci. U.S.A.,* 74, 5118, 1977.

109. **Berendt, M. J. and North, R. T.,** T-cell-mediated suppression of anti-tumor immunity, *J. Exp. Med.,* 151, 69, 1980.

110. **Ershler, W. B., Tuck, D., Moore, A. L., Klopp, R. G., and Kramer, K. E.,** Immunologic enhancement of B16 melanoma growth, *Cancer,* 61, 1792, 1988.

111. **Small, M. and Trainin, N.,** Separation of population of sensitized lymphoid cells into fractions inhibiting and fractions enhancing syngeneic tumor growth *in vivo, J. Immunol.,* 117, 292, 1976.

112. **Small, M.,** Characteristics of the immature cells involved in T-cell-mediated enhancement of syngeneic tumor growth, *J. Immunol.,* 118, 1517, 1977.

113. **Manor, J., Treves, A. J., Cohen, I. R., and Feldman, M.,** Transition from T-cell protection to T-cell enhancement during tumor growth in an allogeneic host, *Transplantation,* 22, 360, 1976.

114. **Treves, A. J., Cohen, I. R., and Feldman, M.,** Suppressor factor secreted by T-lymphocytes from tumor-bearing mice, *J. Natl. Cancer Inst.,* 57, 409, 1976.

115. **Greene, M. I., Fujimoto, S., and Sehon, A. H.,** Regulation of the immune response to tumor antigens. III. Characterization of the thymic suppressor factor(s) produced by tumor bearing hosts, *J. Immunol.,* 119, 757, 1977.

116. **Takei, F., Levy, J. G., and Kilburn, D. G.,** *In vitro* induction of cytotoxicity against syngeneic mastocytoma and its suppression by spleen and thymus cells from tumor-bearing mice, *J. Immunol.,* 116, 288, 1976.

117. **Takei, F., Levy, J. G., and Kilburn, D. G.,** Characterization of suppressor cells in mice bearing syngeneic mastocytoma, *J. Immunol.,* 118, 412, 1977.

118. **Mukherji, B., Wilhelm, S. A., Guha, A., and Ergin, M. T.,** Regulation of cellular immune response against human melanoma, *J. Immunol.,* 136, 1888, 1986.

119. **Mukherji, B., Nashed, A. L., Guha, A., and Ergin, M. T.,** Regulation of cellular immune response against human melanoma. II. Mechanism of induction and specificity of suppression, *J. Immunol.,* 136, 1893, 1986.

120. **Mukherji, B., Guha, A., Loomis, R., and Ergin, M. T.,** Cell-mediated amplification and down regulation of cytotoxic immune response against autologous human cancer, *J. Immunol.,* 138, 1987, 1987.

121. **Yamaguchi, K., Fujimoto, S., and Tada, T.,** Differential activation of cytotoxic and suppressor T-cells against syngeneic tumors in the mouse, *J. Immunol.,* 123, 1653, 1979.

122. **Romerdahl, C. A. and Kripke, M. L.,** Regulation of the immune response against UV-induced skin cancers: specificity of helper cells and their susceptibility to UV-induced suppressor cells, *J. Immunol.,* 137, 3031, 1986.

123. **Elgert, K. D. and Farrar, W. L.,** Suppressor cell activity in tumor bearing mice. I. Dualistic inhibition by suppressor T-lymphocytes and macrophages, *J. Immunol.,* 120, 1345, 1979.

124. **Takashi, K., Ono, K., Hirabayashi, Y., and Taniguchi, M.,** Escape mechanisms of melanoma from immune system by soluble melanoma antigen, *J. Immunol.,* 140, 3244, 1988.

125. **Folkman, J.,** Tumor angiogenesis, *Adv. Cancer Res.,* 19, 331, 1974.

126. **Sidky, Y. A. and Auerbach, R.,** Lymphocyte-induced angiogenesis: a quantitative and sensitive assay of the graft-vs.-host reaction, *J. Exp. Med.,* 141, 1084, 1975.

127. **Auerbach, R., Kubai, L., and Sidky, Y.,** Angiogenesis induction by tumors, embryonic tissue and lymphocytes, *Cancer Res.,* 36, 3435, 1976.

128. **Sidky, Y. A. and Auerbach, R.,** Response of the host vascular system to immunocompetent lymphocytes. Effect of pre-immunization of donor or host animals, *Proc. Soc. Exp. Biol. Med.,* 161, 174, 1979.

129. **Pliskin, M. E.,** Activated lymphoid cells induce vascularization, *Transplantation,* 27, 136, 1979.

130. **Folkman, J., Klagsbrun, M., Sasse, J., Wadzinski, M., Ingber, D., and Vlodavsky, I.,** A heparin-binding angiogenic protein - basic fibroblast growth factor - is stored within the basement membrane, *Am. J. Pathol.,* 130, 393, 1988.

131. **Hadar, E. J., Ershler, W. B., Kreisle, R. A., Ho, S.-P., Volk, M. J., and Klopp, R. G.,** Lymphocyte-induced angiogenesis factor is produced by L3T4+ murine T-lymphocytes, and its production declines with age, *Cancer Immunol. Immunother.,* 26, 31, 1988.

132. **Holmes, F. F. and Hearne, E.,** Cancer stage-to-age relationship: implications for cancer screening in the elderly, *J. Am. Geriatr. Soc.,* 29, 55, 1981.

133. **Goodwin, J. S., Samet, J. M., and Key, C. R.,** Stage at diagnosis of cancer varies with the age of the patient, *J. Am. Geriatr. Soc.,* 34, 20, 1986.

134. **Suen, K. C., Lau, L. L., and Yermakov, V.,** Cancer and old age. An autopsy study of 3535 patients over 65 years old, *Cancer,* 33, 1164, 1974.

135. **Saitoh, H., Shiramizu, T., and Hida, M.,** Age changes in metastatic patterns of renal adenocarcinoma, *Cancer,* 50, 1646, 1982.

136. **Ershler, W. B., Socinski, M. A., and Green, C. J.,** Bronchogenic cancer metastases and aging, *J. Am. Geriatr. Soc.,* 31, 673, 1983.

137. **Schottenfeld, D. and Robbins, G. F.,** Breast cancer in elderly women, *Geriatrics,* 26, 121, 1971.

138. **von Rosen, A., Gardelin, A., and Auer, G.,** Assessment of malignancy potential in mammary carcinoma in elderly patients, *Am. J. Clin. Oncol.,* 10, 61, 1987.

139. **Elwood, J. M. and Godolphin, W.,** Oestrogen receptors in breast tumors: associations with age, menopausal status and epidemiological and clinical features in 735 patients, *Br. J. Cancer,* 42, 635, 1980.

140. **Adami, H.-O., Malker, B., Meirik, O., Persson, I., Bergkvist, L., and Stone, B.,** Age as a prognostic factor in breast cancer, *Cancer,* 56, 898, 1985.

141. **Mueller, C. B., Ames, F., and Anderson, G. D.,** Breast cancer in 3558 women: age as a significant determinant in the rate of dying and causes of death, *Surgery,* 83, 123, 1978.

142. **Berkson, J., Harrington, S. W., Clagett, O. T., Kirklin, J. W., Dockerty, M. B., and McDonald, J. R.,** Mortality and survival in surgically treated cancer of the breast: a statistical summary of some experience of the Mayo Clinic, *Mayo Clin. Proc.,* 32, 645, 1957.

143. **Oates, R. P.,** Forces of mortality among breast cancer patients, *J. Chron. Dis.,* 29, 262, 1976.

144. **McQuire, W. L., Horwitz, K. B., Zava, D. T., Garola, R. E., and Chamness, G. C.,** Progress in endocrinology and metabolism — hormones and breast cancer. Update 1978, *Metabolism,* 27, 487, 1978.

145. **Silvestrini, R., Daidone, M. G., and DiFronzo, G.,** Relationship between proliferative activity and estrogen receptors in breast cancer, *Cancer,* 44, 665, 1979.

Index

INDEX